ST BARTHOLOMEW'S AND THE ROYAL LONDON
SCHOOL OF MEDICINE AND DENTISTRY

WHITECHAPEL LIBRARY, TURNER STREET, LONDON E1 2AD
0171 295 7110

020 7882 7110

4 WEEK LOAN

Books are to be returned on or before the last date below,
otherwise fines may be charged.

Keio University International Symposia
for Life Sciences and Medicine 8

Springer
Tokyo
Berlin
Heidelberg
New York
Barcelona
Hong Kong
London
Milan
Paris

H. Kashima, I.R.H. Falloon,
M. Mizuno, M. Asai (Eds.)

Comprehensive Treatment of Schizophrenia

Linking Neurobehavioral Findings to
Psychosocial Approaches

With 58 Figures

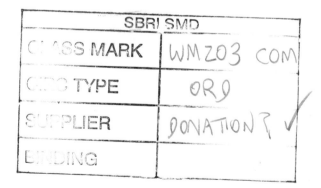
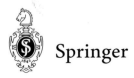 Springer

HARUO KASHIMA, M.D.
Professor, Department of Neuropsychiatry
School of Medicine, Keio University
35 Shinanomachi, Shinjuku-ku, Tokyo 160-8582, Japan

IAN R.H. FALLOON, M.D.
Professor of Psychiatry & Behavioural Science
School of Medicine, University of Auckland
Private Bag 92019, Auckland, New Zealand

MASAFUMI MIZUNO, M.D.
Instructor, Department of Neuropsychiatry
School of Medicine, Keio University
35 Shinanomachi, Shinjuku-ku, Tokyo 160-8582, Japan

MASAHIRO ASAI, M.D.
Guest Professor, Department of Neuropsychiatry
School of Medicine, Keio University
35 Shinanomachi, Shinjuku-ku, Tokyo 160-8582, Japan

ISBN 4-431-70298-9 Springer-Verlag Tokyo Berlin Heidelberg New York

Library of Congress Cataloging-in-Publication Data

Comprehensive treatment of schizophrenia : linking neurobehavioral findings to
psychosocial approaches / H. Kashima . . . [et al.] (eds.).
    p.   ; cm. — (Keio University international symposia for life sciences and medicine ; 8)
    Includes bibliographical references and index.
    ISBN 4431702989 (hard : alk. paper)
    1. Schizophrenia—Congresses. I. Kashima, Haruo. II. Keio International Symposium
for Life Sciences and Medicine (8th : 2000 : Keio Gijuku Daigaku) III. Series.
    [DNLM: 1. Schizophrenia—therapy—Congresses. 2. Neurobehavioral
Manifestations—Congresses. 3. Psychiatry—methods—Congresses. WM 203 C737 2002]
RC514 .C586 2002
616.89′8206—dc21

                                                                2001049886
Printed on acid-free paper

Typesetting, printing, and binding: Best-set Typesetter Ltd., Hong Kong
SPIN: 10778396

Foreword

This volume of the Keio University International Symposia for Life Sciences and Medicine contains the proceedings of the eighth symposium held under the sponsorship of the Keio University Medical Science Fund. As explained in the Opening Remarks by the President of Keio University, the fund was established by the generous donation of Dr. Mitsunada Sakaguchi. The Keio University International Symposia for Life Sciences and Medicine constitute one of the core activities sponsored by the fund, the objective of which is to contribute to the international community by developing human resources, promoting scientific knowledge, and encouraging mutual exchange. Each year, the Committee of the International Symposia for Life Sciences and Medicine selects the most significant symposium topic from applications received from the Keio medical community. The publication of the proceedings is intended to publicize and disseminate the information arising from the lively discussions of the most exciting and current issues presented during the symposium. On behalf of the Committee, I am most grateful to Dr. Mitsunada Sakaguchi, who made the symposia series possible. We are also grateful to the prominent speakers for their contribution to this volume. In addition, we would like to acknowledge the efficient organizational work performed by the members of the program committee and the staff of the fund.

Naoki Aikawa, M.D., D.M.Sc., F.A.C.S.
Chairman
Committee of the International Symposia
for Life Sciences and Medicine

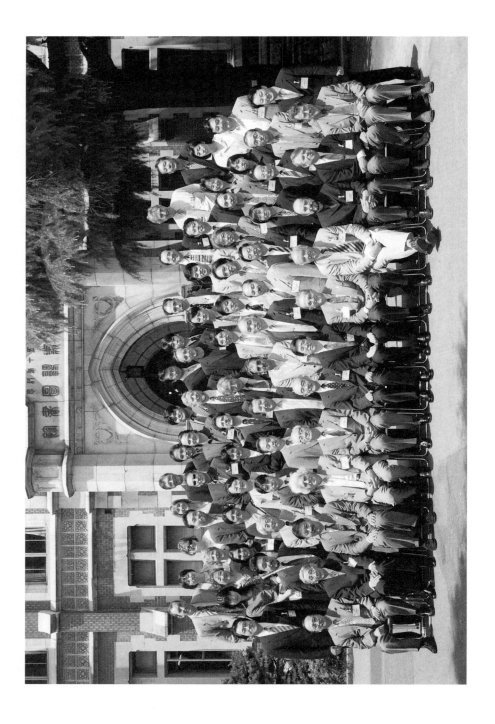

The 8th Keio University International Symposium for Life Sciences and Medicine

First row, from left: Penn, Sarada, Gedye, Berti, Ivarsson, Watanabe, Nemoto, Kobayashi, Kizaki, Miura, Ventura, Catts, Sakuma

Second row, from left: Maeda, Leggatt, Shimodera, Tarrier, Fowler, Mueser, Gräwe, Muramatsu, Oda, Kariya, Ikebuchi, Taira

Third row, from left: Yamashita, Sasane, Shankar, Kim, Roncone, David, Casacchia, Yamaguchi, Harada, Ito, Fujimura, Goto, Akagi, Sugawara

Fourth row, from left: Kim, Oshima, Hayashi, Sakamura, Iseda, Lussetti, Mastroeni, Anzai, Nakatani, Fujii, Nonaka, Kato, Murakami, Mizuno

Fifth row, from left: Niwa, Sakaguchi, Suzuki, Leff, Utena, Asai, Kashima, Liberman, Held, Brenner, Malm, Falloon

Preface

Schizophrenia, the theme of this symposium, is a serious mental disease that can devastate the lives of people who suffer from it and the lives of their families. It typically begins in late adolescence or early adulthood. Although wide variation occurs in the course of the disease, it is basically chronic and sometimes persists throughout the patient's entire life. Patients' pursuit of education and occupational goals are disrupted, and their quality of life is drastically reduced. Schizophrenia occurs throughout the world, and its incidence is rather high, between 0.7%–0.8% of the population. Therefore, better treatment techniques for this serious public health problem are an urgent need in modern psychiatry. Today, thanks to recent progress in the neurosciences, biological studies of schizophrenia, including molecular genetic studies, have been flourishing, and as a result, our knowledge of brain function in this disease has rapidly advanced. However, to understand the behavioral characteristics of schizophrenia and implement effective treatment programs for people with schizophrenia and their families, multifaceted approaches, including psychosocial ones, are most important.

We thank Prof. TORII Yasuhiko, President of Keio University and Chairman of the Keio University Medical Science Fund, and the Committee of the International Symposia for Life Sciences and Medicine, currently chaired by Prof. AIKAWA Naoki and Prof. KANEKO Akimichi, the former chairman, for selecting our proposal of "Comprehensive Treatment of Schizophrenia" as the topic of the 8th Keio International Symposium for Life Sciences and Medicine. We would also like to thank Dr. SAKAGUCHI Mitsunada, an alumnus of the Keio University School of Medicine, for his generous endowment to the Keio University Medical Science Fund. The symposium was held on June 5–7, 2000, in the North Annex (Kita-Shinkan), on the Mita campus of Keio University.

This volume contains a total of 40 papers arranged according to subject area: (1) Neurobehavioral Characteristics, (2) Social Cognition, (3) Expressed Emotion and Psychoeducation, (4) Insight, (5) Pharmacotherapy, (6) Consumer Collaboration, (7) Putting Effective Settings into Practice, (8) Innovations in Practice, and (9) Cognitive Remediation. Our intention has been to cover the variety of approaches reflected in recent clinical progress in the treatment of schizophrenia and allied disorders.

The editors would like to thank all participants for their interesting presentations and stimulating discussions at the conference and for their contributions to the book.

Our thanks are also extended to all members of the audience, to the more than 400 persons who attended the open symposium for family members held on the third day, and to OHIN Hiroshi, SHIMANE Junko, and HOSOKAWA Sachiko, the members of the Symposium Secretariat. Finally, we would like to express our immense appreciation to the staff of Springer-Verlag, Tokyo, for their help and support.

THE EDITORS
KASHIMA Haruo
Ian R.H. FALLOON
MIZUNO Masafumi
ASAI Masahiro

Contents

Part 1 Neurobehavioral Characteristics

Part 2 Social Cognition

Part 3 Expressed Emotion and Psychoeducation

Part 4 Insight

Part 5 Pharmacotherapy

Part 6 Consumer Collaboration

Part 9 Cognitive Remediation

List of Contributors

Opening Remarks

Prof. Yasuhiko Torii
President, Keio University
Chairman, Keio University Medical Science Fund

Distinguished guests, ladies and gentlemen:

On behalf of Keio University, I have the great pleasure of welcoming all the guests and participants to the 8th Keio University International Symposium for Life Sciences and Medicine. I am particularly grateful to the distinguished medical scientists and clinicians who have traveled such long distances to participate in this symposium.

The subject of this year's symposium is "Comprehensive Treatment of Schizophrenia: Linking Neurobehavioral Findings to Psychosocial Approaches."

Although remarkable progress and breakthroughs are reported almost every day in the field of neuroscientific research, it is also true that there still are a large number of people who suffer from schizophrenia. In this regard, I believe that this is indeed an opportune moment to hold a symposium at Keio University on the subject. All the speakers have kindly accepted our invitation to contribute to this symposium on comprehensive treatment of schizophrenia, and I feel certain that this unique meeting will prove both exciting and successful.

In Japan we have 650 universities, including 99 national, 72 municipal public, and 479 private universities. Keio University was founded in 1858 by Yukichi Fukuzawa and is the oldest university in the country. Fukuzawa was a pioneer of enlightenment and modernization in Japan. He was an enlightened man himself, and as a member of the very first mission of the Tokugawa Shogunate government he visited the United States in 1860 and European countries in 1862. He tried to bring to Japan the essence of Western culture, especially the concept and system of medical care, education, and government administration. In 1868, in the midst of civil war, Fukuzawa reorganized his school and named it Keio Gijuku, "Keio" being the name of the era at the time, and the word "Gijuku" meaning "public school."

The School of Medicine was established later, in 1917, with Dr. Shibasaburo Kitasato as its first Dean. Dr. Kitasato was a researcher in the field of microbiology and had spent several years in Germany working with the eminent Dr. Robert Koch. When he returned to Japan, the government was unable to provide him with research facilities, and Dr. Fukuzawa offered him a laboratory which he had built with his own money. This consequently led to the foundation of this medical school, which soon became an institution to reckon with in medical science.

Thus, Keio University had its origins in international exchanges; indeed, international exchanges such as this symposium have been one of the most important academic and social missions of Keio University since its foundation.

This symposium has been organized as one of several projects supported by the Keio University Medical Science Fund. The fund was started with a private donation from Dr. Mitsunada Sakaguchi, an alumnus of the class of 1940 of our medical school. In the fall of 1994, Dr. Sakaguchi donated five billion yen, approximately 50 million dollars, to the university. He expressed the wish that this fund be used to encourage research in life sciences and medicine at Keio University and to promote worldwide progress in life sciences. We fulfilled his wish by launching the Keio University Medical Science Fund in April 1995, and the Fund currently supports four projects, including the International Symposia for Life Sciences and Medicine.

We are now witnessing the dawn of the 21st century and the third millennium. There are many problems that confronted society in the century just past that carry over to the new one. Many new and unknown difficulties await us in this new century. I believe that exploring new horizons in life sciences is one of our most vital tasks at this dawn of the 21st century. It is equally important to ensure that the knowledge gained through such pursuits will be used in a way that brings genuine happiness to humankind.

It is thus more than a pleasure, indeed it is a great honor, for me to be in the midst of so many distinguished medical researchers and clinicians from world-renowned institutions who have gathered here. I am also grateful to the organizing committee, chaired by Dr. Haruo Kashima, for their efforts in ensuring that this symposium will be an auspicious and enjoyable event. I sincerely hope that the symposium will prove to be a worthwhile and profitable experience for you all.

Let me close by wishing all of you gathered here further success in your research and clinical work.

Part 1
Neurobehavioral Characteristics

Keynote Lecture: Life-Oriented Approach to Treatment and Simple Functional Tests for Clinical Practice

HIROSHI UTENA

Summary. Life-oriented treatment was formulated when the Five-Year Project Aimed at Preventing the Relapse of Schizophrenia was introduced at the Gunma University Hospital between 1958 and 1962. A cohort of 140 patients was followed along their life courses. Two guiding aspects were identified: the patients' value-attributions and stress resulting from their environment. The 25-year follow-up is described with special reference to social adjustment. Although the initial aim of relapse prevention failed, the subsequent episodes became shorter and milder. A trend of bifurcation between self-support and hospitalization continued for 20 years and resulted in a dichotomy. To examine the basic mental functions, a low-tech test battery was constructed for clinical use: a simple reaction time is obtained from the time to catch a falling ruler, a mild stress-induced pulse rate difference, at the blood-pressure measurement, and a degree of randomness, from a random number generation test. The markers in combination show an abnormality in 85% of the schizophrenic group compared with 30% for normal controls and correlate with negative symptoms and social adaptability. According to the Baum test, an unusual type of drawing appears frequently in acute cases. This is indicative of a destruction of gestalt formation.

Key words. Life-oriented treatment, Schizophrenia, Long-term study, Low-tech test, Basic mental functions

Introduction

Clinical workers who are engaged in the long-term follow-up study of schizophrenia need to find a comprehensive way of approaching the problem. The bio-psycho-social conception is often emphasized, but a connecting link among the three aspects is not always clear. A comprehensive approach to "life-oriented" treatment and care has emerged in Japan. The life-oriented approach [1] learns from daily experience to build up a harmonious life within one's environment with suitable

Sakamoto Clinic, 1-1-36 Sugasawa, Niiza, Saitama 352-0017, Japan medical support. The strategy of treatment should not simply be called eclectic. It is based on a unitary conception coming from distinct ways of thinking that imply an increasing freedom of choice in living, and the optimism of therapists based upon accurate knowledge of all levels of the complex system in which patients live out their lives.

This review describes two series of studies: one is the long-continuing Project for the Amelioration of Prognosis of Schizophrenia carried on by the Colleagues of Seikatsu-Rinsyo (life clinic), abbreviated as CLC, and the consists of examination of the basic mental functions in daily clinical setting using the simple, low-tech test battery in close collaboration with patients.

The Life-Oriented Approach to Treatment

The life-oriented treatment for schizophrenia was formulated during the development of the Five-Year Project Aimed at Preventing the Relapse of Schizophrenia at the Department of Psychiatry, Gunma University Hospital, between 1958 and 1962. During that period, neuroleptic treatment had just begun to be widely accepted, but it soon became apparent that it was not sufficient to keep the illness on a smooth course. The traditional descriptive symptomatology appeared to be of little use in relapse prevention, and we were unfamiliar with dynamic psychotherapy for schizophrenia at that time. Therefore we were obliged to take practical, experiential, and paradigmatic approaches [2].

The approach of the CLC became gradually directed towards examining the behavior of patients as well as their environments at the time of relapse. The organizer and leader was the late Dr. Yoichi Eguma, Associate Professor in the Department of Psychiatry. The members of the CLC consisted of three generations of psychiatrists who were able to follow up the patients for a very long time. My role as Professor of the Department was in diagnosis, theory, and experimentation. My diagnostic criteria for schizophrenia were rather narrow and were and are almost identical to that of the present-day ICD-10 diagnosis.

The CLC classified patients as active-unstable or passive-stable according to the pattern of their life course. Patients of the active-unstable type persisted in a determined but often inadequate way when managing their life issues, failed in issue management, and relapsed frequently. Patients of the passive-stable type obediently did what they were told to do, and their life courses were relatively stable. When demands from their environment became excessive for them, however, they fell apart and relapse occurred.

Two aspects of the patients' reactions to life events and issues at the time of relapse were distinguished: one aspect was that life events and issues with stress and burdens induced nonspecific schizophrenic reactions, and the other aspect was that the patients' value attributions provoked a person-specific as well as a schizophrenic reaction in response to trivial life events and issues that were somehow related to their concerns with sex, money, social status, or their own physical condition.

Therapeutic techniques were constructed according to the type of life course and the manner of reaction. Learning the way of living of patients by themselves under the therapists' guidance was the main road of the treatment. Support and amelioration of patients' living conditions and circumstances were also considered. Treatment could not be achieved without the support of medication.

The stress-vulnerability model of schizophrenia was accepted as a common understanding among us, and crisis intervention was carried out by homemade techniques.

The subjects of the Relapse-Prevention cohort were 140 schizophrenic patients consecutively discharged from the hospital from 1958 to 1962. They were mainly young, had experienced a first episode, had been hospitalized for six months or less, and were recovered or improved at discharge. In addition, almost all the subjects were living in or close to the prefectural capital city of Maebashi, about 100 km northwest of Tokyo. Almost all belonged to the middle class. There was little population mobility during the follow-up period. The follow-up of the patients was carried out continuously by the CLC until 1997. The results were reported succesively by Utena after 3 years, by Yuasa after 7 years, and by Ogawa and others after 25 and 35 years. In this review, the results of the 25-year follow-up of 130 patients [3] (93% of the total) are reported; 25 patients had died during the period of follow-up.

Figure 1 shows the individual longitudinal courses of the lives of these patients, with special reference to social adjustment, assessed month by month using the five grades of Eguma's Social Adjustment Scale. Each horizontal bar signifies an individual, and the origin point is the start of follow-up. The disease course of each patient is represented by using different shades from white (good) to black (bad) to describe social adjustment. The time scale is in years, and the types of adjustment are described in the footnote. As this figure shows, our initial aim of relapse prevention failed.

Therefore, the CLC had to change the name of the project to Amelioration of Prognosis of Schizophrenia. However, subsequent episodes became much shorter and milder, and their final outcome appeared to be more favorable. The relapse rate gradually decreased and eventually reached a much reduced value after 10 years.

Some notable features may be pointed out. First, a trend of bifurcation between self-support and hospitalization continued for 20 years and eventually resulted in a dichotomy between white and dark on Fig. 1. If community treatment and care were fortified and practiced effectively, the proportion of self-support would become much larger. Second, I named the first decade following the onset of schizophrenia the unstable phase (particularly the initial half); the second decade, the stable phase; and the subsequent years, the calm phase, which included late remission and deterioration as well. The main interest of the CLC had at the beginning been focused on the management of patients' difficulties in the unstable phase, but later the major tasks of the CLC were shifted to the alleviation of the limitation of flexibility of patients in life situations. Third, at the end of the follow-up, 42% of patients were in out-patient service, 31% in in-patient care, and 27% free from drug treatment, respectively. Medical treatment had a role in securing homeostatic stability throughout the course, but psychosocial treatment had more importance in the later phases. The stable phase is a quasi-stationary state in nature, containing a chance for recovery as well as a risk of relapse in the face of various happenings in life. As Pasteur said, "Chance favors only the prepared mind." Therefore, continued preparedness and timely guidance are indispensable.

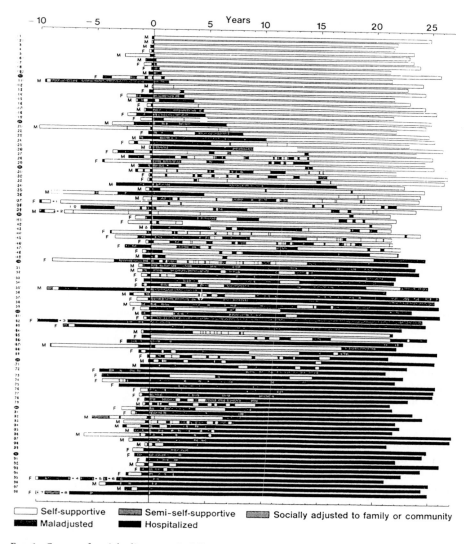

FIG. 1. Course of social adjustment in follow-up of schizophrenia. (From [3], with permission.) In cases 19, 25, and 41, the blank signifies an unidentified grade of Eguma's Social Adjustment Scale. Zero on the X-axis is the start of follow-up on discharge from the index hospitalization

The Low-Tech Test Battery for Examination of Basic Mental Functions

In the past 20 years, various facilities of community service for the psychiatrically disabled have been set up throughout Japan. Outpatient services have been playing a primary and pivotal role in psychosocial treatment and care as well as in medical treatment. At clinics, we patients and therapists need to speak to each other in mutually understandable words. However, it is usually difficult for a patient to accept the opinion of a therapist that he or she has an illness. Since the experience of patients, such as hallucinations and delusions, is a reality for them, even if it is called pathological by outsiders, it can hardly be accepted as a sign or symptom of an illness by the patient. In contrast, it is relatively easy for patients to recognize it as an impairment of their own mental function, such as some kind of distress, anxiety, or sluggishness. This recognition will become more sure when it is presented by the therapist with obvious evidence.

Patients often ask therapists for advice on diverse life issues from trivial to serious, e.g., taking medicine, resting, job seeking, driving a car, getting married, or suicidal impulses. In such instances, therapists are often unable to offer appropriate advice without a mutually understandable basis. This is the reason that a simple, low-tech test battery has been introduced for daily clinical use.

The battery consists of three measurements, each relating to volitional, emotional, and thinking functions, and also contains a qualitative tree-drawing test (Baum Test) for imaginational activity [4–6]. A simple reaction time is obtained by reading the scale on a ruler after the patient catches the falling ruler and converting it into the reaction time (RCT) using Galileo's formula for a falling body: the measurement on the ruler s equals one half of g times t squared, where g is the gravity constant. Thus 20 cm becomes equivalent to 202 ms and 30 cm to 247 ms.

A mild-stress-induced pulse-rate difference (PRD) is obtained at the time of blood pressure measurement. PRD is expressed by the pulse rate during the period while the arm-band pressure is kept at the midpoint between the maximum and the minimum, from which the pulse rate obtained at the wrist prior to blood pressure measurement is subtracted. The flow of thinking is measured during a random-number generation test, in which the patient is asked to write down randomly numbers from 0 to 9 for 1 minute. The degree of randomness (DOR) is calculated using the formula of Murakami, as shown in the footnote of Table 1. DOR denotes a discrepancy between a man-made randomness and a mathematical one, expressing the freedom of choice of thinking by the examinee.

In the first stage of my study [4], 57 chronic schizophrenic patients at an outpatient clinic were examined with respect to RCT and PRD. The patients were in a stable state, and the data were reproducible. The scattergram of the patients and controls revealed that the patients could be classified into three subtypes: usual, slow, and sensitive, with the off-limit lines of mean + 2SD of normal controls. The finding of a delay (25–50 ms) of RCT in the patients as compared with the controls was important in relation to the concept of time cognition as described later. Using the Manchester Scale, an intra-schizophrenic comparison among subtypes was made, which revealed that the sensitive and slow subtypes were significantly correlated with the negative but not with the positive symptoms, as compared with the usual subtype. The abnormal subtypes also showed a correlation with poorer grades of Eguma's Scale. It was surprising that such simple markers could have a relationship with complex social adjustment.

In the second stage of the study [5], another group of mixed, acute and chronic patients at the outpatient clinic were examined with respect to the three markers. The results are shown in Table 2. PRD, RCT, and DOR are independent variables, which means that these markers are derived from three different subsystems of the central nervous system. The differences between schizophrenic and normal groups are sig-

TABLE 1. Low-tech functional test battery

Comments
  Applicable to clinical practice
  Can be used anywhere and anytime and is reproducible
  No need of special instruments
  Time required is less than 10 min
  Allows discussion of data between the patient and the therapist
  Triangulation of the map of mental functions
Methods
  Pulse rate difference during a response to mild stress (PRD)
  Ruler-catching time as a simple reaction time (RCT)
  Degree of randomness of flow of thinking as a random number
    generation test (DOR)

Random number: Nr.
Sequential number: Ns.

$$DOR = \sum_{i=0}^{9} \left| \frac{ni}{Nr} - 0.1 \right| + \sum_{j=9}^{19} \left| \frac{nj}{Nr-1} - \frac{10-|j|}{100} \right|$$

Degree of randomness

$$MRT = \frac{60}{Nr} - \frac{60}{Ns} \quad \text{Mean randomizing time}$$

TABLE 2. Comparison between schizophrenic and normal groups

Variable	Schizophrenic group	Normal controls
No.	52	56
M:F	34:18	30:26
Mean age (yr)	41.7 ± 11.5	40.3 ± 11.5
Duration of illness (yr)	14.6 ± 9.3 (1 − 40)	
PRD (/min)	19.2 ± 12.2	12.0 ± 7.3
RCT (cm)	23.6 ± 3.8	20.5 ± 2.0
DOR	1.136 ± 0.265	0.948 ± 0.172
MRT (s)	0.537 ± 0.246	0.488 ± 0.180
Mean random number (Nr)	55.4 ± 14.3	62.5 ± 13.3
Mean sequential number (Ns)	99.5 ± 20.3	118.5 ± 16.0
Mean dosage (CPZ mg/day)	169.1 ± 119.6	(−)

PRD, pulse rate difference; RCT, ruler catching time; DOR, degree of randomness; CPZ, chlorpromazine

nificant. The mean dosage of antipsychotic drugs is fairly small compared with those in other reports, and it has no relation to the markers.

The off-limit points between normal and abnormal data are set at mean + 1SD of the normal group. For PRD, RCT, and DOR, the data were divided into 0 (normal) and 1 (abnormal). Using the binary numbers, subtypes were classified into eight forms from (000) to (111). Table 3 shows the distribution of subtypes among the schizophrenic and normal groups. As far as the markers are concerned, both groups belong to the same spectrum, and the transition from normal to schizophrenia is continuous. It seems understandable that the normal group contains 40 persons with (000)

TABLE 3. Subtyping and S/N ratio using three markers

Subtype[a]	(000)	(100)	(010)	(001)	(110)	(101)	(011)	(111)	Sum
Schizophrenia (S)	8	5	8	8	4	6	10	3	52
Normal control (N)	40	3	4	4	1	1	3	0	56
S/N ratio	0.20		1.91			4.00		∞	

[b]	LXX (PRD)	xlx (RCT)	xxl (DOR)
[c]	(100), (110), (101), (111)	(010), (110), (011), (111)	(001), (101), (011), (111)
S/N ratio	18/5 = 3.60	25/8 = 3.13	28/8 = 3.50

Markers: Pulse rate difference, reaction time, degree of randomness
[a] In this row, three markers are used. With 0 denoting normal and 1 abnormal, 3-digit markers specify subtypes
[b] Possibility of a particular marker's being attributed to the occurrence of schizophrenia
[c] Including subtypes

and none with (111), but we also find in the schizophrenic group eight patients with (000), of whom four are self-supporting and two are free from drug treatment.

Although a single marker identifies only half of the schizophrenic patients as abnormal, the three markers when used in combination identify 85% of the patients as abnormal, as compared with 30% of normals. Among subtypes, the rate of occurrence of schizophrenia was examined using the ratio of S divided by N, depending upon a number of abnormal marker (1) and its specification. The pace at which schizophrenia occurred was increased additionally with regard to abnormal markers, and each marker was equivalent in this respect. These findings seem to support a multifactor and multistage development hypothesis of schizophrenia. The correlation between markers and symptomatology was examined by using the positive and negative syndrome scale (PANSS). Three markers were strongly correlated with the negative symptoms but not with the positive. DOR was slightly correlated with a subitem of positive symptoms, disorganization of thinking. Since I could not access the positive symptoms from the bottom-up route, I changed my plan to a top-down strategy, and adopted a tree-drawing test (Baum test) as a simple expressive test for imaginational activity. Figure 2 [6] shows samples from these drawings. I distinguished the Baum test data qualitatively into four categories: the usual type (A) and the unusual type, which was divided further into positive (C), negative (B), and combined (D) subtypes. These drawings can be explained by an array of adjectives. Type A is realistic, sketchy, cartoon-like and so on. Figures are more eloquent than words. Interrater reliability of this classification was examined by the use of kappa ($\kappa = 0.634$) indicating fair or good. Table 4 shows that 89% of the normal controls and 32% of the schizophrenic group draw the usual type. Fifty percent of the chronic schizophrenic patients draw the unusual negative subtype, and the acute and relapse-active schizophrenic patients frequently draw the unusual positive subtype.

Figure 3 shows the drawings of three patients with positive symptoms. A postdoctoral fellow in a state of acute psychotic disorder made an HTP (House-Tree-Person) drawing shown at the middle left. The trunks of trees are open and devoid of canopy. At the time of drawing, his binary data were (110). He asked me, "Can I drive a car?"

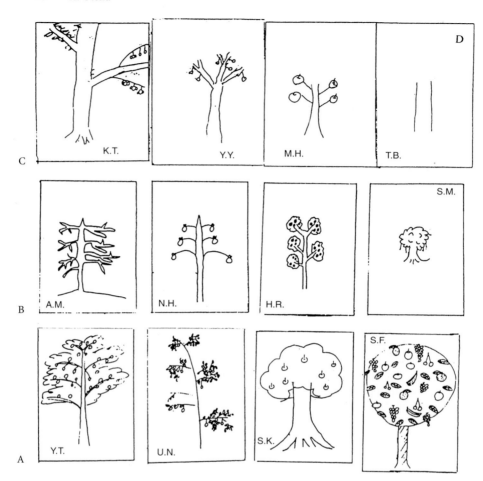

FIG. 2. Categories of Baum drawings (drawn on a postcard-sized paper). **A** Normal, usual type (~00). Realistic, sketchy, cartoon-like, explanatory, illustrative, detailed, luxuriant, etc. **B** Unusual, negative type (~01). Stiff, shrunk, vague, rough, crude, coarse, hazy, etc. **C** Unusual, positive type (~10). Truncated, canopy-less, leaky, chaotic, etc. **D** Unusual, combined type (~11). Combining B and C

and I said, "No, your reaction time is slow." I asked, "What's your feeling now?" He replied, "The three worlds are nothing but expression of the mind." This statement derives from a Buddhist script. After recovery, he drew a normal tree at right with the binary data (000). A 57-year-old professional in an elated state with confused thinking made the drawing at the bottom right. Here we also found a truncated tree without a canopy. He explained the meaning of his drawing with the illustration at left, depicting a monocular apprehension of both the inside and outside of the earth seen simultaneously. His binary data were (001) and his DOR was 1.506. He also said, "Stop the moment, you are beautiful," a quotation from Goethe's *Faust*.

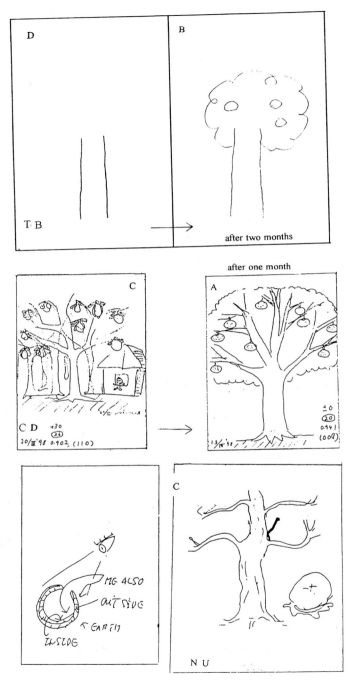

FIG. 3. Drawings by three patients with positive symptoms. Criteria of classification of Baum test (drawn on a postcard-sized paper). **A, B, C, D**: see the legend for Fig. 2

TABLE 4. Baum test: Comparison between normal controls and schizophrenic patients

Phase, stage	Normal controls	Schizophrenic group		Sum
		Chronic, stable	Acute, relapsed	
Mean age (yr)	34 (21–68)	45 (28–60)	36 (20–54)	
Normal, usual type	73 (89%)	17	7	24 (32%)
Unusual, negative type	5 (6%)	24	10	34 (47%)
Unusual, positive type	3 (4%)	1 ⎫ 6	7 ⎫ 9	8 (11%)
Unusual, combined type	1 (1%)	5 ⎭	2 ⎭	7 (12%)
Total sum	82 (100%)	47	26	73 (100%)

My question is, What is the nature of the drawing of the truncated tree without canopy, or How can we grasp the above-mentioned solipsistic state of mind in terms of neuropsychology. When I encountered a drawing consisting of only two perpendicular lines at the top left on the figure, I realized suddenly that it may be due to the destruction of gestalt formation. It has been argued that the gestalt construction may be related to the gamma (25–45 Hz) oscillation of brain activity. Based upon the above-mentioned delay of RCT in patients with schizophrenia, together with other circumstantial evidence, e.g., the apparent movement in Gestalt psychology, the perception of yellow by the fusion of red and green flashes, and the perception of causality (Michotte [7]) etc., I hypothesized a quantal unit of time conception for the duration of 25–50 ms and called it "moment consciousness." It is intriguing to think that the peculiar schizophrenic experiences could be regarded as expressions of disturbance in "moment consciousness" and exert further, profound influences on the long life-course of patients. My hypothesis is described in detail elsewhere [6].

References

1. Utena H (1996) Loss of freedom in mental disorders. Annu Psychoanal 24:131–137
2. Utena H (1996) Studies on relapse, course and outcome of schizophrenia in Japan. Psychiat Clin Neurosci 50:45–49
3. Ogawa K, Miya M, Watarai A, et al (1987) A long-term follow-up study of schizophrenia in Japan—with special reference to the course of social adjustment. Br J Psychiatry 151:758–765
4. Utena H, Miyake Y (1996) Functional subtyping of schizophrenia on the combined use of reaction time and stress response (in Japanese). Seishin Igaku (Clin Psychiatry) 38:127–133
5. Utena H, Miyake Y (1997) Simple psychophysiological tests for the daily clinical use, with special reference to schizophrenia (in Japanese). Seishin Igaku (Clin Psychiatry) 39:801–808
6. Utena H (2000) Brain and mind meet in forms and words (in Japanese). Rinsho-Seishinbyori (Jpn J Psychopathol) 21:205–214
7. Michotte A (1963) La perception de la causalité. English translation by Miles TR, Miles E, The perception of causality. Methuen, London

Efficacy of Semantic Cues in Schizophrenic Patients and Patients with Frontal Lesions from the Standpoint of Neuropsychological Rehabilitation

Haruo Kashima

Summary. Two neuropsychological studies are presented in which the role of verbal or semantic cues in improving the behavioral deficits of patients with schizophrenia and patients with frontal lesions was investigated. In a study of the efficacy of semantic cues in the performance of the Wisconsin Card Sorting Test (WCST), a new modified version of the WCST, the Keio version (KWCST), was administered to patients with chronic schizophrenia and patients with frontal lesions. Instructions for the KWCST are given in two steps in order to make subsequent task performance easier. In the first step, the instructions are the same as in the original WCST, and in the second step, the patients are instructed that the classification category has been changed. In the first step, patients with schizophrenia and patients with frontal lesions had equally poor results on the KWCST, which suggested frontal dysfunction in patients with schizophrenia. However, marked improvement in the score was observed in the patients with schizophrenia in the second step. The study showed that semantic instructions or cues improved the performance on the WCST more effectively in the patients with schizophrenia. The other study investigated impaired verbal regulation of behavior (IVR) IVR is a relatively well-known frontal lobe symptom, but it has not been studied sufficiently. In normal subjects, speech that expresses an action or that is related to it makes performing the action easier. In patients with frontal lesions, however, the facilitating function of words on actions is frequently lost. The occurrence of IVR was investigated during the tasks of the KWCST in patients with schizophrenia and in patients with frontal lesions. About 70% of the patients with frontal lesions and less than 10% of the patients with schizophrenia had IVR. Both studies suggest that verbal or semantic cues given by oneself and/or others improve behavioral deficits more effectively in patients with schizophrenia than in patients with frontal lesions, and they suggest the importance of verbal or semantic approaches in the effective rehabilitation of schizophrenia.

Key words. Schizophrenia, Frontal lobe, Semantic cue, Wisconsin Card Sorting Test, Impaired verbal regulation of behavior

The main theme of this chapter is the cognitive and behavioral rehabilitation of patients with schizophrenia, in which verbal instruction or semantic cues play a

Department of Neuropsychiatry, School of Medicine, Keio University, 35 Shinanomachi, Shinjuku-ku, Tokyo 160-8582, Japan

crucial role. Two neuropsychological studies will be presented, both of which show that semantic cues to control subjects' behavior are much more effective in patients with schizophrenia than in patients with frontal lobe damage. The first study is about the efficacy of semantic cues in the performance of the Wisconsin Card Sorting Test (WCST). The second one is about so-called impaired verbal regulation (IVR) of behavior during the performance of the WCST. In both studies, we used our modified version of WCST, i.e., the Keio version of WCST.

The WCST is a widely used frontal function test and was devised to study concept change or shift of set. In this test the subject is given a pack of cards on which are printed one to four symbols, triangle, star, cross, or circle, in red, green, yellow, or blue. The patient's task is to place them one by one under four stimulus cards according to a principle of classification category that the patient must deduce from the pattern of the examiner's responses to the patient's placement of the cards. For instance, if the classification category is color, the correct placement of a green card is under two green stars, regardless of the symbol or number, and the examiner will respond accordingly. The subject simply begins placing cards and the examiner states whether each placement is correct. After a run of six correct placements in a row, the examiner shifts the classification category, indicating the shift only in the changed pattern of "right" and "wrong" statements.

However, the original version of the WCST is too large and distressing for brain-damaged subjects and is often unavailable. Therefore we devised a new version of the WCST, the Keio version of the Wisconsin Card Sorting Test (KWSCT) [1]. The three main modifications in the KWSCT are smaller number of response cards (48), the order of reaction cards, and the process of giving instructions. We fix the order of reaction cards so as to identify the subject's reaction category completely. The instructions are given in two steps. The instruction of the first step is the same as that in the original version, that is, the instruction of three classification categories. This is the first trial of the KWCST. In the second instruction step, the subject obtains the information that the examiner changes his category after a certain number of correct responses, the second trial. With these modifications, this test can be conducted in most brain-damaged subjects. The instruction in the second step is considered as the verbal or semantic cue, which makes the task much easier, at least for normal subjects.

Efficacy of Semantic Cues in the Performance of the WCST

The first study examined efficacy of semantic cues in the performance of the WCST. Originally the purpose of this study was to investigate frontal dysfunction in patients with schizophrenia. However, the results showed a different pattern from those of frontally damaged subjects. Rather, the results demonstrated that performance of the WCST in patients with schizophrenia was remarkably improved by giving semantic cues.

There were a total of 157 subjects: 53 with schizophrenia (mean age 43.7 years), 30 with frontal lobe damage (mean age 42.6 years) 34 nonfrontally brain-damaged subjects (mean age 42.7 years), and 40 healthy control subjects (mean age 43.4 years). Diagnosis of schizophrenia was according to DSM-III.

Procedure

The KWCST, Wechsler Adult Intelligence Scale (WAIS), and Kraepelin Calculation Test were administered to the subjects. WAIS was selected as a specific test that reflects relatively posterior cerebral functions.

As stated above, in the KWCST, the instructions are given in two steps. The first step is the same as in the original version [2], and in the second step of instruction, the subject obtains the information that the examiner changes his category after a certain number of correct responses [3]. The instruction in the second step is considered the verbal or semantic cue, which makes the task much easier, at least for normal subjects.

Results

As shown in Table 1, in the first trial of KWCST with the first step of instruction, the scores of categories achieved (CA), total errors (TE), and perseverative errors (PE) revealed no significant differences between patients with schizophrenia and the frontal group. The scores of the nonfrontal group were significantly superior to those of patients with schizophrenia and frontal patients. In patients with schizophrenia and in nonfrontal patients, significant correlations were found between the KWCST scores and full IQ. In the WAIS, the frontal group showed significantly higher full IQ than patients with schizophrenia and the nonfrontal group.

As clearly shown in Table 2, in the second trial of KWCST with the second step of instruction, in which the task condition is easier than in the first trial, the scores of categories achieved (CA), total errors (TE), and perseverative errors (PE) improved in patients with schizophrenia and in nonfrontal patients. Notably, the improvement of patients with schizophrenia was so striking that their scores surpassed those of nonfrontal patients. On the other hand, the improvement in the frontal patients was

TABLE 1. First trial of KWCST and IQ

Subjects	CA	TE	PE	IQ
Schizophrenia	2.5	25.5	9.9	76.3
Frontal	2.6	25.4	11.5	92.4
Nonfrontal	3.4	20.2	8.0	72.5
Control	5.4	10.9	1.5	/

KWCST, Keio version of Wisconsin Card Sorting Test; CA, Categories achieved; TE, total errors; PE, perseverative errors

TABLE 2. Second trial of KWCST

Subjects	CA	TE	PE
Schizophrenia	4.5	14.0	2.8
Frontal	3.0	23.7	11.7
Nonfrontal	4.3	17.0	5.1
Control	5.8	8.3	0

CA, Categories achieved; TE, total errors; PE, perseverative errors

TABLE 3. Correlation between KWCST and psychiatric symptoms, IQ, and Kraepelin calculation test in patients with schizophrenia

Test	CA	TE	PE
BPRS			
Nos. 1, 2, 4, 5, 6, 11, 12, 15	−	+	−
Nos. 3, 16	+	+	+
SANS total scores	+	+	+
IQ	+	+	+
Kraepelin Test	+	+	+

BPRS, Brief Psychiatric Rating Scale; SANS, Scale for the Assessment of Negative Symptoms
+ Significant correlation

TABLE 4. Neuropsychological characteristics

Subjects	Improvement in 2nd trial	Dissociation KWCST and IQ	Correlation KWCST and IQ
Schizophrenia	++	−	++
Frontal	−	++	−
Nonfrontal	+	+	−

very little. As shown in Table 3 in the correlation between KWCST and psychiatric symptoms, IQ, and Kraepelin Calculation Test, significant correlations were also found between these KWCST scores and full IQ in patients with schizophrenia, but not in frontal patients.

Table 4 shows summarizes the first study. The results of KWCST differed among patients with schizophrenia, frontal patients, and nonfrontal patients. Frontal patients showed lower scores of KWCST overall, in spite of relatively high IQ, and this may be regarded as a specific dissociation. No significant correlations with full IQ were seen. Most importantly, no improvements were seen in the second trial, despite the easier test condition. In contrast, patients with schizophrenia showed marked improvement in the second trial, no dissociations between KWCST scores and IQ, and high correlation between KWCST scores and IQ. These results demonstrated a marked difference between frontal patients and schizophrenic patients, rather than a resemblance. The frontal dysfunction theory of schizophrenia was not supported in this study. However, the results are most interesting from the viewpoint of the efficacy of verbal instruction or semantic cues in patients with schizophrenia. In patients with schizophrenia, verbal instruction or semantic cues are expected to be more effective than in frontal patients.

Impaired Verbal Regulation of Behavior

The above conclusion is further supported by the second study, on IVR. IVR is a frontal lobe symptom that is been relatively well known but has not been studied in detail [4,5]. In normal subjects, speech that expresses an action or that is related to it makes the performance of the action easier. In patients with frontal lobe lesions, however, the facilitating function of words on the action is frequently lost.

This symptom has also been called the loss of the regulatory role of speech on behavior or dissociation between language and behavior [6]. IVR has been observed and evaluated during tasks of more elementary movement, such as continuous changes among multiple motor acts and drawing multiple figures. The purpose of this study was to examine whether the phenomenon of IVR can be seen even at higher levels of psychological processes. We used the WCST and examined the IVR during the sorting tasks that require concept manipulation in higher orders or levels [7].

The subjects were 38 patients with schizophrenia (mean age 52.1 years), 36 frontally damaged subjects (mean age 57.5 years), 22 nonfrontally brain-damaged subjects (mean age 53.0 years), and 12 healthy control subjects (mean age 49.3 years).

Methods

The KWCST as modified by the authors was used. Among the 48 response cards used in the KWCST, the 13th to 36th cards were utilized for the evaluation of IVR. To test congruence of verbal expression and action, the subject was asked to speak aloud in words the classification category before placing the response card. When the subject's word is correct but the corresponding behavior is incorrect, the performance is considered as IVR, but not vice versa. When the subject's word is incorrect but the behavior is correct, that is not IVR. Only when the subject's word is correct can his or her performance be considered as IVR. Although the definition of IVR is simple, to judge whether the subject's word is correct is not always simple. We strictly defined the following three conditions to judge the subject's word as really correct.

In the first condition, during a series of correct responses, that is, when the classification category of the subject corresponds to that of the tester, the subject may speak aloud the word of that particular classification category. For example, as seen in Fig. 1a, the tester maintained the classification category "color," and the subject continued to place his response cards according to the classification category "color." During this, the subject spoke aloud the word "color" before he placed each response card. The words said in this condition are considered correct.

In the second condition, when the tester switches the classification category, the subject may continue to speak aloud the word of the preceding category. Figure 1b shows an example. Here the classification category "color" had been achieved. According to the manual of our version, one classification category is achieved when six successive correct responses are obtained. The tester then switched to the classification category "figure" without saying it, that is, the tester's category of the seventh card became "figure." The subject is likely to speak aloud "color" at this—the word is judged as correct.

The subject's word is also considered correct in the following condition. After the tester switches to a new classification category, the subject tries to find out the new one. As shown in Fig. 1c, because the subject's classification of the 7th card is wrong, he may speak aloud "figure" or "number" at the 8th card—both are judged as correct, and in addition, if he speaks aloud "figure" at the 9th card, it is also judged as correct.

Although it seems somewhat complicated or perplexing, in this study we considered that the subject said the correct words in these three conditions. Under these

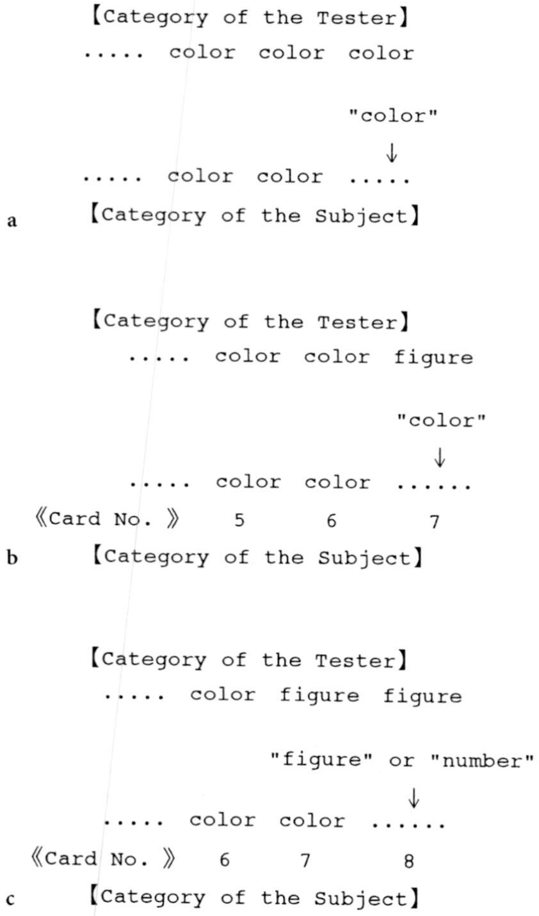

【Category of the Tester】
..... color color color

"color"
↓
..... color color .....
a   【Category of the Subject】

FIG. 1. Definition of impaired verbal regulation of behavior (IVR) **a** Condition 1 under which the words of the subject were judged as correct. **b** Condition 2 under which the words of the subject were judged as correct. **c** Condition 3 under which the words of the subject were judged as correct

【Category of the Tester】
..... color color figure

"color"
↓
..... color color ......
《Card No. 》   5   6   7
b   【Category of the Subject】

【Category of the Tester】
..... color figure figure

"figure" or "number"
↓
..... color color ......
《Card No. 》   6   7   8
c   【Category of the Subject】

TABLE 5. Proportion of subjects with IVR(%) and the frequency of appearance of IVR in each group

Subjects	Proportion of subjects with IVR (%)	Frequency of IVR
Schizophrenia	2/38 (5.3)	0.2
Frontal	25/36 (69.4)	2.35
Nonfrontal	6/22 (27.3)	0.5
Control	0/12 (0)	0

IVR, impaired verbal regulation of behavior

three conditions, disagreement between the classification category used on actually placing the card and the words pronounced was defined as IVR.

Results

Table 5 shows the proportion of subjects with IVR, expressed as percentages of all subjects, and the average numbers of those with IVR. The percentage of subjects with IVR was about 5% in patients with schizophrenia, but 70% in the frontal group. In the nonfrontal group it was slightly less than 30%. IVR occurred significantly more frequently in subjects with frontal lesions than in patients with schizophrenia. The number of subjects with IVR in the frontal group was also significantly higher, about 10 times that in the schizophrenia group. IVR was not observed in the control group. The results clearly demonstrate that in patients with schizophrenia, but not in those with frontal lobe lesions, verbal control of behavior is well preserved. In other words, verbal or semantic cues are likely to work to correct some type of behavioral disturbances in schizophrenic patients.

Those two studies consistently suggested that verbal or semantic cues given by oneself and/or others improve some type of behavioral deficits more effectively in schizophrenic patients than in patients with frontal lesions, which leads to the importance of verbal or semantic approaches in the effective rehabilitation of patients with schizophrenia.

References

1. Kashima H, Handa T, Kato M (1987) Neuropsychological investigation on chronic schizophrenia—aspects of its frontal function. In: Takahashi R, Flor-Henry P, Gluzelier J, Niwa S (eds) Cerebral dynamics, laterality and psychopathology. Elsevier, Amsterdam, pp 337–345
2. Milner B (1973) Effects of different brain lesions on card sorting. Arch Neurol 9:90–100
3. Nelson HE (1976) A modified card sorting test sensitive to frontal lobe defects. Cortex 12:313–324
4. Luria AR (1973) Basis of neuropsychology. Moscow University Press, Moscow
5. Kaczmarek BLJ (1987) Regulatory function of the frontal lobes: a neurolinguistic perspective. In: Perecman E (ed) the frontal lobe revisited. IRBN Press, New York, pp 225–240
6. Luria AR, Homskaya ED (eds) (1996) Frontal lobe and regulation of psychological processes (in Russian). MGU, Moscow
7. Kashima H (1995) Unawareness and impaired verbal regulation in frontal damaged patients (in Japanese). Higher Brain Funct Res 15:181–187

Neuropsychological Investigation of the Effects of Psychiatric Rehabilitation Strategies for Schizophrenia

Masafumi Mizuno and Haruo Kashima

Summary. Several studies have found a relationship between cognitive functioning and social skills in schizophrenia. The results are generally consistent with the hypothesis that poor cognitive functioning contributes to social skill impairment. In a series of studies on the efficacy of social skill training, improvement by training was stressed, but the difficulty of generalization of skills inquired by training is still controversial. The impairments not improved through skill training, however, may provide cues or hints for additional rehabilitation strategies. Several clinical neuropsychological tests, behavioral assessment by rehabilitation evaluation (REHAB), and psychiatric symptoms assessment by the Brief Psychiatric Rating Scale (BPRS) were administered to patients with schizophrenia before and after 22 hours of social skill training (SST) sessions. SST was performed in a day treatment program for outpatients with stable psychiatric symptoms. Trained staffs conducted a 1-hour program every week for a total 22 sessions, in addition to standard psychiatric treatment. The results show that performance on the Idea Fluency Test, which requests as many responses as possible on the uses of objects, was significantly better after the sessions than before the sessions. However, further qualitative analysis of the responses showed that the improvement of the total score on the Idea Fluency Test was due to the increase of task-dependent form responses connected with the regular uses and shapes of the object. Task modification form responses in the Idea Fluency Test that required conversion of viewpoint did not improve. This may in part explain the difficulty of escaping from stereotyped thinking by patients with schizophrenia.

Key words. Schizophrenic disorder, Social functioning, Divergent thinking, Fluency test, SST

It is well known that cognitive impairment is an important feature of people with schizophrenia, who exhibit disabilities that profoundly affect their social functioning [1–5], and a great deal of research has attempted to remedy the cognitive deficits [6–8]. A series of wide-ranging clinical neuropsychological tests was administered before

Department of Neuropsychiatry, School of Medicine, Keio University, 35 Shinanomachi, Shinjuku-ku, Tokyo 160-8582, Japan

and after application of skills training [9,10], but despite the recognition of the importance of cognitive impairment in schizophrenia, the elaboration and development of rehabilitative treatments have not yet borne much fruit. Social skills training is now the most prevalent and one of the most effective rehabilitation techniques used for schizophrenia in Japan. Despite the general efficacy of social skills training in schizophrenia, previous research in the area has not fully demonstrated the mechanisms of its effects on the neurocognitive system. It is necessary to clarify the further specific neurocognitive processes linked with the effect of specific rehabilitation strategies. The present study examined the changes in neurocognitive function before and after social skills training.

Subjects and Methods

The subjects were nine right-handed male outpatients with schizophrenia who regularly participated in day treatment and had stable psychiatric symptoms. Their average age was 31.8 years (range, 26–43), and their mean age at onset was 25.4 years (range, 20–37). Their mean education level was 14.5 years (range, 11–16). The subjects had no known organic impairment, and they were not alcohol or substance dependent. The psychiatric diagnosis was made by their psychiatrists based on ICD-10 Criteria. All of the subjects were treated with neuroleptics, and the mean chlorpromazine equivalent was 209.6 mg (range, 100–350).

All subjects were assigned to a skills training group based on the presence of social skill deficits and problems with interpersonal conflicts, as determined by observations of their everyday life by the staff. The skills training group was conducted by one trained clinical psychologist and another professional coleader. Each group contained about 10 participants. Group sessions lasted about 1 h, and the sessions were held once a week for about 6 months, for a total of 22 sessions. The training focused mainly on interpersonal communication skills, such as "expressing feelings" or "compromise and negotiation," depending on the needs of each individual. Skills training was conducted according to the method outlined by Liberman et al. [11]. It included the following steps: establishing a rationale for learning the skill and its relevance to patients' personal goals, modeling the skill in a role play by the leaders, engaging a patient in a role play to rehearse the skill, providing positive and corrective feedback to the participants, engaging the next patient in a role play, and assigning homework to practice the skill.

Neuropsychological Assessment

Neurocognitive function was assessed by a battery of neuropsychological tests administered before and after the social skills training intervention.

Letter Cancellation Test of Diller et al. [12]

The cancellation test was used to evaluate several functions, including visual scanning, rapid motor response, suppression of reactions, and focus of attention. We constructed a Japanese version of the test of Diller et al., in which the subject must delete a target letter "か (ka)" with a pencil in the right hand. Nine letters were randomly arranged in 6 lines of 52 letters, with each line containing 19 target letters. The correct numbers and the execution time were evaluated.

Stroop Tests [13]

Stroop tests are based on the finding that it takes longer to call out the names of colors of patches than to read the words, and even longer to read the names of colors when they are printed in ink of a different color. The latter phenomenon—the markedly slower naming response when the word is printed in ink of a different color—has been variously interpreted, but it is generally attributed to a response conflict or failure of response inhibition. We used two trials: one requiring naming of the printed colors (Part I), and the other focusing on color words printed in ink of different colors (Part II). Scoring was according to performance on the basis of time.

Wisconsin Card Sorting Test (WCST) (Keio Version) [14]

The WCST tests concept formation and concept change, and the results reflect frontal lobe function. The test uses cards on which one to four red, green, yellow, or blue triangles, stars, crosses, or circles are printed. The subjects are asked to place the cards one by one under four stimulus cards according to a category, color, shape, or number, but the examiner only tells the patients whether their responses are correct, and the patients have to figure out the category the examiner has in mind. In the WCST, patients have a high degree of freedom, and they are under no time restrictions. The WCST was administered twice in this study, and the number of categories achieved (CA), number of perseverative errors (PE), and difficulty of maintaining sets (DMS) scores were compared.

Fluency Test

Three different fluency tests were administered: the word fluency test, idea fluency test, and design fluency test.

In the word fluency test, the examiner asks the patients to say as many words in 60 s as they can think of that begin with a given *kana* (Japanese letter), excluding proper nouns and numbers. We used three *kana* having different frequencies of occurrence in the Japanese language. Category naming was also used. Animal, fruit, and vehicle naming tasks were each performed within 60 s. Fluency tests that require generation of words beginning with the same initial letter give the greatest scope to subjects in seeking a strategy to guide their search for words, and they are most difficult for subjects who cannot develop strategies of their own.

In the idea fluency test [15], the examiner asked the subject to think of as many uses for empty tin cans as possible in 5 minutes. The responses were classified into three groups: task-dependent responses, task-modified responses, and task-independent responses. Task-dependent responses are ideas immediately suggested by a stimulus object, such as its intended or common uses, for example, as an ashtray or a cup. Task-modified responses are ideas generated by considering the object's shape, size, material, and so on, in order to create new uses other than as conventional implements. This type of response requires a change in viewpoint and flexibility of thinking, for example, use of the tin cans as lampshades or toy clogs. Task-

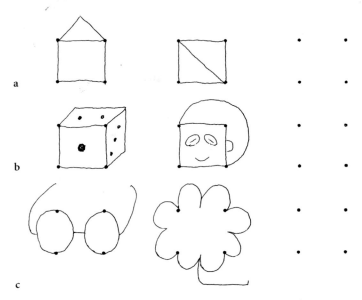

FIG. 1. Examples of responses in design fluency test. **a** Task-dependent responses, **b** task-modified responses, **c** task-independent responses

independent responses are ideas that are perceived from partial characteristics of the object and ignore the characteristics of the tin can as a receptacle. They focus on it as a cavity or a cylindrical form, and use it, for example, as an ornament or a paperweight. This type of response derives from remote conceptions that do not take into account the characteristics of the stimulus.

In design fluency tests [15,16], the examiner requests the subject to create as many pictures as possible in 5 min starting within four dots posted in a square already printed on the paper. The scoring method is the same as that of the idea fluency test. The responses were classified into three groups (Fig. 1): task-dependent responses, task-modified responses, and task-independent responses. Task-dependent responses are designs immediately suggested by the four dots, such as geometrical figures (Fig. 1a). Task-modified responses are designs generated by considering the shape of the four dots, that is, the four dots are on the corners of a square (Fig. 1b). They are, for example, a die, a face, and so on. This type of response requires a change in viewpoint and flexibility of design. Task-independent responses are designs that are generated from partial characteristics of the dots and ignore the characteristics of four dots on the corner as a square form (Fig. 1c). They are, for example, eyeglasses, flowers, and so on.

Other Assessments

The following assessments were administered before and after the skills training to evaluate behavior, psychopathology, and general intelligence levels. REHAB (Rehabilitation Evaluation [17]) was used as the behavior rating scale. It is a 23-item behav-

TABLE 1. Comparison of the Brief Psychiatric Rating Scale (BPRS), Rehabilitation Evaluation (REHAB), and Wechsler Adult Intelligence Test-Revised (WAIS-R) scores of people with schizophrenia before and after social skills training

Test	Before	After	p
BPRS	42.7	36.7	n.s.
REHAB			
Initiation of speech	3.9	2.0	<0.05
Speech clarity	2.3	1.0	<0.05
Amount of speech	2.3	1.9	n.s.
WAIS-R			
VIQ	104.0	108.0	n.s.
PIQ	87.3	93.0	n.s.
FIQ	96.4	102.0	n.s.

VIQ, Verbal Intelligence Quotient; PIQ, Performance Intelligence Quotient; FIQ, Full Intelligence Quotient; n.s., not significant

ior rating scale. Symptoms were assessed before and after skills training by the Brief Psychiatric Rating Scale (BPRS) [18] scored by trained psychiatrists blinded to whether the patients participated in the program. The Wechsler Adult Intelligence Scale-Revised (WAIS-R) [19] was administered before and after social skills training to evaluate general intelligence.

Results

The symptom assessment did not reveal changes after the training program in any parts of the BPRS (Table 1). In the REHAB, the score for initiation of speech (No. 13) improved significantly (before 3.9, after 2.0; $P < 0.05$), and speech clarity (No. 15) also improved significantly (before 2.3, after 1.0; $P < 0.05$). There was no statistically significant improvement in the score for amount of speech (No. 12) after training.

There were no changes in neuroleptic prescriptions between the start and end of the program, and the BPRS scores were unchanged by training.

As shown in Table 2, the results of the neuropsychological assessments showed that mean scores on the attention tests, word and category fluency tests, design fluency test, WAIS-R, and Stroop test did not change after training. The numbers of perseverative errors on the WCST significantly decreased from 5.0 to 2.9 ($P < 0.05$). The total number of responses on the idea fluency test improved significantly (before 9.0, after 12.8; $P < 0.01$), and as shown in Table 3, the numbers of task-dependent-type responses increased significantly, from 5.8 to 9.2 ($P < 0.01$), but there were no increases in the numbers of task-modification-type and task-independent-type responses.

Discussion

In the present study, improvement after skills training was seen in the numbers of perseverative errors on the WCST, the idea fluency test scores, and the sociobehavioral assessment, but not in the assessment of symptoms. All of the participants were

TABLE 2. Comparisons of neuropsychological assessment scores of people with schizophrenia before and after social skills training

Test	Before	After	p
Cancellation test			
Correct responses	110.9	111.4	n.s.
Time (s)	123.4	124.0	n.s.
Stroop test			
Part I	19.3	18.0	n.s.
Part II	27.7	26.6	n.s.
WCST (Keio version)			
CA	3.9	4.2	n.s.
PE	5.0	2.9	<0.05
DMS	1.1	0.7	n.s.
Fluency tests			
Word fluency test			
Letter	28.8	29.5	n.s.
Category	38.5	37.5	n.s.
Idea fluency test	9.0	12.8	<0.05
Design fluency test	11.0	9.8	n.s.

WCST, Wisconsin Card Sorting Test; CA, Categories achieved; PE, perseverative errors; DMS, difficulty of maintaining sets; n.s., not significant

TABLE 3. Comparisons of the idea fluency test scores of people with schizophrenia before and after social skills training

Response	Before	After	p
Total	9.0	12.8	<0.05
Td	5.8	9.2	<0.05
Tm	1.7	1.2	n.s.
Ti	1.4	2.4	n.s.

Td, Task-dependent responses; Tm, task-modified responses; Ti, task-independent responses; n.s., not significant

in a chronic and symptomatically stable stage, and no changes were observed on the BPRS. The WCST score improved in the retest situation, as found by Kashima et al [14].

The total score on the idea fluency test, which reflects fluency of concept production, improved considerably after the training program. The REHAB scores and initiation of speech scores improved significantly (before 3.9, after 2.0; $P < 0.05$), and speech clarity also significantly improved (before 2.3, after 1.0; $P < 0.05$). The results seem to indicate that idea fluency scores can be useful indices for predicting the efficacy of social skills training.

On the other hand, one of the most important aims of the rehabilitation program is to achieve generalization of the trained activities. Our qualitative analysis of the idea fluency data suggested that the increase in response numbers was consistent with the increase in ideas derived from the theme-dependent responses, such as an ashtray or a vessel, which are perceived from the form or characteristics of an empty can. Modified responses, for example, a lampshade or toy clogs for play, which are perceived from the characteristics of the can as a receptacle, could not be found as much in most of the people with schizophrenia, even after the skills training sessions.

The idea fluency test is considered to be a test evaluating divergent thinking. Divergent thinking is a way of thinking to spread through various kinds of courses. It is a thought that demands various information related to the stimuli in sequence. Guilford [20] proposed this form of thinking as one of the factors of creativity. The results of our study suggest that people with schizophrenia have deficits in divergent thinking from a neuropsychological standpoint, and especially that they have difficulty overcoming stereotyped thinking. These difficulties may be related to their inability to solve social problems. Divergent production is part of Guilford's structure-of-intellect model, an attempt to organize all human cognition along three dimensions: thought processes, or operations that can be performed; content, to which operations can be applied; and product, which might result from performing operations on different content categories. Guilford's original conceptualization of divergent thinking has been retained in current creativity theorizing, primarily in the four general categories—fluency, flexibility, originality, and elaboration—into which he grouped them.

In real-life situations, problems and their solutions are very complex, and problem-solving and creative thinking require that intellectual faculties work together. The two are intimately related, because solving problems calls for novel steps in behavior, and this means creative performance.

Nonetheless, initial screening of divergent products (problem-solving capacity) may yield an empirical basis for selecting patients who are most likely to benefit from social and behavioral rehabilitation programs.

References

1. Bellack AS, Morrison RL, Wixted JT, et al (1990) An analysis of social competence in schizophrenia. Br J Psychiatry 156:809–818
2. Mueser KT, Bellack AS, Morrison RL, et al (1990) Social competence in schizophrenia: premorbid adjustment, social skills, and domains of functioning. J Abnorm Psychol 105:271–275
3. Green MF (1996) What are the functional consequences of neurocognitive deficits in schizophrenia? Am J Psychiatry 153:321–330
4. Bellack AS (1992) Cognitive rehabilitation for schizophrenia: Is it possible? Is it necessary? Schizophr Bull 18:43–50
5. Hogarty GE, Flesher S (1992) Cognitive remediation in schizophrenia: Proceed . . . with caution. Schizophr Bull 18:51–57
6. Liberman RP, Green MF (1992) Whither cognitive-behavioral therapy for schizophrenia? Schizophr Bull 90:432–444
7. Penn DL (1991) Cognitive rehabilitation of social deficits in schizophrenia: a direction of promise or following a primrose path? Psychosoc Rehabil J 15:27–41
8. Wallace CJ, Nelson CJ, Liberman RP, et al (1980) A review and critique of social skills training with schizophrenic patients. Schizophr Bull 6:42–63

9. Ikebuchi E, Nakagome K, Takahashi N (1999) How do early stages of information processing influence social skills in patients with schizophrenia? Schizophr Res 35: 255–262
10. Corrigan PW (1991) Social skills training in adult psychiatric populations: a meta-analysis. J Behav Ther Exp Psychiatry 22:203–210
11. Lieberman RP, DeRisi WJ, Mueser KT (1989) Social skills training for psychiatric patients. Pergamon Press, New York
12. Diller L, Ben-Yishay Y, Gerstman LJ, et al (1974) Studies in cognition and rehabilitation in hemiplegia. Rehabil Monogr. 50, New York University Medical Center Institute of Rehabilitation Medicine, New York
13. Dodrill CB (1978) A neuropsychological battery for epilepsy. Epilepsia 19:611–623
14. Kashima H, Handa T, Kato M, et al (1987) Neuropsychological investigation on chronic schizophrenia—aspects of its frontal functions. In: Takahashi R, Flor-Henry P, Gruzelier J et al (eds) Cerebral dynamics, laterality and psychopathology. Elsevier Science Publishers, Amsterdam, pp 337–345
15. Saito H (1996) The reduction of fluency in patients with frontal lobe lesions—a neuropsychological investigation with fluency tests. J Keio Med Soc 73:399–409
16. Jones-Gotman M, Milner B (1977) Design fluency: the invention of nonsense drawings after focal cortical lesions. Neuropsychologia 15:653–674
17. Baker R, Hall JH (1988) REHAB: a new assessment instrument for chronic psychiatric patients. Schizophr Bull 14:97–111
18. Overall JE, Gorham DR (1962) The Brief Psychiatric Rating Scale. Psychol Rep 10: 799–812
19. Wechsler D (1981) WAIS-R manual. Psychological Corporation, New York
20. Guilford JP (1967) The structure of intelligence. The nature of human intelligence. McGraw-Hill, New York, pp 70–249

Coping with Interpersonal Stressors in Schizophrenia

Joseph Ventura[1], Keith H. Nuechterlein[1,2], and Kenneth L. Subotnik[1]

Summary. Although stressful life events can trigger psychotic and depressive symptom exacerbation in schizophrenia, many patients who experience stress do not subsequently relapse. Recent versions of the vulnerability-stress-protective factors model of schizophrenia suggest that coping responses may serve as critical mediating variables. Most of the research on coping behavior in schizophrenia has focused on strategies for dealing with symptoms of the illness rather than with interpersonal stressors. Using the Coping Responses Inventory developed by Moos, we examined how 13 chronic, but clinically stable, schizophrenia outpatients and 11 demographically matched normal subjects responded to a negative interpersonal life event. Cognitively oriented problem-focused approaches ("Think of different ways to deal with the problem") and behaviorally oriented problem-solving strategies ("Make a plan of action and follow it") were used significantly more often by normal controls than by schizophrenic patients ($p < 0.01$). However, the use of cognitive or behavioral avoidance coping did not differ significantly between groups. Whereas normal controls use a wide range of coping behaviors that involves both approach and avoidance responses, the repertoire of coping responses of chronic schizophrenia patients appears, on average, to be relatively more focused on avoidance.

Key words. Schizophrenia, Stress, Coping, Depression

Introduction

Since the publication of the seminal paper on a vulnerability-stress model by Zubin and Spring [1], several versions of such models have been developed to incorporate the latest findings in schizophrenia research [2–6]. Stressful life events, a central feature of these models, have been shown to increase the risk of psychosis [7–9]. It appears that both major and minor life events may be associated with exacerbation of psychotic symptoms [10–12]. In addition, some evidence suggests that the effects

---

[1] Department of Psychiatry and Biobehavioral Sciences, UCLA, 300 Medical Plaza, Room 2240, Los Angeles, CA 90095-6968, USA
[2] Department of Psychology, UCLA, USA

of stress may persist well beyond the cessation of the original stressor [13,14]. Further, neuroleptic medication cannot completely prevent stress-induced increases in dopamine or in psychotic symptoms [15,16], and even when protected by the effects of medication, many patients have residual symptoms and social disability [17]. However, stressful events alone are neither necessary nor sufficient as precursors of psychotic relapse [18,19]. Despite the fact that most clinicians advise their patients to reduce stress to avoid symptoms, some studies and reviews of the literature suggest the relationship between stress and relapse is relatively weak [20,21].

Beyond the role of stressful life events in triggering psychosis in schizophrenia, their role in periods of depression in schizophrenia needs consideration. Several studies show a relationship between stressful life events and exacerbations of depressive symptoms in schizophrenia [22–25]. Although much of this previous research has some methodological weaknesses, recent research with a rigorous experimental design has confirmed earlier findings. A recent well-designed prospective study that used survival analysis techniques showed that stressful life events can trigger depressive exacerbation in patients with recent-onset schizophrenia [26]. These findings suggest that schizophrenic patients who experience undesirable life events may have vulnerability to depression that is similar to the vulnerability of individuals with a primary diagnosis of mood disorder. Thus, stressful events may play an even broader role in schizophrenia than is typically theorized by vulnerability-stress-protective factors models [3,27].

The "dynamic vulnerability formulation" hypothesizes that vulnerability factors interact with and modify each other over time [28]. The dynamic vulnerability perspective implies that a simple bivariate formulation of a stress-relapse relationship in schizophrenia cannot be applied to the majority of schizophrenic patients. Stress might be a sufficient cause for increased psychotic symptoms in some schizophrenic patients, a necessary contributor for others, a trigger of a psychotic episode at one point in time but not at another in the same patient, and totally irrelevant for still other patients. Some individuals with schizophrenia have been hospitalized after seemingly innocuous events, e.g., the local store clerk who befriended one patient moved away precipitously [29]. Yet many schizophrenic patients, as well as many individuals without schizophrenia, have endured severe life events, such as the loss of a family member, without an increase in psychotic symptoms. Furthermore, it has been observed that schizophrenic patients have been hospitalized in the absence of an apparent stressor [30].

The apparent inconsistencies in the reactions of schizophrenic patients to life events can be reconciled by models suggesting that protective factors play a mediating role in the stress-illness relationship. Many schizophrenic patients who experience stressful life events do not relapse, possibly because they mobilize responses that can be termed "successful coping." Several versions of vulnerability-stress models of schizophrenia have emphasized protective factors, such as personal coping skills and positive appraisal of stress [5,27,31,32]. However, most of the research on coping behavior in schizophrenia has focused on patients' strategies for dealing with symptoms of their illness rather than strategies for coping with environmental stressors [33–36].

In research focusing on how individuals in the general community cope with environmental stressors, several different types of coping responses have been characterized. Two types of coping behaviors that are generally considered adaptive have been identified: problem-focused coping behavior and emotion-based coping [37]. Problem-focused coping entails defining a problem, generating possible solutions (strategies), weighing the alternatives, and then taking steps toward changing or reducing the stressful situation. Emotion-based coping is directed at changing the way that one feels about a stressful situation. A third type of coping, avoidance, is generally considered not to be problem-focused. Avoidance coping involves cognitive attempts to avoid thinking realistically about a problem or behavioral attempts to involve oneself in substitute activities [38]. Reducing tension by expressing negative feelings has also been labeled as avoidance coping.

To the extent that schizophrenic patients use similar coping behaviors when dealing with both daily life stressors and symptoms of their illness, studies of coping with symptoms may be informative. The use of multiple coping strategies and the consistent application of one strategy has been associated with successful reduction in psychotic symptoms [33,39]. In addition, studies have found that schizophrenic patients tended to use non-problem-focused methods of coping, e.g., withdrawal from an interpersonal interaction [35,40,41]. Moreover, Böker et al. [35] hypothesized that the successful use of illness coping strategies may alter the course of schizophrenia. Interestingly, the literature on how schizophrenic patients cope with psychotic symptoms suggests that both active and passive strategies are useful.

Effective coping behaviors in patients and their families may change potentially threatening, highly stressful situations into more minor events and thus reduce the risk of relapse [19]. Based on data from a small number of studies, it appears that schizophrenic patients and normal controls may cope with stressful life events differently. Normal controls were found to use more variety in problem-focused coping strategies and reported that their coping efforts were more successful as compared with psychotic patients [42]. In contrast, a majority of patients (62%) reported they often coped with stressful events by using escape/avoidance and distancing behaviors, such as "keeping the problem to myself" [43,44]. Thus, initial evidence suggests that normal controls might use coping behavior that successfully mediates the potentially harmful effects of stress more than do schizophrenic patients.

In this study, we examined whether there were differences in the types of coping strategies used by schizophrenic patients compared with those used by normal controls. We hypothesized that schizophrenic patients use problem-focused coping strategies less often and engage in avoidance coping behavior more often than do controls.

Methods

Participants

The participants were drawn from sample 1 of the Developmental Processes in Schizophrenic Disorders Project [27]. The current sample was composed of 13 outpatients with chronic schizophrenia ($n = 11$) or schizoaffective disorder ($n = 2$). The mean age at the time of assessment was 29.9 years (SD, 5.5), and the mean education was 11.6 years (SD, 1.9). Eleven patients (85%) were male. The distribution of marital status was 69% single, 8% married, and 23% other. The ethnic/racial distribution was 85% Caucasian, 8% Asian, and 8% other. On the Hollingshead Two-Factor Scale [45] of social class, these patients represented the full range, with a mean of 3.1 (SD, 1.1) in the middle class. The 11 normal control subjects were on average 27.8 years old (SD, 5.9) and had an average of 12.4 years of education (SD, 1.7). Nine of the normal subjects (82%) were male. The marital status of the control subjects was 80% single, 10% married, and 10% other. The ethnic/racial distribution was 91% Caucasian, 9% Latino, and 4% Asian. The patients and normal control subjects were statistically comparable with regard to sex, age, education, marital status, and ethnicity. After oral and written information regarding this project had been provided, all subjects gave written informed consent to participate.

Patient participants in the Developmental Processes in Schizophrenic Disorders Project were recruited primarily from four large public psychiatric hospitals in the Los Angeles area during or very shortly after a psychotic episode. A few patients did not require hospitalization and were recruited from referrals to the UCLA Neuropsychiatric Hospital and to the UCLA Aftercare Research Program. The patients met the Research Diagnostic Criteria (RDC) [46] for schizophrenia ($n = 11$) or schizoaffective disorder, depressed type, mainly schizophrenic ($n = 2$). By Diagnostic and Statistical Manual of Mental Disorders, 3rd edition, revised (DSM-III-R) criteria [47], the diagnoses at project entry were schizophrenia ($n = 11$) and schizoaffective disorder ($n = 2$) depressed type.

Procedures

Diagnostic and Screening Procedures

All diagnoses were based on an expanded version of the Present State Examination (PSE) [48] that included items from the Schedule for Affective Disorders and Schizophrenia [49]. All interviewers were trained to minimum standards set by the Diagnosis and Psychopathology Unit of the UCLA Center for Research on Treatment and Rehabilitation of Psychosis (Robert P. Liberman, M.D., Principal Investigator) and entered a quality assurance program to prevent rater drift [50]. Potential normal comparison subjects were screened with the PSE, selected modules from the Structured Clinical Interview for OSM-II (SCID-II), and the Minnesota Multiphasic Personality Inventory (MMPI) to exclude those with major Axis I disorders or schizophrenia spectrum personality disorders. Comparison subjects were eligible for study entry provided there was no family history of a major psychiatric disorder or alcoholism in a first-degree relative. Both groups of participants were required to have no history of head trauma or loss of consciousness for more than 5 min, and no current significant and habitual alcohol or drug abuse.

Clinical Setting

Each patient was assigned a case manager and received individual and group therapy focused on social and independent living skills. This behaviorally oriented therapy was provided within the context of a treatment team at the UCLA Aftercare Research Program. The patient's immediate relatives received education about the illness of schizophrenia. Psychopharmacological treatment was supervised by very experienced clinic psychiatrists and typically included the administration of injectable maintenance antipsychotic medication (fluphenazine [Prolixin] decanoate every 2 weeks). The antipsychotic medication was increased if symptoms worsened and was reduced or otherwise changed if intolerable side effects occurred. In addition, based on clinical need, patients were treated with adjunctive medications (e.g., antidepressants).

Life Events and Coping Assessment Measures

Life Events Schedule. The life events interview consisted of 111 discrete events, of which 102 were adapted from the Psychiatric Epidemiology Research Interview for Life Events (PERI-LE) [51]. Open-ended questions were used to elicit the occurrence of additional life events and to obtain detailed information about each reported event [52]. The life events interview was administered during one of the patient's regular clinic visits. Life events data collection procedures have been described in two previous publications [9,16].

Coping Responses Inventory (CRI). The CRI was administered in an interview-based format and contained 48 items that categorized coping responses into either approach or avoidance coping behavior [53]. Frequency of use of the various coping strategies was rated. The CRI yields two empirically formed clusters. The first is named Approach Coping [54] and consists of items that assess cognitive coping, e.g., "Think of different ways to deal with the problem?" and behavioral coping, e.g., "Did you make a plan of action and follow it?" A second empirical cluster, named Avoidance Coping [54], consists of cognitive avoidance, e.g., "Did you try not to think about the problem?" and behavioral avoidance, e.g., "Did you try to stay away from people in general?" The adult form scales have moderate to high internal consistency (average alpha, .65 for women and .67 for men) and are moderately stable over 1 year (average *r*, .43 for women and .45 for men) [54].

Sampling Procedure

Each patient was assessed once during a regular clinic visit by using the Life Events Inventory to elicit a recent negative stressful life event. Only events that occurred more than 2 weeks, but not more than 2 months before the assessment were included for study. The restriction in time period of the coping assessment was an attempt to standardize the amount of time the subject had to cope with the event. Only negative interpersonal life events that were initiated by the subject were included in this analysis.

Results

The analyses examined whether there were differences in the use of coping behaviors as measured by the CRI in individuals with schizophrenia as compared with normal subjects. To address this issue, we used *t*-tests to contrast the schizophrenic patients and normal comparison subjects on ratings of the frequency of use of problem-focused, approach coping behaviors (cognitive and behavioral) and of avoidance/denial coping behavior (cognitive and behavioral). Normal controls used significantly more approach coping behaviors (cognitive and behavioral) than did the schizophrenic patients (Table 1). Considering the subtypes of problem-focused, approach coping strategies, cognitively oriented strategies and behaviorally oriented strategies were each used significantly more often by normal controls than by schizophrenic patients. In contrast, there were no statistically significant differences in the use of

TABLE 1. A comparison between chronic schizophrenia patients and demographically matched normal controls on the use of approach and avoidance coping behavior in dealing with interpersonal stressors (mean ± SD)

Behavior	Chronic schizophrenia patients ($n = 13$)	Normal comparison subjects ($n = 11$)	p
Approach coping	1.89 ± 0.43	2.45 ± 0.51	0.01
Cognitive approach	2.01 ± 0.57	2.64 ± 0.59	0.02
Behavioral approach	1.76 ± 0.43	2.26 ± 0.51	0.02
Avoidance coping	1.61 ± 0.36	1.85 ± 0.39	0.14
Cognitive avoidance	1.68 ± 0.52	1.96 ± 0.62	0.24
Behavioral avoidance	1.55 ± 0.40	1.75 ± 0.30	0.19

either cognitive or behavioral avoidance coping by schizophrenic patients as compared with normal subjects.

Discussion

Our study of coping behavior in schizophrenia differed from most of the prior related research, which has primarily addressed how patients cope with the symptoms of schizophrenia. Our focus was on how schizophrenic patients cope with real-life interpersonal stressors. The few studies that focused on environmental stressors found that schizophrenic patients often used avoidance strategies in coping with stress [43,44]. Therefore, we anticipated that we would also find that schizophrenic patients would use avoidance coping behaviors more frequently than normal controls. Such avoidance coping is often assumed to be pathological, because in the psychiatric literature avoidance is often noted to be part of the prodrome of an episode of schizophrenia and is also considered to be a feature of a negative symptom.

Our results suggest that the use of avoidance strategies is not necessarily pathological, because their frequency did not differ between the schizophrenic patients and normal subjects. Approach coping behavior and some emotion-based strategies are associated with initial increases in stress (for a review, see Aldwin [55]). Avoidance coping may reduce stress in the short term but may be maladaptive over time, especially in the absence of more active attempts to resolve interpersonal situations that are stressful. Normal subjects appear to differ from schizophrenic patients not in the use of avoidance per se, but in exercising the option of using active problem-focused coping strategies more fully rather than relying extensively on avoidance.

In community samples, a relationship between coping behavior, family/social support, adaptive personality characteristics (as mediating variables), and good psychological and physical health outcomes has been well replicated [56–63]. Unfortunately, relatively few studies have addressed the issue of whether adaptive coping with stressful events also leads to favorable outcomes. Two empirical studies have shown that the use of active problem-focused strategies is associated with a lower risk of relapse in schizophrenia [43,64]. Therefore, we hypothesize that the flexible use of both active and avoidance coping will mitigate against a negative impact of stressful interpersonal situations and result in more favorable outcomes among schizophrenic patients. Considering the central role that stress plays in the exacerbation of psychosis, further study of the mediating effects of coping is certainly warranted.

Manualized social skills training programs have proven to be effective tools for helping schizophrenic patients improve basic interpersonal skills [65] (for a review, see Heinssen et al. [66]). Such interpersonal skills appear to be necessary components of problem-focused coping behavior. Future research should also examine whether training schizophrenic patients in the use of problem-focused coping might improve clinical and functional outcomes.

Acknowledgments. This research was supported by research grants MH37705 (Principal Investigator, Keith H. Nuechterlein, Ph.D.) and MH30911 (Principal Investigator, Robert P. Liberman, M.D.) from the National Institute of Mental Health. The authors wish to thank George Bartzokis, M.D., Craig Childress, M.A., Rosemary Collier, M.S., Rhonda Daily, B.A., David Fogelson, M.D., Sally Friedlob, M.S.W., Debbie Gioia-Hasick, M.S.W., Sun Hwang, M.P.H., Michael Gitlin, M.D., Sandy Rappe, M.S.W., Margie Stratton, M.A., and the patients of the Aftercare Research Program for their contributions to this project.

References

1. Zubin J, Spring B (1977) Vulnerability—a new view of schizophrenia. J Abnorm Psychol 86:103–126
2. Spring B, Coons H (1982) Stress as a precursor of schizophrenic episodes. In: Neufeld RWJ (ed) Psychological stress and schizophrenia. McGraw-Hill, New York, pp 13–54
3. Nuechterlein KH, Dawson ME (1984) A heuristic vulnerability/stress model of schizophrenic episodes. Schizophr Bull 10:300–312
4. Zubin J, Steinhauer SR, Day R, et al (1985) Schizophrenia at the crossroads: a blueprint for the 80s. Comprehen Psychiat 26:217–240
5. Yank GR, Bentley KJ, Hargrove DS (1993) The vulnerability-stress model of schizophrenia: advances in treatment. Am J Orthopsychiat 63:55–69
6. van Os J, Marcelis M (1998) The ecogenetics of schizophrenia: a review. Schizophr Res 32:127–135
7. Brown GW, Birley JLT (1968) Crisis and life change and the onset of schizophrenia. J Health Soc Behav 9:203–214
8. Day R, Nielsen JA, Korten A, et al (1987) Stressful life events preceding the acute onset of schizophrenia: a cross-national study from the World Health Organization. Culture Med Psychiat 11:123–205
9. Ventura J, Nuechterlein KH, Lukoff D, et al (1989) A prospective study of stressful life events and schizophrenic relapse. J Abnorm Psychol 98:407–411
10. Malla AK, Cortese L, Shaw TS, et al (1990) Life events and relapse in schizophrenia. Soc Psychiat Psychiatr Epidemiol 25:221–224
11. Norman RM, Malla AK (1993) Stressful life events and schizophrenia I: a review of the research. Br J Psychiat 162:161–166
12. Norman RM, Malla AK (1993) Stressful life events and schizophrenia II: conceptual and methodological issues. Br J Psychiat 162:166–174
13. Antelman SM, Eichler AJ, Black CA, et al (1980) Interchangeability of stress and amphetamine in sensitization. Science 207:329–331
14. Breier A, Albus M, Pickar D, et al (1987) Controllable and uncontrollable stress in humans, alterations in mood and neuroendocrine and psychophysiological effects. Am J Psychiat 144:1419–1425

15. Breier A (1989) Experimental approaches to human stress research: assessment of neu-robiological mechanisms of stress in volunteers and psychiatric patients. Biol Psychiat 26:438–462
16. Ventura J, Nuechterlein KH, Hardesty J, et al (1992) Life events and schizophrenic relapse during medication withdrawal. Br J Psychiat 161:615–620
17. Bustillo JR, Lauriello J, Keith SJ (1999) Schizophrenia: improving outcome. Harvard Rev Psychiat 6:229–240
18. Brown GW, Harris T, Peto J (1973) Life events and psychiatric disorders: II. The nature of the causal link. Psychol Med 3:159–176
19. Hardesty J, Falloon IRH, Shirin K (1985) The impact of life events, stress, coping on the morbidity of schizophrenia. In: Falloon IRH (ed) Family management of schizo-phrenia. Johns Hopkins University Press Baltimore & London, pp 137–152
20. Hirsch S, Bowen J, Emami J, et al (1996) A one year prospective study of the effect of life events and medication in the aetiology of schizophrenic relapse. Br J Psychiat 168:49–56
21. Rabkin JG (1980) Stressful life events and schizophrenia: a review of the research literature. Psychol Bull 87:408–425
22. Roy A (1980) Depression in chronic paranoid schizophrenia. Br J Psychiat 137:138–139
23. Roy A, Thompson R, Kennedy S (1983) Depression in chronic schizophrenia. Br J Psychiat 142:465–470
24. Chintalapudi M, Kulhara P, Avasthi A (1992) Post-psychotic depression in schizo-phrenia. Eur Arch Psychiat Clin Neurosci 243:103–108
25. Birchwood M, Mason R, MacMillan F, et al (1993) Depression, demoralization and control over psychotic illness: a comparison of depressed and non-depressed patients with a chronic psychosis. Psychol Med 23:387–395
26. Ventura J, Nuechterlein KH, Subotnik KL, et al (2000) Life events can trigger depres-sive symptoms in early schizophrenia. J Abnorm Psychol 109:139–144
27. Nuechterlein KH, Dawson ME, Gitlin M, et al (1992) Developmental processes in schizophrenic disorders: longitudinal studies of vulnerability and stress. Schizophr Bull 18:387–425
28. Nicholson IR, Neufeld RW (1992) A dynamic vulnerability perspective on stress and schizophrenia. Am J Orthopsychiat 62:117–130
29. Meehl PE (1972) A critical afterword. In: Gottesman II, Shields J (eds) Schizophrenia and genetics: a twin vantage point. Academic Press, New York, pp 367–415
30. Beck J, Worthen K (1972) Precipitating stress, crisis theory, and hospitalization in schizophrenia and depression. Arch Gen Psychiat 26:123–129
31. Liberman RP (1986) Coping and competence as protective factors in the vulnerability-stress model of schizophrenia. In: Goldstein MJ, Hand I, Hahlweg K (eds) Treatment of schizophrenia: family assessment and intervention. Springer-Verlag, Berlin, pp 201–216
32. Ventura J, Liberman RP (2000) Stress and psychosis. In: Fink G (ed) Encyclopedia of stress. Vol 3. Academic Press, San Diego, pp 316–325
33. Falloon IRH, Talbot RE (1981) Persistent auditory hallucinations: coping mechanisms and implications for management. Psychol Med 11:329–339
34. Carter DM, Mackinnon A, Copolov DL (1996) Patients' strategies for coping with audi-tory hallucinations. J Ner Ment Dis 184:159–164
35. Böker W, Brenner HD, Wurgler S (1989) Vulnerability-linked deficiencies, psy-chopathology and coping behaviour of schizophrenics and their relatives. Special Issue: Schizophrenia as a systems disorder: The relevance of mediating processes for theory. Br J Psychiat 155(Suppl 5):128–135
36. Wiedl KH, Schottner B (1991) Coping with symptoms related to schizophrenia. Schizophr Bull 17:525–538
37. Lazarus RS, Folkman S (1984) Stress, appraisal, and coping. Springer, New York

38. Moos RH, Schaefer J (1993) Coping resources and processes: current concepts and measures. In: Goldberger L, Breznitz S (eds) Handbook of stress: theoretical and clinical Aspects, 2nd edn. Macmillan, New York, pp 234–257
39. Tarrier N, Beckett R, Harwood S, et al (1993) A trial of two cognitive-behavioural methods of treating drug-resistant residual psychotic symptoms in schizophrenic patients: I. Outcome. Br J Psychiat 162:524–532
40. Cohen CI, Berk LA (1985) Personal coping styles of schizophrenic outpatients. Hosp Commun Psychiat 36:407–410
41. Dittmann J, Schüttler R (1990) Disease consciousness and coping strategies of patients with schizophrenic psychosis. Acta Psychiatr Scand 1990 Oct 82(4):318–322
42. Macdonald EM, Pica S, McDonald S, et al (1998) Stress and coping in early psychosis. Br J Psychiat 172(Suppl 33):122–127
43. Hultman CM, Wieselgren IM, Öhman A (1997) Relationships between social support, social coping, and life events in the relapse of schizophrenia patients. Scand J Psychol 38:3–13
44. Jansen LMC, Gispen-de-Wied CC, Kahn KS (1999) Coping with stress in schizophrenia. Schizophr Res 36(Special Issue):176
45. Hollingshead AB (1957) Two-factor index of social position. Available from August B. Hollingshead, 1965 Yale Station, New Haven, Connecticut
46. Spitzer RL, Endicott J, Robins E (1978) Research diagnostic criteria: rationale and reliability. Arch Gen Psychiat 35:773–782
47. American Psychiatric Association (1987) DSM-III-R: diagnostic and statistical manual of mental disorders, 3rd revision. American Psychiatric Press, Washington, DC
48. Wing JK, Cooper JE, Sartorius N (1974) The measurement and classification of psychiatric symptoms: an instruction manual for the PSE and Catego Program. Cambridge University Press, London
49. Endicott J, Spitzer RL (1978) A diagnostic interview: the Schedule for Affective Disorders and Schizophrenia. Arch Gen Psychiat 35:837–844
50. Ventura J, Liberman RP, Green MF, et al (1998) Training and quality assurance with the Structured Clinical Interview for DSM-IV I/P (SCID). Psychiat Res 79:163–173
51. Dohrenwend BS, Krasnoff L, Askenasy AR, et al (1978) Exemplification of a method for scaling life events: the PERI life events scale. J Health Soc Behav 19:205–229
52. Brown GW, Harris T (1978) Social origins of depression. Free Press: Macmillan, New York
53. Moos RH (1993) Coping Responses Inventory Adult Form Manual. Psychological Assessment Resources, Odessa, FL
54. Moos RH (1997) Coping Responses Inventory: a measure of approach and avoidance coping skills. In: Zalaquett CP, Wood RJ, et al (eds) Evaluating stress: a book of resources. Scarecrow Press, Lanham, MD, pp 51–65
55. Aldwin CM (1994) Stress, coping and development. Guilford Press, New York
56. Folkman S, Lazarus RS (1980) An analysis of coping in a middle-aged community sample. J Health Soc Behav 21:219–239
57. Folkman S, Lazarus RS (1985) If it changes it must be a process: study of emotion and coping during three stages of a college examination. J Personality Soc Psychol 48:150–170
58. Billings AG, Moos RH (1984) Coping, stress, and social resources among adults with unipolar depression. J Personality Soc Psychol 46:877–891
59. Holahan CJ, Moos R (1985) Life stress and health: personality, coping and family support in stress resistance. J Personality Soc Psychol 49:739–747
60. Holahan CJ, Moos R (1986) Personality, coping and family resources in stress resistance: a longitudinal analysis. J Personality Soc Psychol 51:389–395
61. Folkman S, Lazarus RS, Dunkel-Schetter C, et al (1986) The dynamics of a stressful encounter: cognitive appraisal, coping, and encounter outcomes. J Personality Soc Psychol 50:992–1003

62. Holahan CJ, Moos R (1987) The personal and contextual determinants of coping strate-gies. J Personality Soc Psychol 52:946–955
63. Holahan CJ, Moos R (1990) Life stressors, resistance factors, and improved psycho-logical functioning: an extension of the stress-resistance paradigm. J Personality Soc Psychol 58:909–917
64. Pallanti S, Quercioli L, Pazzagli A (1997) Relapse in young paranoid schizophrenic patients: a prospective study of stressful life events, P300 measures, and coping. Am J Psychiat 154:792–798
65. Marder SR, Wirshing WC, Mintz J, et al (1996) Two-year outcome of social skills train-ing and group psychotherapy for outpatients with schizophrenia. Am J Psychiat 153:1585–1592
66. Heinssen RK, Liberman RP, Kopelowicz A (2000) Psychosocial skills training for schizophrenia: lessons from the laboratory. Schizophr Bull 26:21–46

Part 2
Social Cognition

Social Cognitive Problem-Solving Skills in Schizophrenia

CHIYO YAMASHITA, MASAFUMI MIZUNO, and HARUO KASHIMA

Summary. Social cognitive problem-solving skills (SCPS) were studied in patients with schizophrenia and normal volunteers using various measures. The means-ends problem solving procedure (MEPS) was used to assess SCPS; the mini-mental state examination, the Rey auditory verbal learning test (RAVLT), and fluency tests were used to assess molecular neurocognitive deficits. Psychiatric symptoms and general functioning were assessed with the Positive and Negative Symptoms Scale (PANSS) and Global Assessment of Function (GAF), respectively. Fluency tests are measures to evaluate divergent thinking and include the Word Fluency Test and the Idea Fluency Test. Qualitative analysis of responses to the Idea Fluency Test was also conducted. In the entire group with schizophrenia, the relationships among SCPS and symptoms and general functioning were studied. The relationship between SCPS and molecular neurocognitive deficits was studied in patients with higher RAVLT scores. The results indicate that patients with schizophrenia had statistically poorer performance on MEPS. MEPS scores were correlated with GAF but not with any subcategory of PANSS. Regarding molecular neurocognitive deficits, the task-modified responses to the Idea Fluency Test were correlated with MEPS scores in patients with higher RAVLT scores. This suggests that SCPS is related to divergent thinking requiring concept flexibility or conversion of viewpoint in schizophrenia.

Key words. Schizophrenia, Social cognition, Problem solving, MEPS, Fluency

Impaired social functioning or social competence has been regarded as a core aspect of schizophrenia and a major contributor to the social prognosis or quality of life of many people with this disease [1–3]. It has been clinically observed that social dysfunction persists even after positive symptoms have diminished. Poor social competence is thought to be associated with less adequate behavior and vulnerability to relapse [4]. Recently, issues regarding the mechanisms underlying social dysfunction in schizophrenia have received more attention from researchers. In order to more effectively carry out psychiatric rehabilitation programs for social functioning, it is

Department of Neuropsychiatry, School of Medicine, Keio University, 35 Shinanomachi, Shinjuku-ku, Tokyo 160-8582, Japan

important to consider which domains of cognition relate to social functioning and the exact nature of the relationship from various viewpoints. Although many past studies have suggested that certain cognitive deficits are related to social functioning, the results of various studies have not always been consistent [5]. The purpose of this study is to identify molecular cognitive deficits that are related to impaired social functioning.

It is commonly recognized that social functioning is divided into three components: receiving skills, processing skills, and sending skills [6]. Recently, role-play-type tests have become increasingly common in the evaluation of social functioning. These tests can assess three separate components of social functioning in a series of tasks. Furthermore, they have an advantage in evaluating social functioning in situations close to real life in the community. However, in order to see which neurocognitive functions are related to social functioning, it is also necessary to evaluate each component of social functioning in detail. In this study, processing skills were assessed specifically, and relationships between SCPS and neurocognitive deficits in brain dysfunction are discussed.

Methods

Subjects

The subjects were people with an ICD-10 (WHO, 1992) diagnosis of schizophrenia. As controls, age and sex controlled normal volunteers served for this study. All clinical subjects received neuroleptic medication, and the mean haloperidol-equivalent dose was about 8 mg. The Mann-Whitney U test revealed no significant differences in age, sex, or length of formal education between the two groups.

Neurocognitive Assessment

Neurocognitive deficits were assessed by the mini-mental state examination (MMS) [7], the Rey auditory verbal learning test (RAVLT) [8], and fluency tests.

With RAVLT, subjects were instructed to listen to a list of 15 common words read by the examiner. When the examiner finished the list, the subjects were asked to repeat as many of the words as they could remember in any order. The procedure was repeated four more times. The examiner then asked subjects to perform the digit span task. When the subjects finished this task, the examiner asked them to recall as many of the words as possible from the previous word list. The number of words recalled by the subjects after the intervention was taken as the result.

The fluency tests consisted of a letter fluency test, a category fluency test, and an idea fluency test. In the letter fluency test, the examiner asks the subjects to say as many words in 60 s as they can think of that begin with a given *kana* (syllabic letter), excluding proper nouns, numbers, and the same words with different suffixes. In this study, we used three *kana* of varying frequency. In the category fluency test, animals, fruits, and traffic naming tasks were performed within 60 s. In the idea fluency test, the examiner requests that the subject think of as many uses for an empty tin can as possible in 5 min [9]. The responses on the idea fluency test were classified into three subgroups: task-dependent responses, task-modified responses, and task-independent responses. Task-dependent responses are ideas conventionally associated with a stimulus object, such as its intended uses or common uses. Task-modified responses are ideas generated by considering the object's characteristics, such as the shape, size, and material, in order to create new and nonconventional uses. These types of responses require conversion of viewpoint and flexibility of thinking. Task-independent responses are ideas that are perceived from partial characteristics of tin cans and that ignore the receptacle characteristics of cans, such as being a cavity or having a cylindrical form.

Social Cognitive Problem-Solving Assessment

In this study, we focused on social cognitive problem-solving skills (SCPS) as the processing skills of social functioning. We used the Japanese version of the means-ends problem-solving procedure (MEPS) [10] to assess one aspect of SCPS. MEPS consists of vignettes that contain the beginnings and endings of stories. Table 1 shows an example of a MEPS vignette. The beginning presents a hypothetical person who has a problem that is resolved at the end of the story. The subject is instructed to fill in the middle of the story, that is, how the person in the story went about solving the problem.

Responses are scored relative to three factors: means, obstacles, and time. Means are discrete behavioral and cognitive steps that bring the person closer to the presented ending. Obstacles are recognition that something may stand in the way of the goal. Time is taken into consideration, e.g., that it would take some time to solve the problem or that there is an optimal time for a particular strategy to be implemented. The responses were scored in accordance with the MEPS manual. Spivack et al. recommended that the sum of the three factors be considered adequate to create an overall index of means-ends performance [11]. Therefore, the sum was used as the index of performance on MEPS.

Although MEPS has the disadvantage of being a paper and pencil test and therefore less like real life, we selected it for two reasons. First, it is easier to obtain data by MEPS than by role-play-type tests. Second, the study focused on processing skills rather than receiving or sending skills, and MEPS evaluates mainly processing skills. In using MEPS, the problem to be solved is presented in the vignette. Thus, few receiving skills are required. Furthermore, the examiner does not need to evaluate the

TABLE 1. MEPS "Making Friends"

Mr. C. had just moved in that day and didn't know anyone.
Mr. C. wanted to have friends in the neighborhood.
The story ends with Mr. C. having many good friends and feeling at home in the neighborhood.
You begin the story with Mr. C. in his room immediately after arriving in the neighborhood.

MEPS, Means-Ends Problem-Solving Procedure

subject's ability to implement thoughts in real life. Therefore, minimum sending skills are required to perform these tasks.

Symptom and General Functioning Measures

Symptoms were assessed using the Positive and Negative Symptoms Scale (PANSS) [12] to measure the effects of symptoms on SCPS. Global assessment of functioning (GAF) [13] was used to evaluate general functioning.

Procedure

The neurocognitive tasks and MEPS were administered to informed subjects who had agreed to participate in the study. Subjects were also given PANSS and GAF by a psychiatrist. Total testing required 1.5–2 h per subject, and all tests were completed within one week.

Results

Group Differences in SCPS and Neurocognitive Assessments

The mean score of the MMS examination results for the group with schizophrenia was quite good. This indicated that a minimum acceptable level of intelligence was maintained in the examined group. The subjects with schizophrenia demonstrated significantly poorer performance on MEPS, RAVLT, the category fluency test, and the idea fluency test. In the idea fluency test, total responses, task-dependent responses, and task-modified responses were significantly lower in the subjects with schizophrenia.

Association Between SCPS and Symptoms/ General Functioning

The MEPS scores correlated with GAF, but they showed no correlation with any PANSS categories.

Association Between SCPS and Neurocognitive Assessments

In the control subjects, there was no correlation between MEPS scores and neuropsychological test results. This suggests that these functions are independent of each other in the control group.

Subjects with schizophrenia had significantly poorer performance on RAVLT than the controls. In this study, RAVLT was used to evaluate verbal memory. However, other nonspecific factors, such as attention, vigilance, and subject attitude toward tasks, are also considered to possibly affect the results of this test. Since these nonspecific factors influence the results of the fluency tests, it is considered valid to examine the association between MEPS scores and fluency tests in subjects whose RAVLT results were within the normal range. Thus, the subjects whose RAVLT results were equal to or more than the normal RAVLT group were selected from the examined group to assess the association between MEPS scores and fluency test results. In the normal RAVLT group, the mean MEPS score was significantly lower than that of the control group.

MEPS scores correlated only with task-modified responses on the idea fluency test.

Discussion

The results of the present study suggest that processing skills are to some extent related to social functioning, but not to psychiatric symptoms in schizophrenia. The association between MEPS scores and task-modified responses in the idea fluency test suggests that some brain function impairments contribute to impaired SCPS in schizophrenia.

Measures of neurocognitive assessment indicated that subjects with schizophrenia had impaired verbal recall memory and fluency. These findings are consistent with the results of previous studies [14]. Furthermore, the results of this study suggest that in schizophrenia degrees of fluency deficits differ, depending on which kind of fluency is assessed. Specifically, letter fluency and design fluency were relatively well maintained in schizophrenia, as compared with category fluency and idea fluency.

To examine the association between SCPS and fluency tests, we selected subjects whose RAVLT results were within the normal range from among all our subjects with schizophrenia. Since previous studies have suggested RAVLT results to be related to cue perception or acquisition of social skills [15,16], it is necessary to pay attention to the cognitive deficits evaluated by RAVLT. However, we must be careful not to overlook other more specific factors that may contribute to problem-solving skills. As described above, not only verbal memory, but also other nonspecific factors, such as attention, vigilance, and subject attitude toward tasks, could also affect the results of this test. Therefore, it may be difficult to identify specific factors related to social functioning. In order to minimize the effects of these nonspecific factors, the association between SCPS and fluency was assessed only in subjects without impaired RAVLT. Even for the selected subjects, MEPS scores were significantly lower than those of control subjects, and MEPS scores correlated with task-modified responses on the idea fluency test. The idea fluency test is considered to be a test evaluating divergent thinking. Divergent thinking is a way of thinking that is used in answering questions without fixed answers. This thinking process is one of the factors of the structure-of-intellect model proposed by Guilford [17]. The results suggest that people with schizophrenia have certain deficits in divergent thinking, and especially have difficulties in producing ideas requiring concept flexibility or conversion of viewpoints. These difficulties also appear to be related to SCPS disability. Divergent thinking, as evaluated by the idea fluency test, is relatively molecular functioning. According to a previous study, patients with frontal lesions have difficulties with the idea fluency test, especially task-modified responses [9]. Because little evidence is available, we cannot speculate that dysfunction of the frontal lobe contributes to SCPS disability. However, there is a possibility that SCPS disability is based on impairments of molecular cognitive processes in schizophrenia. This supports the findings of previous research [18].

The results of the present study suggest that psychiatric rehabilitation focusing on divergent thinking may be effective. We should also consider the level of each person's neurocognitive deficits in designing rehabilitation programs. For example, in designing a plan for a person with severely damaged cognitive abilities, a molecular-level remediation strategy may initially be required. It is necessary to plan a rehabilitation program for each person that is compatible with his or her unique cognitive function.

This study evaluated only means-ends thinking, one of many factors involved in SCPS skills. Further research is needed to explore the characteristics of other SCPS factors and the association between impaired SCPS and frontal lobe dysfunction. Furthermore, it is also necessary to assess the quality of cognitive deficits in real-life situations.

References

1. Bellack AS, Morrison RL, Mueser KT, et al (1990) Role play for assessing the social competence of psychiatric patients. Psychol Assess 2:248–255
2. Sullivan G, Wells KB, Leake B (1992) Clinical factors associated with better quality of life in a seriously mentally ill population. Hosp Commun Psychiatry 43:794–798
3. Peralta V, Cuesta MJ, de Leon J (1994) An empirical analysis of latent structures underlying schizophrenic symptoms: a four-syndrome model. Biol Psychiatry 36:726–736
4. Bellack AS, Morrison RL, Wixted JT, et al (1990) An analysis of social competence in schizophrenia. Br J Psychiatry 156:809–818
5. Penn DL, Corrigan PW, Bentall RP, et al (1997) Social cognition in schizophrenia. Psychol Bull 121:114–132
6. Donahoe CP, Carter MJ, Bloem WD, et al (1990) Assessment of interpersonal problem-solving skills. Psychiatry 53:329–339
7. Folstein MF, Flostein SE, McHugh PR (1975) "Mini-Mental State." A practical method for grading the cognitive state for the clinician. J Psychiatr Res 12:189–198
8. Lezak MD (1995) Auditory-verbal learning test. Neuropsychological assessment, 3rd edn. Oxford, New York, pp 438–445
9. Saito H (1996) The reduction of fluency in patients with frontal lobe lesions—a neuropsychological investigation with fluency tests. J Keio Med Soc 73:399–409
10. Platt JJ, Spivack G (1975) Manual for the Means-Ends Problem-Solving Procedure (MEPS): a measure of interpersonal cognitive problem-solving skills. Hahnemann Community Mental Health/Mental Retardation Center, Philadelphia
11. Spivack G, Shure MB, Platt JJ (1985) Means-Ends Problem Solving (MEPS): stimuli and scoring procedures. Hahnemann University, Preventive Intervention Research Center, Philadelphia
12. Kay SR, Opler LA, Fiszben A (1991) Positive and Negative Syndrome Scale (PANSS) rating manual. Multi-Health Systems, Toronto
13. American Psychiatric Association (1994) Diagnostic and statistical manual of mental disorders, 4th edn. American Psychiatric Association, Washington, DC
14. Addington J, Addington D (1999) Neurocognitive and social functioning in schizophrenia. Schizophr Bull 25:173–182
15. Kern RS, Green MF, Toomey R (1992) Neuropsychological predictors of skills training for chronic psychiatric patients. Psychiatry Res 43:223–230

16. Corrigan PW, Wallace CJ, Schade ML, et al (1994) Learning medication self-management skills in schizophrenia: relationships with cognitive deficits and psychiatric symptoms. Behav Ther 25:5–15
17. Guilford JP (1967) The structure of intelligence. The nature of human intelligence. McGraw-Hill, New York, pp 70–249
18. Penn DL, van der Does AJ, Spaulding WD, et al (1993) Information processing and social cognitive problem solving in schizophrenia assessment of interrelationships and changes over time. J Nerv Ment Dis 181:13–20

Social Cognition in Schizophrenia

Massimo Casacchia, Monica Mazza, Alessandro De Risio, and Rita Roncone

Summary. This chapter discusses the main operational issues of a peculiar aspect of social cognition, "theory of mind," and its implications in schizophrenia. A brief review of current literature on theory of mind is provided, together with an outline of our department's contribution to this issue in the evaluation of a small sample of people affected by chronic schizophrenia and divided into subgroups according to psychopathological dimensions compared with normal controls. People with chronic schizophrenia and normal IQs have significantly worse performances than normal controls in both first- and second-order theory of mind stories. In first-order stories (a false belief about the state of the world), significant differences were found among psychopathological dimensions. As for second-order stories (a false belief about the belief of another character), one out of four patients subgroups performed worse than the others in one of the four theory of mind stories in our experimental model. Social cognition abilities may be a relevant aspect in social interactions involving people affected by schizophrenia and need to be further investigated in clinical research.

Key words. Schizophrenia, Social cognition, Theory of mind, Neurpsychological measures, Autism

Introduction

A large body of research is focused on the social competence of people affected by schizophrenia. Social cognition is a fundamental ability allowing people to successfully interact with others. This cognitive ability consists in the capacity to understand other people's thoughts and beliefs and includes problem-solving in interpersonal interactions, the ability to maintain adequate interpersonal relations, the ability to express moral judgments, and general communication abilities [1,2].

This ability seems greatly impaired in autistic children and schizophrenic subjects [3,4]. In this paper we will discuss a peculiar aspect of social cognition, theory of mind, and its implications in schizophrenia.

Psychiatric Department, University of L'Aquila, Coppito, Nuovo Ospedale S. Salvatore, 67100 L'Aquila, Italy

Theory of Mind

The difficulty in interpreting other people's mental states found in children with autism and in people affected by schizophrenia may be explained in terms of a unique mental process called *theory of mind*. Such a mechanism, initially described in primates by Premack and Woodruf [5], operates by forming *metarepresentations*, i.e., representations of mental states [6,7], and specifically the attitudes of a character about a certain semantic (for example, believing in something, having some wishes, pretending that . . .). First-order (i.e., making inferences about the state of the world) and second-order (i.e., understanding other characters' mental states) metarepresentations are specific issues of theory of mind processes [6]. Metarepresentational abilities may be operationally assessed by tasks specifically aimed at their measurement.

First-order false belief tasks measure the recognition of a story character's false belief about the world ("Mary thinks that the marble is in the basket"), whereas second-order false belief tasks assess the understanding of the beliefs of a story character about another story character's thoughts ("John thinks that Mary thinks that . . .").

The theory of mind mechanism is modular, i.e., it forms and transforms metarepresentations in a specific domain of knowledge, is inaccessible to introspection [5], is culturally invariant [8], and is determined by an innate cognitive mechanism [9,10].

Theory of Mind and Autism

Theory of mind deficit has been used to explain social deficits in autism [11–13]. Children affected by autism give a strictly literal interpretation of the meaning of words, do not understand metaphors or ironic expressions, and are troubled in beginning a conversation or representing someone's wishes to communicate [14]. They are incapable of spontaneously participating in games based on deception, and such a deficit may stem from a difficulty in interpreting other people's mental states.

Recently, theory of mind abilities of children with schizophrenia, children with high functioning autism, and normally developing children, matched on mental age, verbal mental age, and performance mental age, were compared by Pilowsky et al. [4]. Both clinical groups were matched by chronological age as well, whereas the normally developing children were younger. A fact belief task, a value belief task, a deception task, and a false belief task were administered. Overall, the group with autism passed significantly fewer tasks than the normally developing group, and theory of mind abilities seemed correlated with verbal abilities for individuals with autism. The findings of Pilowsky et al. [4] support the notion of a still limited understanding of theory of mind and support the notion that theory of mind deficits, although more severe in autism, are not unique to autism.

Theory of Mind and Schizophrenia

From the literature, it is generally acknowledged that social withdrawal behavior and flattening of affect in people with autism are similar to social deficits in people with schizophrenia [15]. Cutting and Murphy [16] believe that people affected by schizophrenia are inadequate in acting in social interactions (social ingenuity). Some authors [2,17,18] reformulate social deficits in terms of deficits of willed actions, underlined by a specific brain system including the prefrontal cortex, supplementary motor area, and caudate. A huge body of research postulates that an impairment of the theory of mind mechanism may explain the social interaction deficits in schizo-phrenic subjects [19–25]. Corcoran et al. [19] found that subjects fulfilling DSM-III R criteria for acute schizophrenia performed less well than psychiatric and normal con-trols on task requiring the interpretation of social inferences behind indirect speech (e.g., a child says to his mother, "Please close the window," meaning "I feel cold"). A similar group of acutely ill psychotic patients had a worse performance than controls when requested to understand first-order and second-order false belief tasks [20]. The authors suggest that subjects with negative and positive symptoms have severe diffi-culties in understanding first-order theory of mind tasks, with poor understanding of hints and poor knowledge of conversational rules (e.g., do not give too much or little information to the listener). People with paranoid symptoms (i.e., delusions of refer-ence, delusions of mind reading, persecutory delusions), on the other hand, have a more specific context-dependent deficit. They have difficulties with second-order false belief tasks and have impaired understanding of hints and appropriate levels of polite-ness. These findings were more extensively investigated in a further study [21].

Sarfati et al. [23] postulated that thought and language disorders may reflect a plan-ning deficit in schizophrenic patients, whose ability to attribute mental states to others should be consequently impaired. To avoid problems with language, mental abilities were tested through picture stories. Thought and speech disorganization was found to be linked to impairment of mentalizing abilities.

A recent study by Drury et al. [24] claimed that it is still not clear whether theory of mind deficits in acute psychosis are conceptual in nature or depend on informa-tion-processing limitations. The patients investigated by the authors had multiple and overlapping positive and negative symptoms, and their performance on some of the theory of mind tasks during an acute episode was significantly worse than that of non-schizophrenic patients. Patients with delusion of reference or persecution did not perform significantly worse than patients with negative symptoms on theory of mind tasks. In a study conducted on schizophrenic affective patients and normal controls, Doody et al. [25] found a significant association between negative symptomatology and second-order theory of mind tasks. The evidence of the literature fosters, however, the need to evaluate more accurately how schizophrenic people are able to accomplish theory of mind tasks in relation to their symptom status.

Our Research Contribution

One of our recent studies [26] assessed theory of mind competence in subjects with chronic schizophrenia and investigated whether such competence was related to schizophrenic symptoms, as categorized in the three-dimensional model proposed by Liddle [27]. According to this model, schizophrenic symptoms can be termed as "symptom factors," and three different dimensions are identified. The first dimension, "psychomotor poverty," includes poverty of speech, decreased spontaneous move-ments, and blunting of affect. The second one, "reality distortion," consists of hallucinations and delusions. The last dimension, "disorganization," includes thought disorder, inappropriate affect, and poverty of content of speech. We studied 37 subjects affected by schizophrenia, with a mean length of illness of 7 years and a normal IQ, who were outpatients in our university psychiatric department (September 1997–July 1998). Positive and negative symptoms were assessed by the administration of SAPS and SANS scales [28,29]; a complete neuropsychological battery, including verbal memory and verbal fluency tests [30], the Tower of London test [31], and the Wisconsin Card Sorting Test [32], was administered to all the participants. Social cognition issues were investigated by means of four theory of mind stories, exploring first- and second-order metarepresentations (the Sally and Anne story and the Cigarettes story, the Ice Cream Van task, and the Burglar story) [14].

The sample of schizophrenics was divided according to the triadic domains model of schizophrenia [27]: people with psychomotor poverty ($n = 14$); people with disorganization ($n = 10$), and people with reality distortion syndrome ($n = 13$). In addition to the schizophrenic subjects, 20 normal controls matched for age and education were studied.

The schizophrenic subjects had an overall worse performance in all four theory of mind tasks than normal controls. The thought disorder subgroup had a good performance in first-order stories. The psychomotor poverty subgroup had a poor performance in both first- and second-order stories. As for second-order stories, the psychomotor poverty group was worse than the disorganization subjects and the reality distortion group in the Ice Cream Van task.

Our study showed that people with chronic schizophrenia and normal IQ have significantly worse performances than normal controls in both first- and second-order theory of mind stories [26]. On this issue, data from the literature are contrasting. Corcoran et al. [19] and Frith and Corcoran [20] found that schizophrenic subjects had a worse performance than controls in social inference tasks. Langdon's results [22] show that impaired metarepresentation was not associated with paranoid and other reality distortion symptoms. Our results are consistent with the findings of the first two authors for the performances in the theory of mind stories.

Conclusions

We investigated the relation of different symptom patterns to different impairments of mentalizing abilities in schizophrenic subjects [27]. In our opinion, theory of mind deficit could be considered a selective cognitive function impairment in the psychomotor poverty group, since no significant differences among the three schizophrenic subgroups were found on other neuropsychological tests. Theory of mind deficits could be due to impaired functioning of a specialized cognitive module. More research has to be done to achieve a better understanding of neurocognitive functions involved in mentalizing abilities and symptom expression over time in schizophrenic subjects.

Acknowledgments. Support for the research described in this paper has been provided by a grant from the National Mental Health Project, National Institute of Health, Grant No. 96/Q/T/30, Rome, Italy.

References

1. Taylor EH, Cadet JL (1989) Social intelligence: a neurological system? Psychol Rep 64:423–444
2. Brothers L (1990) The social brain: a project for integrating primate behavior and neuropsychology in a new domain. Concepts Neurosci 1:27–51
3. Penn DL, Corrigan PW, Bentall RP, et al (1997) Social cognition in schizophrenia. Psychol Bull 121:114–132
4. Pilowsky T, Yirmiya N, Arbelle S, et al (2000) Theory of mind abilities of children with schizophrenia, children with autism, and normally developing children. Schizophr Res 42:145–155
5. Premack D, Woodruff G (1978) Does the chimpanzee have a theory of mind? Behav Brain Sci 4:515–526
6. Frith CD (1992) The cognitive neuropsychology of schizophrenia. Lawrence Erlbaum Associates, Hove
7. Frith CD (1994) Theory of mind in schizophrenia. In: David AS, Cutting JC (eds) The neuropsychology of schizophrenia. Lawrence Erlbaum Associates, Hove
8. Avis J, Harris PL (1991) Belief-desire reasoning among Baka children: evidence for a universal conception of mind. Child Dev 62:460–467
9. Leslie AM (1987) Pretence and representation: the origins of "Theory of Mind." Psychol Rev 94:412–416
10. Leslie AM (1994) ToM, ToBy and agency: core architecture and domain specificity. In: Hirschfeld L, Gelman S (eds) Domain specificity and cultural knowledge. Cambridge University Press, Cambridge, UK
11. Baron-Cohen S, Leslie A, Frith U (1985) Does the autistic child have a "Theory of Mind"? Cognition 21:37–46
12. Baron-Cohen S (1992) Out of sight or out of mind? Another look at deception in autism. J child Psychol Psychiatry 33(7):1141–1155
13. Happè F, Frith U (1994) Theory of mind in autism. In: Schopler E, Mesibov G (eds) Learning and cognition in autism. Plenum Press, New York
14. Happè F (1994) An advanced test of theory of mind: understanding of story characters' thoughts and feelings by able autistics, mentally handicapped and normal children and adults. J Autism Dev Disord 24:129–154
15. Forster A, Lewis S, Owen M, et al (1991) Premorbid adjustment and personality in psychosis. Effects of sex and diagnosis. Br J Psychiatry 158:171–176
16. Cutting J, Murphy D (1990) Impaired ability of schizophrenic patients, relative to manics or depressives, to appreciate social knowledge about their culture. Br J Psychiatry 157:355–358
17. Goldberg G (1985) Supplementary motor area structure and function: Review and hypotheses. Behav Brain Sci 8:567–616
18. Passingham RE (1987) Two cortical systems for directing movement. In: Motor areas of the cerebral cortex. Wiley, Chichester, UK, pp 151–161
19. Corcoran R, Mercer G, Frith CD (1995) Schizophrenia, symptomatology and social inference: investigating "theory of mind" in people with schizophrenia. Schizophr Res 17:5–13
20. Frith CD, Corcoran R (1996) Exploring "theory of mind" in people with schizophrenia. Psychol Med 26:521–530
21. Corcoran R, Frith CD (1996) Conversational conduct and the symptoms of schizophrenia. Cogn Neuropsychiatry 1:305–318
22. Langdon R, Michie PT, Ward PB, et al (1997) Defective self and/or other mentalising in schizophrenia: a cognitive neuropsychological approach. Cogn Neuropsychiatry 2(3):167–193

23. Sarfati Y, Hardy-Baylé MC, Besche C, et al (1997) Attribution of intentions to others in people with schizophrenia: a non-verbal exploration with comic strips. Schizophr Res 25:199–209
24. Drury VM, Robinson EJ, Birchwood M (1998) Theory of mind skills during an acute episode of psychosis and following recovery. Psychol Med 28:1101–1112
25. Doody GA, Götz M, Johnstone EC, et al (1998) Theory of mind and psychoses. Psychol Med 28:397–405
26. Mazza M, De Risio A, Surian L, et al (2001) Selective impairments of theory of mind in people with schizophrenia. Schizophr Res 47(2):299–308
27. Liddle PF (1987) The symptoms of chronic schizophrenia: a reexamination of the positive-negative dichotomy. Br J Psychiatry 158:340–345
28. Andreasen NC (1984) Scale for the assessment of positive symptoms (SAPS). University of Iowa, Iowa City, IA
29. Andreasen NC (1984) Scale for the assessment of negative symptoms (SANS). University of Iowa, Iowa City, IA
30. Novelli G, Papagno C, Capitani E, et al (1986) Three clinical tests for the assessment of lexical retrieval and production. Norms from 320 normal subjects in (Italian). Arch Psychol Neurol Psychiatry 47(4):477–506
31. Morice R, Delahunty A (1996) Frontal/executive impairments in schizophrenia. Schizoph Bull 22(1):125–137
32. Heaton RK (1981) A manual for the Wisconsin Card Sorting Test. Psychological Assessment Resources, Odessa, FL

Emotion Perception and Social Functioning in Schizophrenia

DAVID L. PENN

Summary. In this chapter, research is summarized regarding the relationship between measures of emotion perception and indices of social functioning among persons with schizophrenia. In particular, the results of three studies from our social cognition laboratory are reviewed. The findings revealed that better emotion perception skills were associated with more adaptive and less maladaptive ward behavior among inpatients with chronic schizophrenia. In a third study, emotion perception had weak to modest relationships with social skill, as measured with unstructured role plays, among stabilized outpatients with schizophrenia. A similar relationship, albeit weaker, was found in a chronically ill inpatient sample. Overall, these studies suggest that emotion perception skills have a more consistent relationship with ward behavior than with social skills among persons with schizophrenia. Future work needs to address the following issues regarding the relationship between emotion perception and social functioning in schizophrenia: Does emotion perception contribute independent variance to social behavior beyond other social-cognitive measures? Can we develop measures of social cognition and social functioning that are more ecologically valid than those currently in existence?

Key words. Emotion perception, Social cognition, Schizophrenia, Social functioning

Introduction

One of the hallmark characteristics of schizophrenia is impairment in social functioning [1]. Individuals with schizophrenia, relative to both clinical and non-clinical control subjects, demonstrate deficits in social skill [2]. Such deficits are related to more molar indices of functioning, such as behavior in the treatment setting [3] and adjustment in the community [4,5], and have, at best, a modest association with current symptoms [6]. There is also compelling evidence that deficits in social functioning often precede the onset of the disorder [7] and may partially account for the

Department of Psychology, University of North Carolina at Chapel Hill, Davie Hall, CB #3270, Chapel Hill, NC 27599-3270, USA

impoverished social networks often observed for persons with schizophrenia [8]. Thus, the social disability associated with schizophrenia has implications for the development and course of the disorder.

To better understand the social impairments resulting from schizophrenia, researchers have sought to identify the factors that underlie interpersonal deficits. One such factor is cognitive functioning. In particular, verbal memory, vigilance, and executive processing skills have shown a consistent relationship with various indices of social functioning in persons with schizophrenia [9,10]. These relationships have been demonstrated in a variety of samples of persons with schizophrenia, including outpatients [11], chronically ill inpatients [12], and geriatric inpatients [13]. Thus, the relationship between cognition and social behavior is not limited to a particular sub-group of persons with schizophrenia, although it may be stronger in women than in men [14,15].

The foregoing suggests that information-processing skills have a role in support-ing, and perhaps in contributing to, the social behavior of persons with schizophre-nia. However, it would be premature to conclude that cognitive impairments alone account for the social difficulties of persons with schizophrenia. As noted in previous reviews of the literature, research in this area has been "overanalyzed" and "under-powered" [9], and the variance accounted for by cognitive factors in social adjustment is modest, at best [16]. Furthermore, the processing of stimulus information is not limited to nonsocial stimuli, such as numbers, words, and objects [17], but can also involve how one perceives, interprets, and responds to social stimuli [18]. These social stimuli refer to aspects of the self (e.g., how socially skilled one perceives oneself to be), others (e.g., whether someone is angry or sad at a given moment), or the situa-tion (e.g., who is to blame for a negative outcome in a given situation). Known as "social cognition," this area of cognition has also been identified as a potentially crit-ical component of social behavior from a variety of perspectives, including autism, evolutionary biology, and neurophysiology [16,19]. Therefore, social-cognitive processes may play an important role in the social impairments of persons with schizophrenia.

In the last decade, there has been an explosion of research on social cognition in schizophrenia, most notably in the areas of attributional style [20], Theory of Mind (ToM) [21], and emotion perception [22,23]. Interestingly, most of the these studies have examined social cognition from a psychopathology perspective (i.e., how it relates to symptomatology and whether persons with schizophrenia have impair-ments relative to control subjects), with little regard to its relationship with actual social behavior. Thus, scant research has examined how social processing biases or impairments translate into interpersonal deficits.

It is the thesis of this chapter that any discussion of social cognition in schizo-phrenia should be rooted in its implications for social functioning. This will be the approach adopted by this article. Specifically, the focus of this article will be on the ecological validity of one aspect of social cognition, namely, facial affect perception. To achieve this goal, three studies will be reviewed from our research program on social cognition and social functioning in schizophrenia. First, a brief overview of facial affect perception in schizophrenia will be provided. This will be followed by a summary of the aforementioned three studies. The chapter will conclude with a dis-cussion of future research directions.

Facial Affect Perception

Overview

Facial affect perception refers to the ability to recognize the emotional expression in a target's face. There are a number of ways of assessing facial affect perception, but the most common methods are with "identification" and "discrimination" tasks. In a facial affect identification task, the subject is presented with a single stimulus face (for a predetermined duration), and her or his task is to identify the affect expressed (e.g., sadness) from a list of different emotions. In a facial affect discrimination task, the subject is presented with two different target faces simultaneously. The task is to determine if the two faces are expressing the same emotion or different emotions.

An important question in schizophrenia research is whether persons with this disorder have impairments in their ability to identify the emotional expressions of others, and whether such impairments have functional consequences. For example, an individual with schizophrenia who misreads someone's face as being open to conversation, while in actuality the other person is expressing lack of interest, may end up in an aversive encounter. From a diathesis-stress perspective, an increase in aversive or inadequate social encounters may augment stress levels or reduce social support, which could increase the relapse rate. Thus, it is of potential clinical interest to understand the extent of facial affect perception deficits in schizophrenia.

Fortunately, there are a number of excellent reviews on facial affect perception in schizophrenia [22,24]. Based on these reviews, the following conclusions can be made: persons with schizophrenia generally show deficits in facial affect perception (i.e., both identification and discrimination) relative to non-clinical control subjects; persons with schizophrenia typically show deficits in facial affect perception relative to persons with depressive disorder, but the findings are mixed with respect to their impairment relative to control samples with psychotic features (e.g., persons with bipolar disorder); there is a pattern of greater deficits in facial affect perception for negative than for positive facial displays, with impairment perhaps being greatest for the perception of fear [24]; there is some evidence that persons in an acute phase of the disorder perform worse on affect perception tasks than those whose symptoms are in remission [25,26], although if one looks at longitudinal designs, this deficit appears fairly stable [27,28]; the jury is still out regarding whether the facial affect perception deficits are part of a generalized performance deficit [29–32] or specific to decoding only facial emotions [33,34]; there is some evidence for an advantage in facial affect perception in persons with paranoid schizophrenia relative to nonparanoid subtypes (35,36; see [37], for an exception), although these findings need to be replicated before valid conclusions can be drawn.

Facial Affect Perception and Social Functioning

We have published three studies that examined the relationship between facial affect perception and social functioning in schizophrenia [31,38,39]. In the first study [31], we examined the relationship between measures of affect perception (i.e., the Face Emotion Identification Test [FEIT] and the Face Emotion Discrimination Test [FEDT];

TABLE 1. Correlations between results of affect perception tests with social skills and ward behavior (adapted from Mueser et al. [31])

Social functioning	Affect perception tests	
	FEIT	FEDT
Ward behavior		
Social mixing	.45**	.35*
Appropriate behavior	.02	.16
Activity level	.11	.34*
Appearance/hygiene	.61***	.38*
Social skills		
Paralinguistic	.37*	.20
Verbal content	−.04	.06
Overall social skill	.30	.14

* $P < 0.05$; ** $P < 0.01$; *** $P < 0.001$
FEIT, Facial Emotion Identification Test; FEDT, Facial Emotion Discrimination Test

[30]) with two measures of social functioning: Social skill during unstructured role plays and social behavior in the treatment setting, as measured by the Social Behavior Schedule (SBS) [40]. It should be noted that the broader context of this study was to examine the generalized versus specific deficit issue. However, for this chapter, I will focus only on the data relevant to the relationship between emotion perception and social behavior.

The subjects were 28 persons with chronic schizophrenia who had been hospitalized for an average of nine and a half years. The findings showed that both measures of facial affect perception had a fairly consistent association with ward behavior, especially hygiene and grooming (Table 1). However, only performance on the facial affect identification task was related to social skills during the unstructured interactions, albeit weakly.

In a related study [39], we examined the relationship between a battery of social-cognitive tasks, which included facial affect perception (measured by Ekman's pictures of facial affect) [41] and social behavior in the treatment setting, as measured by the Nurse's Observation Scale for Inpatient Evaluation [42]. Like the research participants in the first study, the research participants in this study were inpatients with chronic schizophrenia, although their length of hospitalization was typically less than two years. Correlational analyses revealed that facial affect perception was significantly associated only with indices of adaptive ward behavior (i.e., social competence, social interest, and neatness) (Table 2). Interestingly, as in the first study, facial affect perception had the strongest relationship with hygiene and grooming. Conversely, the association of facial affect perception with maladaptive ward behavior was not significant, although in the expected direction.

Finally, in the third study [38], we examined the relationship between multiple measures of social perception, including facial affect perception (i.e., the FEIT and FEDT),

TABLE 2. Correlations between facial affect identification
and ward behavior (adapted from Penn et al. [39])

Ward behavior	Facial affect identification
Adaptive behavior	
Social competence	.37*
Social interest	.34*
Neatness	.54**
Maladaptive behavior	
Irritability	−.25
Psychoticism	.07
Psychomotor retardation	−.30

* $P < 0.05$; ** $P < 0.01$ (Bonferroni corrected)

TABLE 3. Correlations between results of emotion perception tests and social skill variables (adapted from Ihnen
et al. [38])

Social skills	Emotion perception tests	
	FEIT	FEDT
Overall social skill	.44**	.17
Speech fluency	.08	.12
Speech clarity	.50***	.29
Affective expressiveness	.32*	.07
Gaze	.29	.39**
Involvement	.34**	.18
Number of questions asked	.09	.08

* $P < 0.06$; ** $P < 0.05$; *** $P < 0.01$

with social skill in a sample of clinically stabilized outpatients with schizophrenia.
Social skill was again measured with a pair of unstructured role-plays. The results
revealed that performance on the emotion identification test, but not the discrimination test, was significantly associated with various indices of social skill (e.g., overall
social skill) (Table 3). It should be noted, however, that the significant correlations
were only modest in size and did not remain significant after the Bonferroni correction was employed.

Given the small number of studies in this area, conclusions regarding the association between facial affect perception and social functioning in schizophrenia are
preliminary. At this point, however, the following can be concluded: (1) facial affect
identification is significantly associated with social behavior in the treatment setting
among inpatients with chronic schizophrenia and modestly associated with social
skill among stabilized outpatients; and (2) evidence for an association between facial
affect discrimination and social functioning is limited to social adjustment in the
treatment setting. However, it is not clear why the association between facial affect
perception and social functioning appears more consistent for facial affect identification than discrimination. It is possible that facial affect identification tasks are better
at tapping into the types of skills more likely to be used in everyday life; identifying

how a particular person is feeling is a more common task than determining whether two people are feeling the same emotion or different emotions. However, this is clearly an issue for future investigators to consider.

Concluding Remarks and Future Directions

In this article, our work on the association of facial affect perception with social functioning in persons with schizophrenia was reviewed. The results suggest a correlational relationship between these domains. However, the strength of the association is modest, at best. Furthermore, we have no evidence of how these relationships change over time or whether they are stronger in some subgroups of patients with schizophrenia versus others. These are issues that need to be addressed in future research.

There are a number of additional unanswered questions that should be explored. First, does improvement in affect perception correspond to improvement in actual social behavior? Two recent studies have shown that performance on affect perception tasks can be improved with either remediation-type strategies [43] or atypical neuroleptics [44]. Therefore, the next step is to determine whether such improvements generalize to social functioning. Second, do other social-cognitive tasks contribute independent variance to social behavior beyond that of affect perception skills? In essence, this is a reprisal of the "generalized" versus "specific" deficit issue, only the question now is whether facial affect perception is a unique feature of social cognition or merely reflective of general social-cognitive impairment. This issue can be addressed by research that includes multiple social-cognitive measures (e.g., affect perception, Theory of Mind, attributional style, etc.) in a multiple regression design predicting social competence.

Finally, a critical future step is to examine social behaviors that have a conceptual link to the social-cognitive process in question. The series of studies reviewed in this article could be criticized for conducting only a generic assessment of affect perception and social functioning relationships. In fact, one could argue that, given the types of social behaviors measured, it is not surprising that the relationships were only modest in strength. Specifically, the role-plays used in this research were brief (three minutes) and involved research confederates who were trained to be emotionally neutral (to ensure standardized performance). Therefore, these role-plays may have limited the number of affective cues available to decode, thus reducing the likelihood that perception of facial affect will have an association with social behavior. This raises the issue of how the association between affect perception and social skill would change if the confederates were trained to consistently demonstrate a particular emotion across role-plays, clearly an issue for future research to investigate. In other words, the challenge for future research is to develop social tasks that represent behavioral translations of the social-cognitive processes in question. This type of work has already been done in the area of autism. For example, the functional significance of Theory of Mind (ToM) deficits in children with autism has been assessed by examining their response to an experimenter who dropped "hints" about needing assistance (e.g., carrying a lot of books into a room while commenting on how heavy they are) [45]. Such tasks will provide us the best opportunity to examine social cognition and its potential impact on the behavior of persons with schizophrenia.

Finally, we need to move beyond laboratory-based social-cognitive tasks to those based more on ongoing social behavior. Thus, rather than assessing emotion perception with static faces presented on videotape, a more ecologically valid way would be to investigate how persons with schizophrenia respond to persons demonstrating different emotional expressions during actual social encounters. The current social-cognitive tasks used to assess emotion perception, attributional style, and Theory of Mind, are generally sterile and do not engage the subject in a personal, affective way. This may be because such tasks were developed with a focus on understanding the underlying psychopathology of schizophrenia, rather than the functional significance of these constructs. Ironically then, the current pool of social-cognitive tasks stands the risk of falling victim to the same problems that plague nonsocial stimuli [16]. Therefore, we need to develop social-cognitive tasks that are engaging, personally relevant, and emotionally meaningful. Then, and only then, can we develop valid social-cognitive models of schizophrenia and their potential impact on social behavior.

References

1. American Psychiatric Association (1994) *Diagnostic and statistical manual* (4th edition). Washington, DC
2. Bellack AS, Morrison RL, Wixted JT, et al (1990) An analysis of social competence in schizophrenia. Br J Psychiatry 156:809–818
3. Penn DL, Mueser KT, Doonan R, et al (1995) Relations between social skills and ward behavior in chronic schizophrenia. Schizophr Res 16:225–232
4. Bellack AS, Morrison RL, Mueser KT, et al (1990) Role-play for assessing the social competence of psychiatric patients. Psychol Assess 2:248–255
5. Halford WK, Hayes RL (1995) Social skills in schizophrenia: assessing the relationship between social skills, psychopathology, and community functioning. Soc Psychiatr Psychiatr Epidemiol 30:14–19
6. Glynn SM (1998) Psychopathology and social functioning in schizophrenia. In: Mueser KT, Tarrier N (eds) Handbook of social functioning in schizophrenia. Allyn & Bacon, Boston, pp 66–78
7. Amminger GP, Pape S, Rock D, et al (1999) Relationship between childhood behavioral disturbance and later schizophrenia in the New York high-risk project. Am J Psychiatry 156:525–530
8. Macdonald EM, Jackson HJ, Hayes RL, et al (1998) Social skill as a determinant of social networks and perceived social support in schizophrenia. Schizophr Res 29:275–286
9. Green MF (1996) What are the functional consequences of neurocognitive deficits in schizophrenia? Am J Psychiatry 153:321–330
10. Penn DL, Corrigan PW, Racenstein JM (1998) Cognitive factors and social adjustment in schizophrenia. In: Mueser KT, Tarrier N (eds) Handbook of social functioning in schizophrenia. Allyn & Bacon, Boston
11. Addington J, Addington D (1999) Neurocognitive and social functioning in schizophrenia. Schizophr Bull 25:173–182
12. Penn DL, Mueser KT, Spaulding WD, et al (1995) Information processing and social competence in chronic schizophrenia. Schizophr Bull 21:269–281
13. Harvey PD, Sukhodolsky D, Parrella M, et al (1997) The association between adaptive and cognitive deficits in geriatric chronic schizophrenic patients. Schizophr Res 27:211–218
14. Mueser KT, Blanchard JJ, Bellack AS (1996) Memory and social skills in schizophrenia: the role of gender. Psychiatry Res

15. Penn DL, Mueser KT, Spaulding WD (1996) Information processing, social skills, and gender in schizophrenia. Psychiatry Res 59:213–220
16. Penn DL, Corrigan PW, Bentall RP, et al (1997) Social cognition in schizophrenia. Psychol Bull 121:114–132
17. Corrigan PW, Toomey R (1995) Interpersonal problem solving and information processing in schizophrenia. Schizophr Bull 21:395–403
18. Fiske ST, Taylor S (1991) Social cognition, 2nd edn. McGraw-Hill, New York
19. Silverstein SM (1997) Information processing, social cognition, and psychiatric rehabilitation in schizophrenia. Psychiatry 60:327–340
20. Bentall RP. Social cognition and delusional beliefs. In: Corrigan PW, Penn DL (eds) Social cognition in schizophrenia. American Psychological Association, Washington, DC (in press)
21. Corcoran R. Theory of mind and schizophrenia. In: Corrigan PW, Penn DL (eds) Social cognition in schizophrenia. American Psychological Association, Washington, DC (in press)
22. Hellewell JSE, Whittaker JF (1998) Affect perception and social knowledge in schizophrenia. In: Mueser KT, Tarrier N (eds) *Handbook of social functioning in schizophrenia*. Allyn & Bacon, Boston, pp 197–212
23. Mandal MK, Pandey R, Prasad AB (1998) Facial expressions of emotions and schizophrenia: a review. Schizophr Bull 24:399–412
24. Edwards J, Jackson HJ, Pattitson P (2001) Emotion recognition via facial expression and affective prosody in schizophrenia: a methodological review. Manuscript submitted for publication
25. Cutting J (1981) Judgement of emotional expression in schizophrenia. Br J Psychiatry 139:1–6
26. Gessler S, Cutting J, Frith CD, et al (1989) Schizophrenic ability to judge facial emotion: a controlled study. Br J Clin Psychol 28:19–29
27. Addington J, Addington D (1998) Facial affect recognition and information processing in schizophrenia and bipolar disorder. Schizophr Res 32:171–181
28. Gaebel W, Wolwer W (1992) Facial expression and emotional face recognition in schizophrenia and depression. Eur Arch Psychiatry Clin Neurosci 242:46–52
29. Bellack AS, Blanchard JJ, Mueser, KT (1996) Cue availability and affect perception in schizophrenia. Schizophr Bull 22:535–544
30. Kerr SL, Neale JM (1993) Emotion perception in schizophrenia: specific deficit or further evidence of generalized poor performance? J Abnorm Psychol 102:312–318
31. Mueser KT, Doonan R, Penn DL, et al (1996) Emotion recognition and social competence in chronic schizophrenia. J Abnorm Psychol 105:271–275
32. Salem JE, Kring AM, Kerr SL (1996) More evidence for generalized poor performance in facial emotion performance in schizophrenia. J Abnorm Psychol 105:480–483
33. Heimberg C, Gur RE, Erwin RJ, et al (1992) Facial emotion discrimination: III. Behavioral findings in schizophrenia. Psychiatry Res 42:253–265
34. Penn DL, Combs D, Ritchie M, et al. Emotion recognition in schizophrenia: further investigation of generalized versus specific deficit models. J Abnorm Psychol (in press)
35. Kline J, Smith JE, Ellis HC (1992) Paranoid and nonparanoid schizophrenic processing of facially displayed affect. J Psychiatr Res 26:169–182
36. Lewis SF, Garver DL (1995) Treatment and diagnostic subtype in facial affect recognition in schizophrenia. J Psychiatr Res 29:5–11
37. Mandal MK, Rai A (1987) Responses to facial emotion and psychopathology. Psychiatry Res 20:317–323
38. Ihnen GH, Penn DL, Corrigan PW, et al (1998) Social perception and social skill in schizophrenia. Psychiatry Res 80:275–286
39. Penn DL, Spaulding WD, Reed D, et al (1996) The relationship of social cognition to ward behavior in chronic schizophrenia. Schizophr Res 20:327–335

40. Wykes T, Sturt E (1986) The measurement of social behaviour in psychiatric patients: an assessment of the reliability and validity of the SBS. Br J Psychiatry 148:1–11
41. Ekman P (1976) Pictures of facial affect. Consulting Psychologists Press, Palo Alto, CA
42. Honigfeld R, Klett JC (1966) NOSIE-30: A treatment sensitive ward behavior scale. Psychol Rep 19:180–182
43. Penn DL, Combs D. Modification of facial affect perception deficits in schizophrenia. Schizophr Res (in press)
44. Kee KS, Kern RS, Marshall BD, et al (1998) Risperidone versus haloperidol for perception of emotion in treatment-resistant schizophrenia: preliminary findings. Schizophr Res 31:159–165
45. Sigman M, Ruskin E (1999) Continuity and change in the social competence of children with autism, Down syndrome, and developmental delays. Mon Soc Res Child Dev 64:1–142

Social Skills Training for Schizophrenia: Research Update and Empirical Results

Volker Roder, Hans D. Brenner, Daniel Müller, Marc Lächler, Rosa Müller-Szer, and Peter Zorn

Summary. This multicenter study compared the effectiveness of three newly developed social skills training programs (experimental groups) with that of a conventional, general social skills training program (control group) in terms of social functioning, cognitive abilities, and psychopathology. These new social skills programs focus on rehabilitation topics that are especially relevant for schizophrenia patients and also include specific cognitive interventions. Patients with a diagnosis of schizophrenia or schizoaffective disorder were included in the study and assigned to residential, vocational, recreational, or general social skills training groups by significant matching variables. The first three months of therapy (treatment phase) were followed by a three-month aftercare phase. To date, 112 patients participating in the vocational, recreational, and general social skills training groups have been evaluated. Higher global treatment effects (effect sizes) were obtained, especially for the treatment phase, on almost all dependent variables in both experimental groups as compared with the control group. Treatment effects in all groups further increased during the aftercare phase. Analyses of variance and covariance indicated significantly greater improvements in some cognitive variables for the control group and higher symptom reduction for both experimental groups. The findings suggest that the specifically targeted social skills training programs contribute to better transfer and generalization effects. The results also indicate that psychopathology can be decisively reduced by the new programs. In view of these favorable effects, this new era of social skills training programs might replace more conventional programs in the future.

Key words. Schizophrenia, Social skills training, Cognitive-behavioral therapy, Rehabilitation

Introduction

Against the background of vulnerability-stress models [1], the present-day treatment and rehabilitation of schizophrenia patients consists principally of pharmacotherapy, sociotherapy, and modern behavioral therapy approaches. Contemporary compara-

Psychiatric Services, University of Berne, Bolligenstr. 111, 3000 Berne 60, Switzerland

tive studies have empirically demonstrated the superiority of coping-oriented behavioral therapy methods, which address the problems arising in day-to-day living over dynamic insight-oriented psychotherapies [2,3]. Four main approaches can be distinguished in the area of cognitive-behavioral therapy intervention: cognitive training for elementary information-processing deficits [4], cognitive therapy for persistent positive symptoms [5,6], psychoeducation and behavioral family therapy [7–10], and social skills training (SST) [11–14].

Three eras of methodology have been instrumental in the development and refinement of social skills training procedures [15]. Initially, around 40 years ago [16], social skills training was conducted indirectly, i.e., through operant conditioning (token economy programs). These interventions generally led to reliable empirical results and succeeded in activating patients with negative symptoms and in (re-)establishing social behavior. Today this approach usually is limited to patients with a very low level of social functioning, severe negative symptoms, and resistance to other therapeutical interventions. During the second era in the early 1970s, "social learning" through the use of role-playing was introduced. This technique was utilized to improve both "molecular" skills, such as eye contact and fluency of speech and gestures, and "molar" skills, such as assertiveness and expression of variety of emotion [17]. The review of the Schizophrenia Patient Outcomes Research Team (PORT) [18] states that there is strong empirically based supporting evidence for the acquisition and maintenance of these social skills [19]. Moderate supporting evidence for the efficacy of this era of social skills training is recorded for generalization and social adjustment. Only weak supporting evidence was found in psychopathology. The results obtained with regard to vocational adjustment and quality of life, however, proved contradictory. The intervention programs of the third and youngest era represent an extended development of the second era. By focusing the training on rehabilitation domains that are particularly relevant for individuals with schizophrenia and incorporating a specific problem-solving approach into the skills-training enterprise, modern practitioners now have at their disposal an arsenal of techniques that can significantly improve the course and outcome of schizophrenia. Liberman and coworkers [20–22] were among the first to develop highly standardized therapy modules for the treatment of deficits in social skills, including, for example, the domains of disorder self-management, community re-entry, work, and leisure (SILS modules [Social and Independent Living Skills]). The application of these modules appears far more effective than either occupational therapy or group therapy, particularly in terms of the generalization of skills and social adjustment [19,22–24]. Two of these therapy modules, Medication Management and Symptom Self-Management, have been translated into German, adapted to cultural and social differences, and favorably evaluated [25,26]. However, because of the inherent Anglo-American socioeconomic and cultural context, the goals and content of residential, vocational, and recreational skills training proved not to be readily applicable to European conditions.

The current status of research on rehabilitation in general, and on residential, vocational, and recreational rehabilitation in particular, is thus unsatisfactory. Despite the emphasis in the literature on the importance of providing schizophrenia patients with specific community skills training, there is a lamentable paucity of research on these issues and a lack of empirical data to evaluate the efficacy of such measures in terms of outcome and relapse prevention. Although several publications in the international literature of the past 15 years deal with vocational, residential, and recreational reha- bilitation, most of these studies do not fulfil the scientific criteria for treatment research, for a variety of reasons. Quite often the reader encounters a heterogeneity of nosological groups, a lack of scientific research design (experimental and control groups), no defined intervention methods (time, frequency, treatment, therapists), and nonspecified statistical standard values (mean, standard deviation) for age, IQ, edu- cation, duration of illness, and duration of hospitalization.

Moreover, standardized controlling instruments have not been employed in most cases, nor have the investigators focused on key variables, such as social functioning and adaptation, cognitive abilities, and psychopathology. Thus, a cross-comparison of the results of the different studies is hardly feasible. Furthermore, the use of cognitive-behavioral therapy methods has not been explicitly mentioned in any of these studies. Nevertheless, an overview clearly indicates that most of the applied interventions effectuated some improvement. However, the impact on social role func- tioning, cognitive abilities, psychopathology, relapse rates, and the course of the dis- order still remains largely uninvestigated. In this context, the necessity of conducting further investigative controlled studies with appropriate designs and an adequate number of subjects becomes obvious. These new training approaches should bridge the still existing gap between cognitive-behavioral therapy methods and general reha- bilitation topics, especially in the areas of residential, vocational, and recreational activities. Against this background, the scope of the social skills training subprogram of the Integrated Psychological Therapy (IPT) for Schizophrenia Patients has been expanded. This subprogram of the IPT represents an approach of the second era of SST and was conceptualized during the 1980s by our research group [11,27,15]. We developed three new cognitive social skills programs for residential, vocational, and recreational topics [28], which were evaluated in pilot studies with single-case exper- imental designs and in two preliminary studies in 1991. As the results demonstrated the importance of these domains in the treatment of patients, a comparative evalua- tion of the programs was conducted.

Methods

Patient Sample and Design of the Multicenter Study

Subjects were recruited from eight psychiatric institutions (five in Switzerland, two in Germany, and one in Austria), all of which offer a comparable standard of care in the areas of pharmacotherapy, sociotherapy, and work therapy. The following selection criteria were applied: diagnosis of a schizophrenic or a schizoaffective disorder accord- ing to ICD-10 (F20, F25 [29,30]; history of three or more previous hospitalizations; age between 20 and 50 years; average intelligence according to the short form of the Wech- sler Intelligence Test (WIP) [31]; continuous deterioration in the following areas of psychosocial functioning over the past 24 months: housing, work, leisure, and social skills (Global Assessment of Functioning Scale (GAF), DSM-IV [32]) and the need for therapy in these areas. Evidence of excessive substance abuse or organic brain syn- drome (double diagnosis patients) constituted exclusion criteria. The study follows an intergroup design and was aimed at the evaluation of treatment effects by using repeated measurements. The experimental groups received one of the three new programs (residential, vocational, or recreational skills training), while the control group was offered general social skills training and problem-solving training according to the IPT. Within the framework of social skills methodology, programs of the third era were compared with a program of the second era. Subjects were assigned to the different treatment groups according to the following matching variables: duration of hospitalization, psychopathology (Brief Psychiatric Rating Scale, BPRS [33]), daily dose of neuroleptics when starting therapy, motivation (Therapy Motivation Questionnaire, FPTM [34]), and IQ (WIP [31]). Each group was offered a three-month treatment phase with two group sessions (90 minutes each) and one individual session (30 minutes) a week, followed by a three-month aftercare phase with one group session a week and one biweekly individual session. The follow-up interval was one year after entry in the study. Assessment instruments were applied at four different intervals: before and after treatment (T1 and T2), at the end of the aftercare phase (T3), and after the follow-up (T4). We anticipated that better results would be achieved in the experimental groups regarding an improvement in general social abilities and psychopathology. In addition, we expected better generalization and transfer effects in the experimental groups in specific areas of social functioning, such as housing, work, and leisure. The new programs and the general social skills and problem-solving training were expected to be equally effective with regard to cognitive parameters.

Assessment Instruments

The instruments used in the study can be classified into measures of cognitive abilities, social functioning, and psychopathology. The measures of cognitive abilities were the: Number Connecting Test, ZVT ([35]; test) to assess speed of cognitive performance; the Continuous Concentration Test, KVT ([36]; test) to assess sustained concentration over a longer period of time; and the Attention-Stress Test, d2 ([37]; test) to assess discrimination task performance and speed of information processing. Social functioning was measured by the following instruments: the Global Assessment of Functioning Scale, GAF (DSM-IV [32]; expert rating) to assess the general level of psychosocial role functioning (psychological, social, and vocational level of functioning, social behavior, social adjustment); the Social Interview Schedule, SIS ([38,39]; self-rating) to assess psychosocial adjustment and social behavior (areas: residential and job adjustment, economic situation, leisure and recreational behavior, and contacts in and outside the family. Assessment covers the following aspects for each area: real-life situations, satisfaction with different social roles, and role performance); the Disability Assessment Schedule, DAS-M ([40,41]; expert rating) to assess social impairment (residential, vocational and recreational adjustment, general social behavior); and the Intentionality Rating Scale, InSka, Subscales I and V ([42]; expert rating) to assess initiative and motoric impulse. Psychopathology was evaluated by the Brief Psychiatric Rating Scale, BPRS ([33,43]; expert rating) to assess psychopathological symptoms; the Scale for the Assessment of Negative Symptoms, SANS ([44]; expert rating) to assess negative symptoms; and the Scale for the Assessment of Well-Being, BF-S ([45]; self-rating) to assess well-being as perceived by the patient. Motivation for participation in the group and motivational influences during therapy were measured by the Therapy Motivation Questionnaire, FPTM ([34]; self-rating).

Treatment Programs for Residential, Vocational, and Recreational Skills

Each of the new cognitive-behavioral therapy programs focuses on sensitizing the patients to their needs, options, and skills (cognitive and emotional skills training); helping them to make a decision in any one of these three areas; providing support in putting the decision taken into action (practical implementation of skills); and teaching them how to anticipate difficulties and to solve concrete problems that might occur in the new residential, vocational, or leisure-time situation. All three programs have the same structure, which on the whole allows for flexible behavior and problem analysis. Four different formats of therapeutic intervention can be distinguished: group therapy, individual therapy, in vivo exercises, and homework assignments. Each group of patients is treated with only one therapy program. The following cognitive-behavioral techniques are employed: problem and behavior analysis, modeling, role-playing, cognitive restructuring, problem-solving, brainstorming, decision training, positive reinforcement, positive connotation, structuring, covert learning, self-control, self-verbalization and self-reinforcement, cognitive rehearsal, coaching, coping techniques, etc. Detailed and highly standardized therapy manuals are available for all three therapy programs.

Data Analysis

In the analysis of the data, we did not expect to find marked between-group differences, because the experimental condition consisted of treatment groups with specific social skills training, and the second era SST had already been well evaluated [11]. The estimation of sample size was therefore based on the expected medium effect sizes for two-tailed analysis of variance (ANOVA) for repeated measurements ($f = 0.25$), with a generally accepted statistical power of 0.80 at an alpha level of significance (two-sided) of 5% [46,47].

Data analysis had five main steps. *Data reduction*: By means of factor analysis, we empirically investigated the theoretical demarcation of three levels of deficits (psychopathology, cognitive deficits, and social deficits). We then exploratively combined the 16 corresponding dependent variables to factors. This statistical approach seemed tenable because the 16 variables within the three levels differed considerably in regard to theoretical conceptualizations and empirical significance. The individual factors were subsequently subjected to an analysis of reliability. *Effect sizes*: These are calculated for all factors as dependent variables in order to describe the course over the four measurement points [48]. Effect sizes for each group were defined by the difference in the means of two measurement points for the reference group divided by the standard deviation of the whole sample at baseline. According to Cohen [46], effect sizes can be generally categorized as small (0.2), medium (0.5), and large (0.8). *Inferential statistics*: For inferential statistics, the results of each of the 16 dependent variables distributed over the factors were transformed into standardized z-values, and the mean z-values were built for each factor. The comparability of the four therapy groups at baseline with regard to the individual factors was assessed by one-way ANOVA and subsequent Scheffé tests. The course over the measurement points (T1 to T4) was analyzed for significant main effects and interactions by two-tailed ANOVA for repeated measurements. *Differential analysis of social skills acquisition*: To obtain a more detailed picture of the changes in social functioning of each group, we combined the items of the two dimensions "management/coping" and "satisfaction" of the Social Interview Schedule (SIS) for vocation, living accommodation, recreation, and general social skills. *Moderator variables*: An assessment of the impact of potential moderator variables, such as medication or therapy motivation, on outcome was performed by comparing patients receiving typical with those receiving atypical neuroleptic medication. Therapy motivation was rated according to the results of a scale for the assessment of therapy motivation [34].

Results

Results for the vocational, recreational, and control groups (social skills) are available for the treatment (T1–T2) and aftercare phases (T2–T3).

Patient Characteristics and Grouping

Seventy-two subjects participating in either a recreational or a vocational group, as well as 40 controls (IPT: social skills training of the second era), have been included in data analysis thus far. The following results are therefore based on a total current sample of 112 subjects. Demographic and clinical characteristics are presented in Table 1.

No significant differences (ANOVA) were evident for IQ, duration of hospitalization, daily dose of neuroleptics, psychopathology, or motivation. However, the groups differed in age and duration of illness. In order to control for possible influences of age and duration of illness on the treatment results, these variables were included as covariates in further statistical analysis. The three treatment groups did not differ in the ratio of men to women (Pearson chi-square test).

TABLE 1. Overview of patient characteristics (means ± SD) ($n = 112$)

Characteristic	Experimental groups ($n = 72$)		Control group ($n = 40$)
	Recreational ($n = 44$)	Vocational ($n = 28$)	Social skills ($n = 40$)
Age	35.7 ± 7.6	33.0 ± 7.0	31.1 ± 7.2
IQ (WIP)	102.5 ± 15.9	102.5 ± 10.9	100.1 ± 8.5
Duration of hospitalization (mo)	19.4 ± 32.0	8.3 ± 10.4	14.6 ± 17.7
Duration of illness (yr)	9.5 ± 6.1	5.8 ± 3.9	5.7 ± 5.3
Daily dose of neuroleptics (chlorpromazine values)	355.8 ± 235.5	285.4 ± 211.2	383.5 ± 306.6
Psychopathology (BPRS/SANS; z-values)	0.06 ± 0.83	0.18 ± 0.79	0.2 ± 0.79
Motivation (FPTM total score)	106.9 ± 12.9	108.5 ± 9.7	102.4 ± 11.6

Dropouts

From the whole sample of 112 patients taking part in the study, 17 dropped out, giving a dropout rate of 15.2% (8 men and 9 women). The dropout rates did not differ significantly between groups (Pearson chi-square test). The reason for dropping out for nine patients was an increase in the symptom level with or without concomitant psychotic relapse. Four patients were discharged from the psychiatric institution because of marked psychosocial improvements, two patients found a job, one met with an accidental death, and one was excluded from the study because of irregular attendance at the sessions.

Data Reduction

The 16 variables were grouped by varimax-rotated factor analysis into the following five factors, which explain a total variance of 69.3%: Factor 1, "speed of information processing," includes the variables d2 (number of signs), d2 (number of correct signs), ZVT, and KVT (speed performance). Factor 2, "maintenance of concentration," includes both KVT variables "concentration" and "accuracy." Factor 3, "social interest and social integration," consists of DAS-M and GAF, two SANS scores (abulia/apathy and anhedonia), and both InSka scores "motoric impulse" and "initiative." Factor 4, "social well-being and psychosocial coping," includes both SIS dimensions "management/coping" and "satisfaction," together with Bf-S. Finally, Factor 5, "psychopathology," combines the BPRS and three further SANS scores (affective flattening, alogia, and attention). The item composition of each factor was determined by an analysis of reliability (Cronbach's alpha coefficients), which was considered satisfactory.

Effect Sizes

The effect sizes compared at baseline (T1) with the measurement points after treatment (T2) and at the end of the aftercare phase (T3) are presented in Fig. 1 for each group.

With the exception of psychopathology, the effect sizes for the treatment phase (T1–T2) are generally rather small, increasing to medium effects when the baseline and aftercare phase are compared. With the exception of a minimal deterioration in psychopathology for the control group, all these effects indicate improvements. The two factors representing cognitive functioning show non-uniform results. The control group improved most on the speed factor (T1–T2: ES = 0.38, T1–T3: ES = 0.63), whereas effects on the concentration factor remained comparatively small (T1–T2: ES = 0.08; T1–T3: ES = 0.24). The results for the vocational group show an almost opposite tendency: improvements on the speed factor are weaker for these patients (T1–T2: ES = 0.27; T1–T3: ES = 0.36), whereas on the concentration factor this group's performance was clearly superior to that of the controls (T1–T2: ES = 0.49; T1–T3: ES = 0.61). The recreational group showed generally weaker but more homogeneous results on the cognitive level. Developments on the level of social functioning vary among the three comparison groups. On the factor "social integration," all patients improved until the end of the aftercare phase. However, the effect sizes for the recreational and control groups are larger throughout in comparison to the vocational group. The

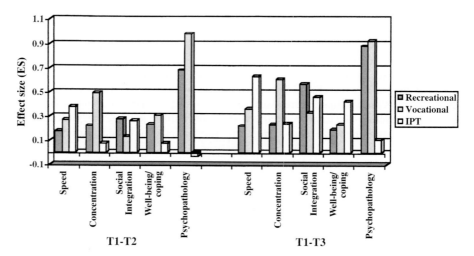

FIG. 1. Effect sizes of the five factors (treatment phase, T1–T2; treatment phase and aftercare phase, T1–T3)

recreational group reached the largest effect size on this factor (T1–T3: ES = 0.57). On the factor "well-being/coping," the effects for the three comparison groups are somewhat ambiguous due to the results of the control group. The effect size for the control group was the smallest after treatment (T1–T2: ES = 0.08) but the largest at the end of the aftercare phase (T1–T3: ES = 0.42). The overall strongest effects were obtained on the factor "psychopathology." However, these large effects were limited to the experimental groups (vocational: T1–T2, ES = 0.98; T1–T3, ES = 0.92; recreational: T1–T2, ES = 0.68; T1–T3, ES = 0.88). The control group showed small positive effect sizes at the end of the aftercare phase (T1–T3: ES = 0.11), after a slight deterioration during treatment (T1–T2: ES = −0.03). As a next step, the effect sizes for the five factors were combined in order to obtain an overview of the global therapy effects (Fig. 2).

During treatment, small global effects were revealed for the control group (ES = 0.15) and medium effects for both experimental groups (recreational: ES = 0.32; vocational: ES = 0.43). All groups continued to improve during the aftercare phase. The difference in the global effect size between the experimental and control groups diminished at T3 with values at a medium level. However, the treatment effects at this point are still larger for both experimental groups (vocational: ES = 0.49; recreational: ES = 0.42; control: ES = 0.37).

Inferential Statistics

Data were examined by one-way ANOVA for differences at baseline, including age and duration of illness as covariates. This analysis yielded significant between-group differences on the factor "social integration" ($F = 3.83$; $P = 0.02$). Subsequent Scheffé tests showed that participants in the recreational group were more impaired on this level

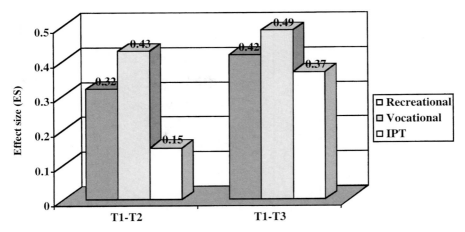

Fig. 2. Mean effect sizes of the five factors (treatment phase, T1–T2; treatment phase and after-care phase, T1–T3)

than those in the vocational group. However, the covariates did not prove to have significant influence on any of the five factors. The course over the three measurement points was examined in all groups for the five factors by ANOVA for repeated measurements. In the case of significant main effects, we subsequently checked the difference in means between two measurement points (T1–T2; T1–T3) by one-way ANOVA. Age and duration of illness were once again included as covariates, but no significant influences were found for any of the five factors. Although the calculation of the means of the z-transformed values of the five factors is considered conservative, and therefore smaller effects would be expected, we nonetheless obtained significant interaction effects in three of the five factors (Table 2).

On the cognitive level, a highly significant interaction was found for the factor "speed" ($F = 3.32$; $P = 0.01$). An ANOVA was performed to specify this effect. Improvement was significantly higher in the control group from T1 to T3 compared with the recreational group ($F = 6.05$; $P = 0.00$, Scheffé test). On the level of social functioning, a significant main effect "group" ($F = 4.26$; $P = 0.01$) as well as a significant interaction effect ($F = 3.21$; $P = 0.01$) was found for the factor "social integration." During the period T1–T3, improvement was significantly higher for the recreational group than for the vocational group ($F = 4.59$; $P = 0.01$, Scheffé test). However, the baseline level of the vocational group was significantly higher than that of the recreational group. To determine whether the effects in the recreational group could be attributed to the different baseline levels of the three groups, these baseline levels were included as covariates in the ANOVA. A significant influence of the different baseline levels could be confirmed. Therefore, neither a significant group effect nor a significant interaction effect in reference to the factor "social integration" was ascertainable. On the psychopathological level, a highly significant interaction effect ($F = 6.98$; $P = 0.00$) was found as a result of the greater improvement in both experimental groups as compared with the control group (T1–T2: $F = 15.21$, $P = 0.00$; T1–T3: $F = 10.09$, $P = 0.00$, Scheffé test). With regard to type I errors by multiple testing (ANOVA), the

TABLE 2. Results of ANOVA for repeated measurements: interaction effects of the five factors (means ± SD)

Factor	Recreational group (n = 44)			Vocational group (n = 28)			IPT group (n = 40)			ANOVA	
	T1	T2	T3	T1	T2	T3	T1	T2	T3	F	P
Speed	.03 ± .89	−.11 ± .92	−.14 ± .76	.05 ± .76	.07 ± .91	.01 ± .89	−.07 ± .76	.03 ± .63	.14 ± .68	3.32	.01
Concentration	.05 ± .91	.04 ± .95	−0.4 ± 1.0	−.02 ± 1.1	.08 ± .98	.07 ± .97	.08 ± .98	−.07 ± 1.0	.00 ± 1.0	0.69	n.s.
Social integration	−.27 ± .73	−.20 ± .80	−.14 ± .76	.33 ± .72	.23 ± .61	.17 ± .71	.04 ± .67	.06 ± .75	.04 ± .83	3.21	.01
Well-being/ coping	−.08 ± .73	−.03 ± .70	−.12 ± .80	.07 ± .80	.18 ± .74	.05 ± .80	.04 ± .82	−0.8 ± .79	.10 ± .89	0.97	n.s.
Psychopathology	−.06 ± .83	.12 ± .79	.18 ± .80	−.18 ± .79	.29 ± .64	.12 ± .59	.20 ± .79	−.33 ± .88	−.34 ± 1.0	6.98	.00

T1, T2, T3: Points of assessment

level of significance of $\alpha = 0.05$ would be reduced to $\alpha' < 0.003$ after Bonferoni correction.

Differential Analysis of Social Skill Acquisition

In a first step, both SIS dimensions "management/coping" and "satisfaction" in the areas of vocation, recreation, and general social skills—six variables in total—were examined for baseline differences by one-way ANOVA. No significant baseline differences between the groups were found. In a second step, paired-samples t-tests for within-group comparisons of baseline with T2 and T3 were conducted for all six variables. Only the recreational group showed significant improvements on the dimension "management/coping" in the area of recreation during the entire therapy interval (T1–T2: $T = 3.41$, $P = 0.00$; T1–T3: $T = 3.08$, $P = 0.00$). On the other hand, significant improvements in the dimension "satisfaction" were found only in the vocational group in the vocational area (T1–T2; $T = 2.38$; $P = 0.02$). General social skills on the dimension "management/coping" improved significantly for both the control group (T1–T2: $T = 2.93$, $P = 0.00$; T1–T3: $T = 2.83$; $P = 0.00$) and the vocational group (T1–T2: $T = 3.43$, $P = 0.00$). For all other variables, no significant within-group effects were found.

Moderator Variables

Motivational Influences over the Course of Treatment

The FPTM [34] was assessed at all measurement points in order to detect possible motivational influences moderating the treatment effects. Neither the total score, nor one of the six subscales (degree of mental suffering, symptom-generated attention from others, hope, denial of mental distress, initiative, knowledge) proved significant with regard to baseline differences (ANOVA). ANOVA for repeated measurements yielded a significant main effect on the scale "knowledge" ($F = 3.66$; $P = 0.03$). Subsequent least significant difference (LSD) tests revealed a significantly higher motivation to acquire illness-specific knowledge in both the experimental groups as compared with the control group.

Medication

To determine whether the variation in effects was dependent upon medication, patients were divided into two groups, of which one received typical and the other atypical neuroleptic medication. Five patients received no neuroleptic medication for the duration of the study. In the remaining sample, 52% were treated with typical and 48% with atypical neuroleptics. No between-group differences were found in patient characteristics (t-tests for independent samples), and patients with typical and atypical medication were equally distributed according to the three treatment groups (Pearson chi-square test). The five factors were examined for between-group differences by two-tailed ANOVA for repeated measurements. On the level of cognitive functioning, a significant main effect ($F = 5.26$; $P = 0.02$) could be found for the factor "concentration" (Fig. 3).

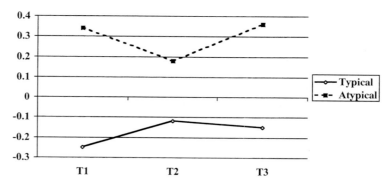

FIG. 3. Z-values of the factor, "concentration" for typical and atypical neuroleptics

Subsequent *t*-tests for independent samples yielded significant between-group differences at T1 ($T = 2.78$, $P = 0.00$) and at T3 ($T = 2.03$, $P = 0.04$), the group receiving atypical medication having better scores on the factor "concentration" at both baseline and T3.

Discussion

Improvements in social functioning were found for both conventional training in general social skills (IPT of the second era, control group) and the newly developed SST of the third era in the specific areas of vocation and recreation (experimental groups). The effects over the three-month treatment phase must be regarded as rather modest. However, social functioning further improved during the aftercare phase, so that six months after the beginning of treatment, moderate to high effects for all groups were obtained on this level. Moreover, the results indicate better social coping and social well-being for those patients who participated in an experimental group. In addition, notable results were obtained in a differential analysis of the Social Interview Schedule (SIS [38,39]). On the one hand, the vocational group rated the satisfaction with their vocational status significantly higher after treatment. On the other, we found higher scores in the recreational group at treatment and aftercare phase with regard to social management, social competence, and social coping in the recreational area. These findings indicate that the patients in the vocational or recreational groups had higher satisfaction or improved coping capacities in precisely those areas that had been focused upon during treatment. Consequently, it would seem that the newly developed SST achieved a transfer and generalization of acquired social skills to daily life.

Whereas several studies posit that positive and negative symptoms have only minimal influence on the patients' ability to benefit from social skills training [49–52], it seems that negative symptoms can influence the generalization of acquired social skills in a negative way [17]. In the present study, patients participating in the newly developed SST had a significant reduction of negative symptoms. According to Smith et al. [17], these reductions of symptoms could have been a supporting factor with regard to the obtained generalization effects of these patients. For both experimental groups, we found high treatment effects on the factor "psychopathology" in the treatment as well as in the aftercare phase. The control group showed no significant symptom reduction after treatment, and only a small reduction at the end of the aftercare phase was found. We assume that these positive effects in the experimental groups can be ascribed to the direct and focused way of dealing with goal-oriented contents highly relevant to daily life, and that this in turn generated a greater tangible significance of the therapy goals for the participants in these groups. So far our data on social functioning as well as on the symptom level support the view that greater attention to narrow but vitally important areas of social functioning in schizophrenia can lead to better outcomes as compared with general social skills training [17].

Finally, we found positive effects on the level of cognitive functioning. Attentional tests revealed small to medium improvements in all treatment groups up to the end of the aftercare phase. These results confirm findings of previous studies showing that IPT can affect improvement in cognitive functioning [4] and indicate that the newly developed SST can produce similar positive outcomes on the cognitive level. With regard to attentional processes, it must be borne in mind that many complex social situations, such as carrying on a conversation, make high demands on attentional processing [53]. Although previous studies do not support the hypothesis of a directly pervasive influence of improved cognitive functions on a more complex level of behavior (as originally postulated by Brenner [54]), the improvement of cognitive deficits in schizophrenia patients seems to be a necessary but not exclusive precondition for socially competent behavior [55]. Green [56] states that attentional deficits can predict the acquisition of narrowly circumscribed social skills, whereas results predicting functioning on a more global, generalized social level, such as community functioning, are still outstanding. Further data analysis will prove whether such relations can be found. With regard to medication, our results suggest that patients receiving atypical neuroleptics are more capable of maintaining concentration. This result is in accordance with previous studies [57,58] suggesting favorable influences of atypical neuroleptic medication on cognitive functions.

In summary, we found higher global treatment effects on all dependent variables for both experimental groups as compared with the control group, especially for the treatment phase. Global treatment effects further increased during the aftercare phase in all groups, whereas the difference between the treatment and aftercare phases is highest in the control group. This finding indicates that in comparison with general social skills training, the newly developed SST prime focus on specific social skills in narrowly defined areas, such as vocation or recreation, can lead more rapidly to improvements in social, cognitive, and psychopathological parameters. In addition, this result clearly shows that the treatment sessions during the aftercare phase of 12 weeks, although less intensive, contribute to further improvements, which points to the necessity of longer-term therapy to achieve satisfying treatment effects. Our data therefore support the assumption of Mueser et al. [19] that if SST is to be effective, it must be provided for extended periods of time. The follow-up data will show whether enduring benefits have been achieved.

Finally, some critical aspects should be mentioned. We did not use a design with randomization. Despite the resulting methodological limitations, we decided to carry out a matching procedure to secure the participation of the different centers in the study. Including natural settings in therapy research offers some advantages in comparison to academic sites. First, patients can be treated in their "natural environments." Second, longer sample sizes can be included in research designs within a short time. Finally, rapid distribution and successful implementation of new effective treatment approaches are easier. It also must be pointed out that the course of illness and the rehabilitation status of the patients before, during, and after treatment have an influence on the therapeutic goals. Therefore, we are evaluating these variables for a period of two years before starting and after termination of therapy and we will try to include them in statistical analyses. A further critical aspect is that different therapists treated the various groups. However, by using highly standardized manual-based therapies and regular supervision sessions, we tried to obviate possible sources of bias.

Acknowledgments. We would like to thank the following institutions for their participation in the project: Switzerland: Psychiatric University Hospital Zurich, Extern Psychiatric Services Liestal, Psychiatric Hospital Rheinau, Psychiatric Hospital Wil; Germany: Private Psychiatric Hospital Dr. med. Kurt Fontheim/Liebenburg, Psychiatric Hospital Haar/Munich; Austria: Institute of Psychotherapy Vienna. This project is supported by Grant No. 32-45577.95, Swiss National Science Foundation.

References

1. Nuechterlein KH, Dawson ME, Ventura J, et al (1994) The vulnerability / stress model of schizophrenic relapse: a longitudinal study. Acta Psychiatr Scand 89:58–64
2. Scott JE, Dixon LB (1995) Psychological interventions for schizophrenia. Schizophr Bull 21:621–630
3. Mojtabai R, Nicholson RA, Carpenter BN (1998) Role of psychosocial treatment in management of schizophrenia: a meta-analytic review of controlled outcome studies. Schizophr Bull 24:569–587
4. Olbrich R, Mussgay L (1990) Reduction of schizophrenic deficits by cognitive training. An evaluative study. Eur Arch Psychiatry Neurol Sci 239:366–369
5. Vauth R, Stieglitz RD (1993) Psychologische Interventionsmöglichkeiten bei persistierendem Wahn und persistierenden akustischen Halluzinationen bei schizophrenen Patienten. Psychiatrische Praxis 20:211–217
6. Chadwick P, Birchwood M, Trower P (1996) Cognitive therapy for delusions, voices and paranoia. John Wiley & Sons, Chichester, England
7. Kieserg A, Hornung WP (1996) Psychoedukatives Training für schizophrene Patienten: (PTS). Ein verhaltenstherapeutisches Behandlungsprogramm zur Rezidivprophylaxe. Tübingen, Germany, dgvt-Verlag
8. Bäuml J (1994) Psychosen aus dem schizophrenen Formenkreis: Ein Ratgeber für Patienten und Angehörige. Springer-Verlag, Berlin
9. Hahlweg K, Feinstein E, Müller U, et al (1989) Family management programmes for schizophrenic patients. Prevention of relapse and modification of familial communication patterns. In: Brenner HD, Böker W (eds) Schizophrenia as a systems disorder. Br J Psychiatry 155(Suppl 5):112–116
10. Hahlweg K, Dürr H, Müller U (1995) Familienbetreuung schizophrener Patienten. Beltz, Weinheim, Germany

11. Brenner HD, Hodel B, Roder V, et al (1992) Treatment of cognitive dysfunctions and behavioral deficits in schizophrenia. Schizophr Bull 18:21–26
12. Roder V, Eckman TA, Brenner HD, et al (1990) Behavior therapy. In: Herz MI, Keith SJ, Docherty JP (eds) Handbook of schizophrenia. Vol 4. Psychosocial treatment of schizophrenia. Elsevier Science Publishers, Amsterdam, pp 107–134
13. Liberman RP, Massel HK, Mosk MD, et al (1985) Social skills training for chronic mental patients. Hosp Commun Psychiatry 36:396–403
14. Liberman RP (1998) International perspectives on skills training for the mentally disabled. Int Rev Psychiatry 10:5–8
15. Roder V, Brenner HD, Kienzle N, et al (1997) Integriertes Psychologisches Therapieprogramm (IPT) für schizophrene Patienten, 4. überarbeitete Auflage. Beltz, Weinheim, Germany
16. Cohen, R, Florin I, Grusche A, et al (1973) Dreijährige Erfahrung mit einem Münzsystem auf einer Station für extrem inaktive, chronisch schizophrene Patienten. Z Klini Psychol 2:243–277
17. Smith ET, Bellack AS, Liberman RP (1996) Social skills training for schizophrenia. Review and future directions. Clin Psychol Rev 16:599–617
18. Lehmann AF, Steinwachs DM (1994) Literature review: treatment approaches for schizophrenia. Schizophrenia Patient Outcomes Research Team (PORT), University of Maryland, Baltimore
19. Mueser KT, Wallace CJ, Liberman RP (1995) New developments in social skills training. Behav Change 12:31–40
20. Liberman RP, Kopelowicz A, Smith TE (1999) Psychiatric rehabilitation. In: Sadock BJ, Sadock VA (eds) Comprehensive textbook of psychiatry, 7th edn Lippincott Williams & Wilkins, Baltimore, pp 3218–3245
21. Liberman RP, Eckman TA (1989) Dissemination of skills training modules to psychiatric facilities. Overcoming obstacles to the utilisation of a rehabilitation innovation. In: Brenner HD, Böker W (eds) Schizophrenia as a systems disorder. Br J Psychiatry 155(Suppl 5):117–122
22. Liberman RP, Wallace CJ, Blackwell G, et al (1993) Innovations in skills training for the seriously mentally ill: the UCLA social and independent living skills modules. Innov Res 2:43–60
23. Marder SR, Wirshing WC, Mintz J, et al (1996) Two-year outcome of social skills training and group psychotherapy for outpatients with schizophrenia. Am J Psychiatry 153:1585–1592
24. Wallace CJ (1998) Social skills training in psychiatric rehabilitation: recent findings. Int Rev Psychiatry 10:9–19
25. Brenner HD, Waldvogel D, Wäber M, et al (1988) Therapieprogramm zum eigenverantworlichen Umgang mit Medikamenten bei chronisch psychisch Kranken. Schweiz Z Med Medizin Technik 11:15–20
26. Schaub A, Behrendt B, Brenner HD (1998) A multi-hospital evaluation of the medication and symptom management modules in Germany and Switzerland. Int Rev Psychiatry 10:42–46
27. Brenner HD, Roder V, Hodel B, et al (1994) Integrated psychological therapy for schizophrenic patients. Hogrefe & Huber, Seattle, WA
28. Roder V, Jenull B, Brenner HD (1998) Teaching schizophrenic patients recreational, residential and vocational skills. Int Rev Psychiatry 10:35–41
29. Dilling H, Mombour W, Schmidt MH (1991) Internationale Klassifikation der Krankheiten in der 10. Revision (ICD-10). Huber, Berne
30. World Health Organisation (1993) The ICD-10 classification of mental and behavioural disorders. Psychiatric Adaption. WHO, Geneva
31. Dahl G (1986) Reduzierter Wechsler-Intelligenztest (WIP). Testzentrale der Schweizer Psychologen, Huber, Berne

32. American Psychiatric Association (1994) DSM-IV: Diagnostic and Statistical Manual of Mental Disorders, 4th edn Washington, DC
33. Overall JE, Gorham DR (1962) The Brief Psychiatric Rating Scale. Psychol Rep 10:799–812
34. Schulz H, Nübling R, Rüddel H (1995) Entwicklung einer Kurzform eines Fragebogens zur Therapiemotivation. Verhaltenstherapie 5:89–95
35. Oswald WD, Roth E (1978) Der Zahlen-Verbindungs-Test (ZVT). Hogrefe, Göttingen, Germany
36. Abels D (1961) Konzentrations-Verlaufs-Test (KVT). Hogrefe, Göttingen, Germany
37. Brickenkamp R (1975) Aufmerksamkeits-Belastungs-Test (Test d2). Hogrefe, Göttingen, Germany
38. Clare AW, Cairns VE (1978) Design, development, and use of a standardized interview to assess social maladjustment and dysfunction in community studies. Psychol Med 8:589–604
39. Hecht H, Faltermaier A, Wittchen HU (1987) Social Interview Schedule (SIS). Materialien zur Klinischen Pschologie und Psychotherapie. Roderer, Regensburg, Germany
40. World Health Organization (1987) Disability Assessment Schedule. Geneva
41. Jung E, Krumm B, Biehl H, et al (1989) Mannheimer Skala zur Einschätzung sozialer Behinderung. Beltz, Weinheim, Germany
42. Mundt C, Fiedler PA, Pracht B, et al (1985) InSka (Intentionalitätsskalen) ein neues psychopathometrisches Instrument zur quantitativen Erfassung der schizophrenen Residualsymptomatik. Nervenarzt 56:146–149
43. CIPS Collegium Internationale Psychiatriae Scalarum (1981) Internationale Skalen für Psychiatrie. Beltz, Weinheim, Germany
44. Andreasen NC (1981) Scale for the Assessment of Negative Symptoms (SANS). University of Iowa City
45. Zerssen D (1976) Die Befindlichkeits-Skala. Beltz, Weinheim, Germany
46. Cohen J (1988) Statistical power analyses for the behavioral sciences. Erlbaum, Hillsdale, NJ
47. Bortz J, Döring N (1995) Forschungsmethoden und Evaluation. Springer-Verlag, Berlin
48. Smith ML, Glass GV (1977) Meta-analyses of psychotherapy outcome studies. Am Psychol 752–760
49. Eckman TD, Wirshing SR, Marder RP, et al (1992) Technique for training schizophrenic patients in illness self-management: a controlled trial. Am J Psychiatry 149:1549–1555
50. Munroe-Blum H, McCleary L (1995) RCT: social treatments for schizophrenia: 12 month findings. Schizophr Res 15:221
51. Mueser KT, Kosmidis MH, Sayers MD (1992) Symptomatology and the prediction of social skills acquisition in schizophrenia. Schizophr Res 8:59–68
52. Douglas MS, Mueser KT (1990) Teaching conflict resolution skills to the chronically mentally ill. Social skills training groups for briefly hospitalized patients. Behav Modif 14:519–547
53. Spaulding WD, Reed D, Poland J, et al (1996) Cognitive deficits in psychotic disorders. In: Corrigan PW, Yudufsky SC (eds) Cognitive rehabilitation for neuropsychiatric disorders. American Psychiatric Press, Washington, DC, pp 129–166
54. Brenner HD (1987) On the importance of cognitive disorders in treatment and rehabilitation. In: Böker W, Brenner HD (eds) Psychosocial treatment of schizophrenia. Huber, Toronto
55. Hodel B, Brenner HD (1994) Cognitive therapy with schizophrenic patients: conceptual basis, present state, future directions. Acta Psychiatr Scand 90:108–115
56. Green MF (1996) What are the functional consequences of neurocognitive deficits in schizophrenia? Am J Psychiatry 153:321–330

57. Goldberg TE (1995) Cognitive effects of atypical neuroleptics: a double blind study of risperidone and clozapine. Paper presented at the Second Mount Sinai Schizophrenia Conference, New York, April 1995
58. Green MF (1998) Schizophrenia from a neurocognitive perspective. Allyn and Bacon, Boston

Part 3
Expressed Emotion and Psychoeducation

Keynote Lecture:
Relatives' Expressed Emotion:
From Measurement Technique
to Practical Help for Families

JULIAN LEFF

Summary. The measurement of Expressed Emotion (EE) has proved to be one of the most useful predictive tools in psychiatry. It is associated with the outcome of schizophrenia, mania, depressive neurosis, eating disorders, child abuse, post-traumatic stress disorder, and alcoholism. Numerous studies on schizophrenia have shown that the association between EE and outcome is independent of culture and language, indicating the universality of patients' psychological responses to emotional relationships. On this scientific basis, programs have been developed to work with families to alter the patients' emotional environment. Evaluation of these programs has been carried out by a series of randomized, controlled trials. The results of these trials have been consistent, showing that when family work is added to maintenance with antipsychotic drugs, the relapse rate is reduced by one half over two years. In order to make the skills of family work available, national training networks have begun to be established in Britain, and are successful in equipping community psychiatric staff with the necessary skills. However, trained workers are finding it difficult to put their expertise into practice. This problem may be overcome by involving managers in the initial stages of the training.

Key words. Schizophrenia, Family, Emotions, Therapy, Training

Introduction

The measurement of Expressed Emotion (EE) was developed by Brown and Rutter [1] and modified by Vaughn and Leff [2] to assess emotional relationships in families with a member suffering from schizophrenia. Subsequently the measure of EE has been found to predict the course of a variety of psychiatric conditions, including mania, depressive neurosis, eating disorders, child abuse, post-traumatic stress disorder, and alcoholism. These associations suggest, but do not prove, that each of these disorders, whatever their biological basis, is responsive to the social environment. The most convincing proof of a causal connection would be the demonstration that altering the

Institute of Psychiatry, De Crespigny Park, London SE5 8AF, UK family's emotional attitudes to the patient led to a modification of the course of the condition. So far, proof of this nature has been established for schizophrenia, mania [3], and depressive neurosis [4], but by far the strongest evidence relates to schizophrenia.

Family Interventions for Schizophrenia

In the 1970s, three programs of family interventions were initiated by groups in the USA and the UK. The first was headed by Michael Goldstein at the University of California in Los Angeles, which became the center of such research in the USA, two further studies being conducted there. Goldstein's study [5] established the pattern for this type of research. It was a randomized, controlled trial in which all patients were maintained on neuroleptic medication, and in addition the experimental group received family intervention while the control group was given care as usual for the individual patient. During a six-month follow-up, no experimental patient relapsed, compared with 48% of control patients. This dramatic result was published while two other trials were in progress, those of Falloon's group [6] and Leff's group [7]. Falloon's trial was also conducted in Los Angeles, and Leff's trial was carried out at the Institute of Psychiatry in London. The latter followed on directly from the naturalistic studies of EE and schizophrenia, a line of research that had been pursued in the Social Psychiatry Unit at the Institute of Psychiatry over several decades [8–10]. Leff's group mounted their intervention primarily to tackle the question of the direction of cause and effect in the association between relatives' EE and relapse of schizophrenia. It was of course recognized that the trial would also be testing the efficacy of the intervention in altering the emotional environment in the home, but this was considered to be secondary to the scientific issue concerning causality. Although the other trials emerged from the background of the EE research, they all had the primary aim of evaluating the efficacy of family interventions.

All the early trials of family intervention had relatively small numbers of subjects, taking place in the era before power calculations became obligatory. Nevertheless, the differences in relapse rates between experimental and control patients were so large that statistical significance was attained. The first three trials were followed by others of similar design by Hogarty's group in Pittsburgh [11], Tarrier's group in Manchester [12], and another study in Los Angeles, which was the first to utilize ordinary clinicians as opposed to being conducted by a specialized research team [13]. Alongside this body of research from the USA and the UK must be set two studies conducted in China [14,15]. This surprising development was promoted by Michael Phillips, a Canadian psychiatrist who has been working in China for the past ten years and has a particular interest in EE research.

The results of these trials are displayed in Fig. 1, which shows a striking consistency in the relapse rates of experimental and control patients. The standard length of follow-up has been nine months, continuing the tradition of the naturalistic studies. However some of the researchers have followed up patients after one year, whereas in the trial by Xiong and colleagues the period was 18 months, which accounts for the unusually high relapse rates in their groups of patients. Four of the studies also included a two-year follow-up, which revealed that the relapse rates continued to rise

FIG. 1. Relapse rates in randomized, controlled trials of family interventions plus medication against medication alone. All trials had a 9-month follow-up, except that by Xiong, where the follow-up was 18 months. *Black blocks*, medication alone; *white blocks*, medication plus family intervention

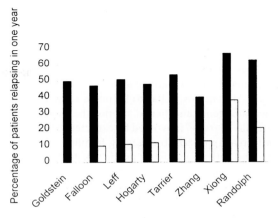

over time in both experimental and control patients, but that the significant advantage of family interventions was still demonstrable [16–19].

It is clear from Hogarty's account of his team's two year follow-up [18] that he was disappointed at the rising relapse rate over time, indicating that the intervention did not prevent relapse but only postponed it for a while. However, the value of this effect should not be disregarded. The time over which negative symptoms recover is much more protracted than that for positive symptoms. If relapses occur frequently, with only short intervals in between, the patient has insufficient time to recover from the negative symptoms, and social functioning remains severely impaired.

The fact that the findings of the Chinese trials are commensurate with those of the British and American studies is of considerable importance. It suggests that family interventions can succeed in a wide variety of settings, regardless of cultural variations in family structure and function.

Unsuccessful Interventions

There have been several trials of family interventions that have not demonstrated their efficacy. There are useful lessons to be learned from these studies. An early study in Hamburg [20] offered families psychodynamic group therapy. The patients from several families joined one group while their relatives formed a separate group. The failure of this form of therapy to make any impact on the course of the patients' illness suggests that psychodynamic group therapy is an ineffective treatment for schizophrenia.

A different set of problems was encountered by McCreadie's group in Scotland [21]. Over a number of years, they have studied the total known population of people with schizophrenia in a defined catchment area. At one stage they offered a family intervention to all patients who were living with relatives. About half the families refused the help offered on the grounds that they were coping all right or that they did not need treatment themselves. This raises two issues: the first is that it is preferable to offer help at a point of crisis when the patient has relapsed or is causing a disturbance at home. It is well recognized that many patients seal over their psychotic experiences once they have recovered. There is a similar response in families who do not wish to face the challenges of professional intervention once the situation has returned to its previous state, however unsatisfactory that may be. The other issue is the way in which help is offered to families. The now discredited theory that families cause schizophrenia alienated many relatives from professionals and left them suspicious of therapists' intentions. It has to be made crystal clear that families are not considered to be pathogenic and hence are not the focus of treatment. For this reason the term "family therapy" is avoided by experienced professionals working in this field. A more effective approach to engaging families is to offer them help to improve conditions for the patient, making it explicit that the patient's illness is something they need to learn to cope with but that they are not responsible for causing.

McCreadie's study also illustrates the importance of appropriate training of the therapists. Of the two therapists who worked with the Scottish families, one had received no formal training, whereas the other had been trained in family therapy, but not in the specific skills required for families with a schizophrenic member. The nature of these skills will be discussed in detail below.

A trial in Australia [22] employed well-trained therapists who ran group sessions for relatives, but the number of sessions was limited to 10. The failure to have an impact on the patients' relapse rate is most likely due to the relatively restricted therapeutic input. At the end of the course, the relatives were eager to partake in more sessions, reflecting their awareness of unmet needs. It is evident that a long-term illness like schizophrenia renders brief interventions inappropriate.

A trial conducted in the Netherlands was unusual in including patients from both high-EE and low-EE homes [23]. Although patients with high-EE relatives did benefit from the intervention compared with a control group, those from low-EE families actually had a higher relapse rate than their controls. This surprising finding suggests that the intervention had a negative effect on the low-EE families. Although side effects are constantly in the mind of the physician prescribing drugs, the possibility that social interventions might have side effects is rarely considered. Since this result has only been recorded from a single trial, it needs to be treated with caution, but it may require the recognition by clinicians of the distinction between high-EE and low-EE families. It would be too daunting to expect every clinical team to include a trained rater of EE, but this is not necessary, since there are some simple rules of thumb for the recognition of high-EE families [24]. These include families in which there are frequent arguments leading to physical violence, families who call in the police because they cannot control the patient, patients who are known to be taking their medication but who relapse once a year or more frequently, and relatives who constantly contact the staff for advice and reassurance.

The Content of Family Interventions

Each of the interventions evaluated in the above controlled trials has been given a different name by the team using it. The terms include Behavioural Family Therapy [6], Psychoeducation [11], and Family Work for Schizophrenia [24]. This apparent diversity illustrates one of the problems in evaluating social therapies. Unlike drugs, they are difficult to standardize, and even the provision of treatment manuals does not ensure conformity. Comparison of three of these manuals [24–26] reveals a considerable degree of similarity in the interventions described. This was confirmed recently when the World Schizophrenia Fellowship brought together Falloon, Leff, and McFarlane to produce a consensus statement on the content of family interventions. Half a day was sufficient for these experts to reach agreement on the essential ingredients and to draw up a document [27].

Education

Education about the nature of schizophrenia, the symptoms, course, and treatment and management is seen as an essential basis to work with families, as it is for professional carers. However, education is much more than the simple provision of information. Information is not emotionally neutral: the term schizophrenia is surrounded by a penumbra of negative connotations derived from the media and from the grim images projected by the asylums. Relatives need time to come to terms with the diagnosis, to absorb the facts about the illness, and to learn effective coping strategies. Education is a process that continues throughout work with the family. There is a tendency for professionals to feel that they have discharged their obligations to the family by offering a couple of sessions in which they provide information about schizophrenia, perhaps encouraged by the term "psychoeducation." This is far from the truth.

Problem Solving

Life with a person suffering from schizophrenia gives rise to many problems: how to respond when the patient says he is the saviour of the world, how to get the patient out of bed, how to persuade her to have a bath, how to stimulate an interest in anything other than watching television; these are just a few examples. A structured technique for tackling problems has been developed within cognitive psychology. This is a straightforward sequence of steps that families can learn. However, therapeutic skill is required to guide the family to choose a small problem to start with. Big problems feel more pressing but are less likely to yield to a problem-solving approach when the family is still inexperienced with this technique.

Resolving Conflicts

Disagreements between family members on how to manage the problems make it very unlikely that solutions will be found. Conflicts may also arise between the patient and the carers. Therapists need to listen to the various viewpoints and seek a resolution through compromise. Anger, anxiety, and guilt expressed by family members should be dealt with in a sensitive way. Anger can often be reframed as caring. Carers need to be encouraged to take time off from the caring role and do something outside of the home that they will enjoy.

Improving Communication

High levels of anxiety and anger in family members lead to interruptions and talking over each other. They fail to listen to others, and the person with schizophrenia is often ignored and excluded from the conversation. The intervention consists of ways of regulating the dialogue so that each person gets an equal opportunity to contribute and no one is left out. The therapist also promotes active listening.

Developing Realistic Expectations

It is hard for relatives to accept that the negative symptoms of schizophrenia have a long time course. They are naturally anxious to see the patients resume a normal life as soon as possible, but this can put a considerable strain on the person recovering from an episode of illness. On the other hand, some relatives become resigned to patients' inactivity, particularly after many years of illness. The therapist needs to help relatives to adjust their expectations to a realistic level, given the patient's disabilities and the stage of the illness.

Dealing with Loss

Schizophrenia can so alter peoples' behavior and thinking that they appear as strangers to those who know them. This metamorphosis is especially painful for parents and partners of the patient, who will need help in mourning the loss of the person they used to know. Parents also experience another loss: the hopes and expectations they nourished for their child. Therapists need to assist them to work through the associated grief, otherwise they cling to unrealistic aspirations that can never be fulfilled. Successful grief work enables carers to develop realistic targets that the patient has the capacity to achieve.

Modes of Delivering Family Interventions

Engagement

The questions of how to engage families and how best to deliver the interventions arise from considerations of efficiency. An efficacious treatment is of little usefulness if it is unacceptable to families. All the existing programs begin with education sessions. This is a logical starting point but has other advantages in terms of engagement. Carers are eager to obtain information about a condition that can be quite baffling. In the past, professional attitudes to carers were strongly influenced by the myth that families caused schizophrenia. As a result, they excluded carers from consultations about the patient and from the treatment process. This illogical behavior not only angered and frustrated carers, it denied them the information they needed to do their best for the patient. Some carers are aware of that legacy of the past and are understandably wary of professional attitudes of blame towards them. Therefore, providing them freely with information and with plenty of time to ask questions is greatly appreciated and helps to establish a therapeutic relationship between carers and professionals.

Working in the Home

Both Leff's and Falloon's teams [24,25] provided most of their programs in the family's own home. This is an effective way of engaging families, since they are usually grateful that professionals are prepared to make the effort to come to them. Furthermore, it is difficult for them to refuse access to their home, whereas failing to attend an appointment at the clinic is an effortless way of opting out of a therapeutic program. There are some problems associated with home visiting.

Health professionals in some countries have no tradition of making home visits, and it is difficult to institute a practice that has no institutional precedent. Another issue is the conflict between coming to a family's home to work and being in the position of a guest. Families are often grateful for the professionals' visits and offer food and drink. Although it would be rude to refuse their hospitality completely, it is necessary to establish boundaries between what is acceptable and what is excessive and undermines the working relationship.

Relatives' Groups

Self-help organizations for users and carers naturally meet in groups, and this format has a therapeutic function. Some of the professional programs have adopted this format for the education component. For example, Hogarty's team started their intervention with a "survival skills workshop" attended by several families, in which information about schizophrenia was presented [26]. Other teams have delivered the entire program to groups rather than individuals. In the first trial by Leff and colleagues [7], a relatives' group was run in parallel with family sessions in the home. Patients were excluded, but low-EE relatives were invited to the group as well as the high-EE experimental relatives. The aim was to discover from the low-EE relatives what coping strategies they used and to encourage the high-EE relatives to learn from them. In their second trial [28], families were randomized to a relatives' group or to sessions in the home. It turned out that almost half the relatives assigned to the group failed to attend even a single session. Not surprisingly, very little change occurred in the emotional atmosphere in these families over the course of the trial, and the patients had a high relapse rate. This led Leff and colleagues to recommend that a relatives' group should not be offered on its own, but that staff should retain the flexibility to visit families in their homes if they found the group unacceptable.

Groups have the obvious advantage of enabling two staff members to provide help to several families at the same time. Most groups of this kind cater to six to eight families, representing an efficient way of delivering interventions. Furthermore, Leff and colleagues [29] found that the relatives'group was more effective in reducing EE than family sessions. One program, run by McFarlane in the USA, is based exclusively on the group format [30]. His team compared groups for relatives only with multiple family groups, which included the patients. They found that the multiple family groups were more effective in reducing the relapse rate. This interesting result requires replication by another team before influencing practice. Although groups continue to be run by voluntary organizations for users and carers, such as the National Schizophrenia Fellowship in the UK, few clinical teams have established these on a permanent basis. This brings us to the issue of implementation.

Implementing Family Interventions

Family interventions for schizophrenia are supported by a strong scientific evidence base [31], yet there are few clinical services that offer them as a routine. It is important to explore the reasons for this if the situation is to be changed. The most obvious problem is the lack of promotion by an organization with a commercial interest in the product. Pharmaceutical companies spend vast sums of money promoting their drugs, because the potential return from the market is enormous. Although schizophrenia affects only 1% of the population, most patients fall ill in early adulthood and have to remain on medication for the rest of their life. A pharmaceutical company is delighted if their product guarantees 10% more improvement than a drug made by a rival company. Family work added to medication cuts the relapse rate of schizophrenia to 50% over two years compared with medication alone. This would be an enormously powerful selling point for a company marketing family work, but it is not a commercial product.

Another issue is that to prescribe a drug, the doctor simply writes its name on a prescription. Family interventions cannot be prescribed in this way. It is necessary to have a pool of trained people available. The most notable attempt to solve this problem has been the Thorn Initiative in the UK [32]. Once the value of family interventions was firmly established, it was recognized that a national network of training centers needed to be set up. A cascade model was chosen in which trainees would come to a central training course and, having completed the course, would establish a local training course in their own service. The two national centers were situated in Manchester and London and offered a nine-month course run one day per week. The course is modular, with family work being taught in one module, while the others cover assertive community treatment and cognitive interventions for psychotic symptoms. Initially only community psychiatric nurses were accepted as trainees, but now the course is open to staff from any discipline related to psychiatric care. Selected trainees undergo a further three months of training to equip them as trainers and to enable them to run their own training course. Over one thousand individuals have now completed the training, and six satellite centers have been established, with a further six close to becoming functional.

Evaluations of the training have shown that trainees gained significant increases in their knowledge and positive changes in their attitudes to family work [33]. A randomized, controlled trial of the effectiveness of Thorn-trained staff has recently been completed and demonstrated that the trainees were able to produce as much change in the family emotional atmosphere as the originators of the intervention [34]. Equipping staff with the necessary skills overcomes a major barrier to implementation but does not guarantee that the trained staff will be able to put into practice what they have learned.

Barriers Within the Service

A few surveys have been conducted of the experiences of community staff when they have tried to introduce working with families into their clinical setting [35–37]. They all concur in finding that the top-ranking problems were integration of the work with their existing caseload and allowance of time from the service to undertake the intervention. Both these problems stem from a lack of understanding by the managers of community staff that the trained workers need to be relieved of some of their regular clinical responsibilities in order to work with families. Fadden [35] found that staff members who were most successful in putting their training into practice were able to use a large number of creative strategies to overcome the difficulties encountered. They were also more willing to see families in their own time, to work outside the usual hours, to be proactive in engaging families, and to work with a cotherapist. Finding a cotherapist clearly has resource implications, but the work is difficult and demanding and the support of a colleague is essential.

Fadden concluded that it was necessary to attempt to change the systems in which the trainees worked in order to overcome these barriers. This approach was adopted by McFarlane and colleagues [30], who began their program with a one-day orientation that included both administrators and senior clinicians. All the modern interventions with families are based on forming an alliance with family members in which they are treated as equal partners. McFarlane's group applied this approach to establishing relations with local administrators, who were included in decision making from the beginning, consulted about problems related to the conduct of the project at their own and other sites, and invited to participate in training sessions. The same strategy was then used to maintain a collegial relationship with new supervisors, providing a model for their relationships with their trainees and the administrators of the services in which they were providing training.

Conclusions

Over the course of forty years, a measurement tool for research, relatives' EE, has stimulated the development of a new and efficacious social intervention for schizophrenia. The success of this endeavor is firmly based on forming a therapeutic alliance with the family. Training programs have been established, and the necessary skills and expertise will soon be available on a national basis in the UK. However, the integration of this technique into routine clinical practice requires the formation of an alliance with the local health administrators and managers. Hence, what has been learned about the functioning of the family as a system needs to be applied to the local system of health care in order to make this effective form of help available to all those who could benefit from it.

References

1. Brown GW, Rutter M (1966) The measurement of family activities and relationships: a methodological study. Hum Relations 19:241–263

2. Vaughn C, Leff JP (1976) The measurement of expressed emotion in families of psychiatric patients. Br J Soc Clin Psychol 15:157–165
3. Miklowitz DJ, Hooley JM (1998) Developing family psychoeducational treatments for patients with bipolar and other severe psychiatric disorders: a pathway from basic research to clinical trials. J Marital Fam Ther 24:419–435
4. Leff J, Vearnals S, Brewin CR, et al (2000) The London Intervention Trial: An RCT of antidepressants versus couple therapy in the treatment and maintenance of depressed people with a partner: clinical outcome and costs. Br J Psychiatry 177:95–100
5. Goldstein MJ, Rodnick EH, Evans JR, et al (1978) Drug and family therapy in the aftercare treatment of acute schizophrenia. Arch Gen Psychiatry 35:169–177
6. Falloon IRH, Boyd JL, McGill CW, et al (1982) Family management in the prevention of exacerbations of schizophrenia: a controlled study. N Engl J Med 306:1437–1440
7. Leff JP, Kuipers L, Berkowitz R, et al (1982) A controlled trial of social intervention in the families of schizophrenic patients. Br J Psychiatry 141:121–134
8. Brown GW, Carstairs GM, Topping G (1958) Post hospital adjustment of chronic mental patients. Lancet ii:685–689
9. Brown GW, Birley JLT, Wing JK (1972) Influence of family life on the course of schizophrenic disorders: a replication. Br J Psychiatry 121:241–258
10. Vaughn C, Leff JP (1976) The influence of family and social factors on the course of psychiatric illness: a comparison of schizophrenic and depressed neurotic patients. Br J Psychiatry 129:125–137
11. Hogarty GE, Anderson CM, Reiss DJ (1986) Family psychoeducation, social skills training, and maintenance chemotherapy in the aftercare treatment of schizophrenia: I. One-year effects of a controlled study on relapse and Expressed Emotion. Arch Gen Psychiatry 43:633–642
12. Tarrier N, Barrowclough C, Vaughn C, et al (1988) The community management of schizophrenia: a controlled trial of a behavioural intervention with families to reduce relapse. Br J Psychiatry 153:532–542
13. Randolph ET, Eth S, Glynn SM (1994) Behavioural family management. Outcome of a clinic-based intervention. Br J Psychiatry 164:501–506
14. Zhang M, Wang M, Li J (1994) Randomised control trial of family intervention for 78 first-episode male schizophrenic patients: an 18-month study in Suzhou, Jiangsu. Br J Psychiatry 165(Suppl 24):96–102
15. Xiong W, Phillips MR, Hu X (1994) Family-based intervention for schizophrenic patients in China: randomised controlled trial. Br J Psychiatry 165:239–247
16. Falloon IRH, Williamson M, Razani J (1985) Family versus individual management in the prevention of morbidity of schizophrenia: I. Clinical outcome of a two-year controlled study. Arch Gen Psychiatry 42:887–896
17. Leff JP, Kuipers L, Berkowitz R, et al (1985) A controlled trial of social intervention in the families of schizophrenic patients: two year follow-up. Br J Psychiatry 146:594–600
18. Hogarty GE, Anderson CM, Reiss DJ (1987) Family psychoeducation, social skills training and medication in schizophrenia: the long and the short of it. Psychopharmacol Bull 23:12–13
19. Tarrier N, Barrowclough C, Vaughn C, et al (1989) Community management of schizophrenia: a two-year follow-up of a behavioural intervention with families. Br J Psychiatry 154:625–628
20. Köttgen C, Sonnichsen I, Mollenhauser K, et al (1984) Results of the Hamburg Camberwell Family Interview Study. 1-III. Int J Fam Psychiatry 5:61–94
21. McCreadie RG, Phillips K, Harvey JA, et al (1991) The Nithsdale schizophrenia surveys VIII: Do relatives want family intervention—and does it help? Br J Psychiatry 158:110–113
22. Vaughan K, Doyle M, McConaghy N, et al (1992) The Sydney intervention trial: a controlled trial of relatives' counselling to reduce schizophrenic relapse. Soc Psychiatry Psychiatr Epidemiol 27:16–21

23. Linszen D, Dingemans P, Van Der Does JM, et al (1996) Treatment, expressed emotion and relapse in recent onset schizophrenic disorders. Psychol Med 26:333–342
24. Kuipers L, Leff J, Lam D (1992) Family work for schizophrenia: a practical guide. Gaskell, London
25. Falloon IRH, Boyd JL, McGill CW (1984) Family care of schizophrenia. Guilford, New York
26. Anderson CM, Reiss DJ, Hogarty GE (1986) Schizophrenia in the family: a practitioner's guide to psychoeducation and management. Guilford, New York
27. World Schizophrenia Fellowship (1998) Families as partners in care. World Schizophrenia Fellowship Strategy Document
28. Leff J, Berkowitz R, Shavit N, et al (1989) A trial of family therapy. v. A relatives' group for schizophrenia. Br J Psychiatry 154:58–66
29. Leff J, Berkowitz R, Shavit N, et al (1990) A trial of family therapy versus a relatives' group for schizophrenia, two year follow-up. Br J Psychiatry 157:571–577
30. McFarlane WR, Dunne E, Lukens E, et al (1993) From research to clinical practice: dissemination of New York State's Family Psychoeducation Project. Hosp Commun Psychiatry 44:265–270
31. Pharoah FM, Mari JJ, Streiner D (1999) Family interventions for schizophrenia (Cochrane Review). In: The Cochrane Library, Issue 3. Oxford, Update Software
32. Gamble C (1995) The Thorn Nurse Training Initiative. Nursing Standard, 9:31–34
33. Leff J, Gamble C (1995) Training of community psychiatric nurses in family work for schizophrenia. Int J Men Health 24:76–88
34. Leff J, Sharpley M, Chisholm D, et al (2001) Training community psychiatric nurses in schizophrenia family work: A study of clinical and economic outcomes for patients and relatives. J Men Health 10:189–197
35. Kavanagh DJ, Piatkowska O, Clarke D (1993) Application of cognitive-behavioural family intervention for schizophrenia in multi-disciplinary teams: what can the matter be? Aust Psychol 28:181–188
36. Fadden G (1998) Research update: psychoeducational family interventions. J Fam Ther 20:293–309
37. Butterworth CAB, Baguley I, Fahy K, et al (in press) Bringing into clinical practice skills shown to be effective in research settings: a follow-up of the "Thorn" training in psychosocial family interventions for psychosis

Expressed Emotion Studies in Japan

Shinji Shimodera[1], Shimpei Inoue[1], Yoshio Mino[2], and Hirokazu Fujita[1]

Summary. The Camberwell Family Interview (CFI) for the measurement of Expressed Emotion (EE) was introduced in Japan in 1990. In the 10 years since then, many EE studies have been conducted in Japan. In this report, 13 Japanese EE studies written in English are reviewed. Japanese EE studies can be classified into two groups: those that used the CFI and those that used the Five-Minute Speech Sample (FMSS). These two groups consisted of two fields of schizophrenia and mood disorders. In Japanese, the prediction of recurrence by using EE measured by the CFI and the FMSS has been shown to be more accurate in mood disorders than in schizophrenia, as shown in a prior study by Vaughn and Leff (1976). From an intercultural viewpoint, Japanese critical comments (CCs), which are the main components of EE, were different from those of the English in their distribution and contents. Positive symptoms were the most frequent comments (34%) and negative symptoms were not so frequent (11%) in a schizophrenic CFI study. No marked difference was found in the optimal cutoff point of CC in patients with schizophrenia and mood disorders between Japan and Western countries, but CCs were less frequent in Japanese families.

Key words. Expressed Emotion, Family, Japan, Schizophrenia, Mood disorders

Introduction

In Japan, mental health services emphasize a hospital-oriented approach to treatment, with most patients being admitted [1]. Community care resources are gradually increasing, but many discharged patients have no choice except to return to their families. As a result, compared with Western societies, Japanese families with their close ties can exert a greater influence on their discharged relatives. In addition, inadequate information about illness is provided to patients and their families. Thus, EE research in Japan is expected to have an important role in preventing schizophrenic relapse and improving communication from specialists to the general population.

---

[1] Department of Neuropsychiatry, Kochi Medical School, Kohasu, Oko-cho, Nankoku, Kochi 783-8505, Japan
[2] Department of Hygiene and Preventive Medicine, Okayama University Medical School, 2-5-1 Shikata-cho, Okayama 700-8558, Japan

Expressed Emotion (EE) studies have been conducted in various countries during the last decades [2–4]. The EE status of families of patients with schizophrenia has been found to be a good predictor of relapse [5]. The subjects of EE studies were widened to mood disorders [6,7], senile dementia [8], and eating disorders [9], and those developments were remarkable. In schizophrenia, various types of psychoeducation were reported [10–12].

The first Japanese report of EE written in English was published by Otsuka et al. [13] in 1994, and since then 13 studies conducted in Japan have been published in English [4,13–24].

Methods

Of the 13 reports, EE assessment was conducted by the Five-Minute Speech Sample (FMSS) [25] in 3, by the Camberwell Family Interview (CFI) [26] in 8, and both methods in 2. We classified these studies into five groups: EE and social adjustment of schizophrenia [13,17], EE and the course of schizophrenia [4,16,18], EE and the course of mood disorders [15,24], inter-rater reliability and validity of different methods of assessing EE [21], and factors related to high EE [19,22].

EE and Social Adjustment of Schizophrenia

There were two reports in this group. Katz Adjustment Scales (KAS) [27] were used to evaluate the social functioning in both. Otsuka et al. [13] investigated the relationship between the sectional KAS score and the EE evaluated by the FMSS. High-EE relatives evaluated the patients' performance of social activities as rather low and showed strong dissatisfaction with the patient's leisure activities [13]. Inoue et al. [17] conducted a nine-month cohort study using CFI. The results were different from those of Otsuka et al. [13]. There were no differences in the baseline KAS score between high- and low-EE groups [17]. In the high-EE group, the levels of performance of both socially expected activities and free-time activities declined slightly at follow-up [17]. In contrast, those in the low-EE group improved, and the increase in the level of performance of socially expected activities was significant [17].

EE and the Course of Schizophrenia

This was the main topic of the original EE studies. The relapse rates of patients in the high-EE groups were significantly higher than those of patients in the low-EE groups in the nine-month and two-year cohort studies [4,18]. The nine-month and two-year relapse risks of patients in the high-EE groups were 58% and 71%, respectively [4,18]. The risks in low-EE groups were 21% and 37%, respectively [4,18]. EE remained a good predictor for schizophrenic relapse over a two-year course in Japan [18]. However, a significant difference shown over the two years could be due to the strong association between EE and relapse occurring in the first nine months [18].

Uehara et al. [16] investigated the relationship between nine-month relapse of outpatients with schizophrenia and EE evaluated by the FMSS. The results suggested that the FMSS is suitable for use as a convenient instrument to measure EE, although it showed more false-positive results [16]. They recommended that borderline EE of the FMSS might have to be regarded as high EE [16].

EE and the Course of Mood Disorders

Uehara et al. [15] reported a relationship between EE assessed by FMSS and the six-month outcome in outpatients with major depression. The rate of nonremission increased in response to the level of criticism, from pure low-EE (31.0%), to border critical (60%), to EOI (75.0%), and then to high critical (100%) [15]. Multiple logistic regression analysis showed that the level of criticism and a past history of depression were significant predictors of poor outcome ($P < 0.05$) [15].

Mino et al. [24] investigated the nine-month relapse risks of patients with mood disorders, including bipolar disorders, in high- and low-EE groups. Subjects with three or more critical comments or an EOI score of 3 or higher were regarded as belonging to high-EE groups, and the others as belonging to low-EE groups. Their relapse risks were 83.3% and 19.2%, respectively, and the relapse risk ratio was 4.3, with a 95% confidence interval of 1.8 to 12.2 [24]. The values of the validity parameters were the highest, and the cut-off points were similar to those in other countries [24].

Inter-rater Reliability and Validity of Different Methods of Assessing EE

The original CFI requires three to four hours to conduct, but Vaughn and Leff [26] succeeded in abbreviating the process without losing any of the significant factors. Recently, the shortened form of the CFI was applied in EE studies. In Japanese EE studies, inter-rater reliability of a short CFI evaluated both schizophrenia [14] and mood disorders [23]. In the study of schizophrenia [14], the kappa values for EE, CC, EOI, and Positive Remarks were over 0.8, with the exception of Warmth, which was 0.56. On the contrary, the kappa values for CC, Hostility, and EOI were 0.4 to 0.7, and the reliability of EE ratings in mood disorders was not high in Japan [23]. In comparison with EE ratings in schizophrenia, the reliability of EE ratings in family members of patients with mood disorders was questionable. The primary reason for this poor reliability was that EE ratings based on CFI were originally designed for schizophrenia [23]. In family members of patients with mood disorders, the distributions of all EE subscales were closer to 0, and their ranges were small in Japan [23]. Probably for these reasons, the kappa value was considered to be smaller than in schizophrenia [23].

Magana et al. [25] attempted to shorten the interview time. They instructed the family to speak for five minutes about their family member (the patient), and evaluated the results based on the FMSS [25]. In the EE study of schizophrenia, the validity of the FMSS in comparison to the CFI was conducted in Japan [21]. The sensitivity level for the assessment of the FMSS versus the CFI was 53.8%, and the specificity was

65.2% [21]. In this study, sensitivity was 92.3% and specificity was 52.2% on the CFI when borderline low-EE subjects were included in the high-EE group [21]. Borderline low-EE subjects may have to be included in the high-EE group to improve the validity of EE assessment [21].

Factors Related to High EE

Shimodera et al. [22] evaluated the association between family distress assessed by the General Health Questionnaire (GHQ) [28] and EE in schizophrenia. The GHQ score was higher in the high-EE group that was determined by both the CFI and FMSS [22]. Japanese family distress was also closely associated with the EE classification as prior Western studies [29], and the EE classification by CFI more markedly reflected family distress than FMSS [22].

EE level evaluated by the FMSS was high among relatives who thought the patient was belligerent, negativistic, unstable, or helpless [13]. The relationship between the EE and the severity of the patient's symptoms was not parallel, but the difference of the most common CC type depended on the cultural background [19]. Although Kuipers et al. reported that about 70% of CC was directed toward negative symptoms, only 11% of the comments in the Japanese sample were in this area [30]. Positive symptoms were the most frequently commented on (34%) in the Japanese samples [19]. Although the reason was not clear, Japanese families tolerate negative symptoms, and the delay of psychoeducation might be related to this [19]. There is a considerable amount of social stigma against mental illness in Eastern Asian societies, including Japan, and because of this, there is tendency to delay seeing a doctor [19]. In other words, families tolerate negative symptoms only when positive symptoms are so bad as to cause mental and physical injury to others [19]. The result of this kind of coping behavior may be that there is a high tolerance for negative symptoms, with little CC made against them [19]. The second reason is that there has been little educational approach by specialists to patients and their families in traditional psychiatric practice in Japan. Consequently, there are still many families who do not view the hallucinations and delusions of their mentally ill family members as an illness, with the result that they exhibit critical behavior toward these symptoms [19].

Discussion

Japanese EE reports are not many but do contain a lot of recent topics. In psychoeducation programs, not only patients but also family should be supported to help improve the distress as caregivers.

The effects of EE on the course of schizophrenia and mood disorders are not different among cultures. Expressing criticism in the CFI interview might be considered shameful by Japanese relatives. However, no marked difference was found in the optimal cut-off point of CC in patients with schizophrenia and mood disorders between Japan and Western countries. Even so, CCs were less frequent in Japanese families.

Finally, the limitations of this study are discussed. Although Japanese EE studies written in English were reviewed in this study, there are many well-investigated Japanese EE studies written in Japanese. Therefore, we should review more Japanese EE studies to know the cultural background.

References

1. Mino Y, Kodera R, Bebbington P (1990) A comparative study of psychiatric services in Japan and England. Br J Psychiatry 157:416–420
2. Brown GW, Birley JL, Wing JK (1972) Influence of family life on the course of schizophrenic disorders: a replication. Br J Psychiatry 121:241–248
3. Vaughn CE, Leff JP (1976) The influence of family and social factors on the course of psychiatric illness: a comparison of schizophrenic and depressed neurotic patients. Br J Psychiatry 129:125–137
4. Tanaka S, Mino Y, Inoue S (1995) Expressed emotion and the course of schizophrenia in Japan. Br J Psychiatry 167:794–798
5. Bebbington P, Kuipers L (1994) The predictive utility of expressed emotion in schizophrenia: an aggregate analysis. Psychol Med 24:707–718
6. Hooley JM, Orley J, Teasdale JD (1986) Levels of expressed emotion and relapse in depressive patients. Br J Psychiatry 148:642–647
7. Okasha A, El Akabawi AS, Snyder KS (1994) Expressed emotion, perceived criticism, and relapse in depression: a replication in an Egyptian community. Am J Psychiatry 151:1001–1005
8. Bledin KD, Maccarthy B, Kuipers L, et al (1990) Daughters of people with dementia expressed emotion, strain and coping. Br J Psychiatry 157:221–227
9. Blair C, Freeman C, Cull A (1995) The families of anorexia nervosa and cystic fibrosis patients. Psychol Med 25:985–993
10. Leff J, Kuipers L, Berkowitz R, et al (1982) A controlled trial of social intervention in the families of schizophrenic patients. Br J Psychiatry 141:121–134
11. Falloon IR, Boyd JL, Mcgill CW, et al (1982) Family management in the prevention of exacerbation of schizophrenia: a controlled study. N Engl J Med 306:1437–1440
12. Tarrier N, Barrowclough C, Vaughn C (1988) The community management of schizophrenia: a controlled trial of a behavioural intervention with families to reduce relapse. Br J Psychiatry 153:532–542
13. Otsuka T, Nakane Y, Ohta Y, et al (1994) Symptoms and social adjustment of schizophrenic patients as evaluated by family members. Acta Psychiatr Scand 89:111–116
14. Mino Y, Tanaka S, Tsuda T, et al (1995) Training in evaluation of expressed emotion using the Japanese version of the Camberwell Family Interview. Acta Psychiatr Scand 92:183–186
15. Uehara T, Yokoyama T, Goto M, et al (1996) Expressed emotion and short-term treatment outcome of outpatients with major depression. Compr Psychiatry 37:299–304
16. Uehara T, Yokoyama T, Goto M, et al (1997) Expressed emotion from the five-minute speech sample and relapse of out-patients with schizophrenia. Acta Psychiatr Scand 95:454–456
17. Inoue S, Tanaka S, Shimodera S, et al (1997) Expressed emotion and social function. Psychiatry Res 72:33–39
18. Mino Y, Inoue S, Tanaka S, et al (1997) Expressed emotion among families and course of schizophrenia in Japan: a 2-year cohort study. Schizophr Res 24:333–339
19. Shimodera S, Inoue S, Tanaka S, et al (1998) Critical comments made to schizophrenic patients by their families in Japan. Compr Psychiatry 39:85–90
20. Mino Y, Inoue S, Shimodera S, et al (1998) Expressed emotion of families and negative/depressive symptoms in schizophrenia: a cohort study in Japan. Schizophr Res 34:159–168

21. Shimodera S, Mino Y, Inoue S, et al (1999) Validity of a five minute speech sample in measuring expressed emotion in the families of persons with schizophrenia in Japan. Compr Psychiatry 40:372–376
22. Shimodera S, Mino Y, Inoue S, et al (2000) Expressed emotion and family distress in relatives of patients with schizophrenia in Japan. Compr Psychiatry 41:392–397
23. Mino Y, Shimodera S, Inoue S, et al (2000) Evaluation of expressed emotion (EE) status in mood disorders in Japan: Inter-rater reliability and characteristics of EE. Psychiatry Res 94:221–227
24. Mino Y, Shimodera S, Inoue S, et al (2001) Expressed emotion of families and the course of mood disorders: a cohort study in Japan. J Affect Disord 63:43–49
25. Magana AB, Goldstein MJ, Karno M, et al (1986) A brief method for assessing expressed emotion in relatives of psychiatric patients. Psychiat Res 17:203–212
26. Leff J, Vaughn C (1985) Expressed emotion in families. Guilford Press, New York, pp 26–62
27. Katz MM, Lyerly SB (1963) Methods for measuring adjustment and social behavior in the community: I. Rationale, description, discriminative validity and scale development. Psychol Rep 13:503–535
28. Kitamura T, Sugawara M, Aoki M (1989) Validity of the Japanese version of the GHQ among antenatal clinic attendants. Psychol Med 19:507–511
29. Barrowclough C, Parle M (1997) Appraisal, psychological adjustment and expressed emotion in relatives of patients suffering from schizophrenia. Br J Psychiatry 171:26–30
30. Kuipers L, Leff J, Lam D (1992) Family work for schizophrenia: a practical guide. Gaskell, London, p 33

Family Psychoeducation with Schizophrenic Patients and Their Families from the Viewpoint of Empowerment

Junichiro Ito[1], Iwao Oshima[2], Kazumi Tsukada[3], and Hiraku Koisikawa[3]

Summary. We evaluated the effectiveness of psychoeducational intervention in the families of schizophrenic patients. Eighty-five schizophrenic patients admitted to Kounodai Hospital were randomly assigned to receive either multiple family psychoeducational interventions (intervention group) or routine treatment alone (control group). EE (Expressed Emotion) scores and Brief Psychiatric Rating Scale (BPRS) scores were monitored prospectively, and the dosages of antipsychotics were also measured retrospectively when all of the interventions had finished. In the nine months of follow-up after discharge, family psychoeducation significantly decreased the risk of psychotic relapse, not only in the high-EE group but also in the total group. The rate of high Emotional Overinvolvement (high EOI) was decreased significantly in the intervention group, and the total dosage of antipsychotics during hospitalization was also significantly decreased in the intervention group. These findings suggest that psychoeducation resulted in greater protection of the patients against psychotic relapse than routine treatment alone. A remarkable decrease in EOI of relatives and decrease in the total antipsychotic dosages of the patients could be the indices of the change in the relationships between the patients and their relatives. An experience of empowerment in the program could have a positive influence on interpersonal relations within the family.

Key words. Psychoeducation, Schizophrenia, Expressed emotion, Empowerment, Psychiatric rehabilitation

[1] Department of Psychiatric Rehabilitation, National Institute of Mental Health, 1-7-3 Kohnodai, Ichikawa, Chiba 272-0827, Japan
[2] Department of Mental Health, Graduate School of Medicine, University of Tokyo, 7-3-1 Hongo, Bunkyo-ku, Tokyo 113-0033, Japan
[3] Department of Psychiatry, Kohnodai Hospital, National Center of Psychiatry and Neurology, 1-7-1 Kohnodai, Ichikawa, Chiba 272-0827, Japan

Introduction

The Japanese psychiatric system has four negative characteristics. The first is the hospital-centered treatment system. There are still over 300 000 inpatients in psychiatric hospitals, and the average length of stay for patients is over 400 days. The second is paternalism on the part of psychiatrists and other staff members. Mentally disordered people and their families are considered to be too weak and incapable to cope with their own problems. The third is the lack of psychosocial resources in the community. The fourth is the forced burden on families. Many psychiatrists require families of mentally disordered people to take care of them at home. In addition, the Mental Health Act forces families to take the role of guardianship for the patients with very little opportunity to obtain necessary information or resources for caring for their ill family member.

We initiated a psychoeducational multiple-family group program as a catalyst to improve these conditions. In developing the groups, we referred to the studies conducted by W. McFarlane and others [1]. In the process of conducting the psychoeducational group, we were able to implement concepts such as community-based treatment, consumer-centered collaborative work, supporting self-help and self-advocacy activity, and increasing the competence of families.

The Structure of the Psychoeducational Group

We have two basic attitudes in the psychoeducational family group. One is consumer centered: we believe that the consumers and their families have the right to obtain the information they need, and we also believe that they have enough strengths and resources to cope with their difficulties. The other is the attitude that both patients and their families need support. These attitudes have been informed by research on Expressed Emotion (EE).

Our Psychoeducational Group meets at the Kounodai Hospital, which is located in the National Center of Neurology and Psychiatry. The meetings take place once a month. The meetings are semiclosed and continue for a total of 10 sessions. Two different components constitute this group program. One is a lecture in which we offer information about disease, treatment, and social welfare. About 30 or 40 family members listen to the lecture together in one large room. The other is a group session that is solution focused [2] and interactive. As members are readily able to take part in small groups, we divide the participants into several groups of about nine members each. Nurses, psychologists, social workers, and psychiatrists take part in this group program as staff members.

The Process of the Psychoeducational Group

The goal of the lectures is to share information necessary for families living with schizophrenic patients. Neither families nor patients have enough opportunity to get such information in their daily treatment relationships. Information on etiology, models for helping the understanding of schizophrenia, the course and prognosis of the disease, effects and side effects of medication, disability, and rehabilitation systems that they can use are included in the contents of the lecture. The lectures are kept very simple and concise. A pamphlet containing a lot of visual information such as figures and tables assists the families to understand the lectures.

In the solution-focused interactive group, we aim at increasing members' cooperative power to solve their problems. Members who want to find the solution to their own problems can talk about their experiences, get help in choosing appropriate goals, listen to many reflective comments of other members, and finally select ideas that are useful to solve their problems. At the same time, the members can experience helping the other members by recounting in the group how they coped with problems in their own lives.

By constructing or finding solutions in the process, the group enhances feelings of self-efficacy, increases the sense of personal control, and instills skills and capabilities essential for coping with daily life. These gains lead to empowerment among family members.

Gaining knowledge about the disease, treatments, and resources is very important when families start to take part in the group. The sense of safety and the feeling that they are not alone are necessary for families to maintain their motivation to take part in the group. On the basis of these feelings, they can collaborate in finding solutions to their problems. When families can reduce their difficulties and help each other to advocate for themselves, the style of the group can gradually shift to that of a peer support group. Sometimes families begin to manage to group work in their own styles.

Psychoeducational Multiple Family Group Trial, 1996–1997: A Brief Report

We report here a randomized controlled trial of a psychoeducational multiple-family group, which was conducted during 1996 and 1997.

Subjects and Methods

The subjects were patients who were admitted to the inpatient treatment unit of Kounodai Hospital for over 20 days between June 1996 and July 1997. They were diagnosed with schizophrenia according to ICD-10 and were between 15 and 65 years old.

TABLE 1. Sociodemographic and clinical characteristics of subjects

Characteristic	Psychoeducational group	Control	P
n	43	42	
Male/female	19/24	15/27	NS
HEE/LEE	18/25	16/26	NS
Mean age (yr)	33.1	34.0	NS
Mean number of hospital admissions	2.7	3.0	NS
Mean duration of illness (mo)	109.5	69.2	NS

HEE, High Expressed Emotion; LEE, Low Expressed Emotion; NS, not significant

The subjects lived with their families or had family members who helped them with daily living. We obtained agreement from the subjects and their family members to participate in the research when they were admitted to the hospital.

The subjects were randomly assigned to the psychoeducational multiple-family group combined with routine treatment, or to the control group, in which only routine treatment was carried out. Routine treatment consisted of medication, electric convulsive therapy, and supportive care in the admission wards.

Results [3], [4]

There were no significant differences between the two groups in the ratio of male to female, ratio of EE of relatives, average age, mean number of hospital admissions, or mean duration of illness.

Table 2 shows the types of family members who participated in the research. Although mothers predominated, there were no significant differences between the groups.

Figure 1 compares the relapse rates in the two groups at 9 months after discharge. In the subjects whose families were assessed as high EE on their admission, the relapse rate of the psychoeducational group was 11%, which was significantly lower than the

TABLE 2. Relatives who participated in the research

Relative	Psychoeducational group	Control	P^a
Father	6	4	
Mother	28	28	
Spouse	6	7	
Others	3	3	
Total	43	42	.926

$^a \chi^2$ test, two-tailed

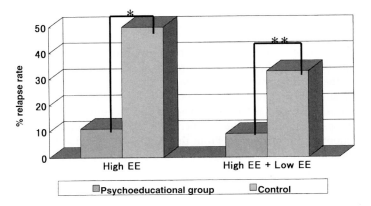

FIG. 1. Comparison of the relapse rates at 9-month follow-up after discharge in psychoeducational group vs. control. EE. Expressed Emotion. $^*p < .05$, $^{**}p < .01$; Fisher's exact test, two-tailed

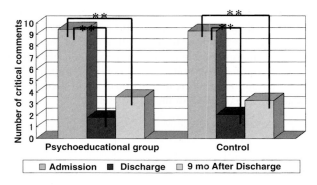

FIG. 2. Change in Critical Comments during the research. **$p < .01$ (t-test)

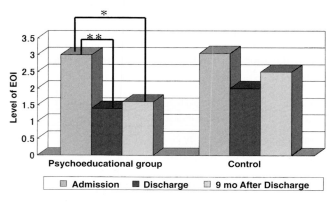

FIG. 3. Change in emotional overinvolvement (EOI) during the research. **$p < .01$, *$p < .05$ (t-test)

control group's rate of 50%. When the total group of patients was examined, the relapse rate of the psychoeducational group was 9%, which was also significantly lower than the control group's rate of 33%.

Figure 2 shows the change in the mean value of Critical Comments (CC) of the family who were assessed as High CC on admission. In both the experimental and the control groups, we found that the number of CC was lower not only at discharge but also at 9 months after discharge. From this result, it seems that the lowering of CC does not account for the therapeutic effect of the psychoeducational group.

However, we obtained a different result for Emotional Overinvolvement (EOI). Figure 3 shows the change in the mean value of EOI of the families who were assessed as High EOI on admission. In the psychoeducational group, EOI was significantly lowered both at discharge and at 9 months after discharge, although there were no significant changes in the control group.

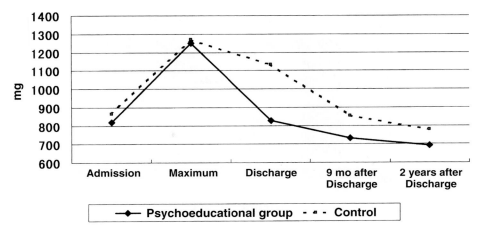

FIG. 4. Change in the amount of medication (conversion into chlorpromazine)

The lowering of EOI was one of the major effects of the participation of the families in the psychoeducational group. The lowering of EOI had already happened while the patients were hospitalized. Changes were noted after families took part in the group for only two or three sessions following hospitalization, since the psychoeducational program was held only once a month, and the mean number of hospitalization days was about 90. That is, changes in EOI were generated in the very early stages of the family psychoeducational program.

Figure 4 shows another result of the family psychoeducational group. This figure compares the change of medication doses between two groups. Medication doses are converted into chlorpromazine by the authorized conversion table. We found that doses could be reduced earlier in the psychoeducational group than in the control group during the hospitalization.

Figure 5 shows the differences in the maximum doses of medication prescribed and doses prescribed at discharge between the two groups. It shows that the amount of medication was significantly reduced in the psychoeducational group as compared with the control group during hospitalization. No differences between the two groups were observed on the rating of psychotic symptoms by the Brief Psychiatric Rating Scale (BPRS). This evidence suggests that despite the existence of psychotic symptoms, positive changes in the patient–family interaction had been generated in the early stages of the psychoeducational group.

Conclusions

In the multiple-family psychoeducational groups, it is important for the families to gain a sense of self-affirmation and self-efficacy and feelings of safety. The results of our research indicate that changes in EOI and medication doses were generated in the early stages of the group program. This suggests that the families in the group were able to change their situation by using the power of the group before they had devel-

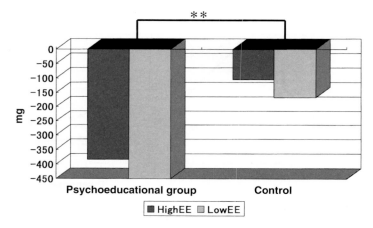

FIG. 5. Difference in the amount of medication at the maximum and at discharge (conversion into chlorpromazine. **Analysis of variance; $p < .01$). EE, Expressed Emotion

oped enough competence to cope with their difficulties. Through experiences such as being accepted by the members and trying to construct solutions in cooperation with other members, families were able to enrich their sense of self-affirmation and self-efficacy and feelings of safety in the early stages of the group. Such gains from the group enabled families to shift their interactions with their own family members to those that are more calm and comfortable. In addition, their small success in shifting the interactions activated the group further. The psychoeducational multiple-family group is an effective and useful treatment in the field of psychiatric rehabilitation. It can protect patients against psychotic relapse and contribute to the empowerment process among families.

References

1. McFarlane WR, Lukens E, Link B, et al (1995) Multiple-family groups and psychoeducation in the treatment of schizophrenia. Arch Gen Psychiatry, 52:679–687
2. Berg IK (1994) Family based services: a solution-focused approach. W. W. Norton, New York
3. Tsukada K, Ito J, Oshima I, et al (2000) Effects of family psychoeducation on clinical outcome of schizophrenic patients and family expressed emotion. J of Chiba Medicine 76:67–73
4. Koishikawa H, Tsukada K, Tomiyama M, et al (2000) Effects of family psychoeducation on medication doses of schizophrenic patients. Psychiat Neurol Jap 102:1061–1066

Part 4
Insight

The Psychopathological Foundation of Insight in Schizophrenia

YOSHIHARU KIM

Summary. The description of psychiatry, especially that for schizophrenia, has been based upon two roots. One is to delineate the diagnostic contour of an illness, and the other is to clarify the content: in other words, extension versus intension-oriented description. The diagnostic concept of schizophrenia inherited from Kraepelin through Schneider to the current *Diagnostic and Statistical Manual of Mental Disorders*, 4th edition (DSM-IV) belongs to the former, whereas the concept of psychosis proposed by Jaspers, which contains as its components the loss of insight together with incomprehensibility, belongs to the latter. Because the DSM-IV does not consider any discussion on the intension of a disease, the concept of psychosis or insight finds no place in this system. Nevertheless, the concept of insight still has considerable importance: first, it is still strongly held by psychiatric clinicians, as our study has demonstrated; second, it has a heuristic value for future research in the cognitive dysfunction in schizophrenia, in that insight is related to the self-monitoring function whose disturbance plays an essential role in schizophrenia.

Key words. Insight, Schizophrenia, Psychosis, Awareness, Subjective

Introduction

Throughout the history of the modern development of psychiatry, especially in the nineteenth and early twentieth centuries, the lack of insight has been regarded as one of the important features of psychosis. Even before Jaspers, who defined psychosis as a condition that lacked insight into illness, some outstanding authors had claimed this concept as the central characteristic of psychotic disorders.

However, the notion of insight, or the lack of it, is hardly mentioned in the modern nomenclature of diagnostic systems, such as the *Diagnostic and Statistical Manual of Mental Disorders*, 4th edition (DSM-IV). Its criteria or comments for the diagnosis of schizophrenia do not mention insight. So, where has insight gone? Has it stopped serving as the key element of psychosis? What is strange is that there has been

National Institute of Mental Health, National Center of Neurology and Psychiatry, 1-7-3 Kohnodai, Ichikawa, Chiba 272-0827, Japan

no argument regarding whether or not to discard the lack of insight from the diagnostic concept of schizophrenia.

To speak more precisely, the lack of insight was involved not in the disease concept, such as schizophrenia, but in the psychotic nature of certain mental phenomena. The discussion on the nature of psychosis, apart from the nosological definition of psychotic disorders, was most vividly promoted by Jaspers, who wrote the huge volume of the *General Psychopathology*. It was rather roughly incorporated by Schneider in the categorical classification of psychotic disorders. He used the notion of psychosis, whose nature was essentially phenomenological, not categorical, as the basic division between the disorders that show delusion or hallucination and those that do not have such experiences of unusual meanings. His emphasis was on the division within the realm of psychoses not attributable to somatic diseases of schizophrenia and affective disorders.

From that time on, nosological efforts were dedicated to the definition of schizophrenia, and especially to its differential diagnosis from affective disorders. When we think of the fact that the DSM since its third version has inherited the basic notion of psychotic disorders from Schneider, it may be no wonder that the DSM focuses on how to differentiate schizophrenia from other psychotic, particularly affective, disorders rather than on how to clarify its psychotic nature.

This can be stated in other words: whereas the nosological definition of schizophrenia concerns the extension of the illness, phenomenological debates on its psychotic nature concern the intension. The aim of the DSM is to draw correct lines of extension between various disorders, and it tends to regard the extension as the definition of nosological category. As the DSM became the world-wide standard of psychiatry, use of the extension-oriented criterion as the definition of psychiatric disorders moved from premise to consensus.

However, does the intension-oriented understanding of psychosis no longer attract the interest of contemporary psychiatrists? Do they, or do we, manage our work without any understanding or knowledge of what happens inside the psychotic disorders? To resume the topic of insight, do we treat patients with schizophrenia without relying on the notion of its loss?

Clinicians' View of Insight

To confirm this point, the author and Professor A.S. David of the Institute of Psychiatry performed a questionnaire survey on the extent to which the loss of insight is admitted by current psychiatrists, as well as how their attitude toward the notion of insight is influenced by differences in culture, education, or training. We sent a questionnaire to randomly selected psychiatrists in London and Japan. We received a reply from 104 of 200 Japanese psychiatrists and 111 of 310 British psychiatrists. The results showed that approximately 95% of the responders included, to a varying degree, any type of insight disturbance in the definition of schizophrenia, with the Japanese responders being slightly more positive for it. This demonstrated that the notion of insight is still widely held by contemporary clinicians both in Japan and the UK.

Interestingly enough, most responders answered that they preferred to use diagnostic systems such as the DSM and the *International Classification of Diseases* (ICD), which do not include the loss of insight as the definition of schizophrenia. It seems that the clinicians have dual systems of diagnosis of schizophrenia: one is the DSM-like system and the other is based on the traditionally constructed understanding of the nature of psychotic disorders.

Such a dual system of diagnosis is not actually a very new one but has been inherited from Schneider's classification, which is the root of the current diagnostic notion of schizophrenia. As already mentioned, he proposed two important dichotomous classifications: one between psychoses and nonpsychoses and the other between schizophrenia and the other psychoses. The first-rank symptoms were proposed as the definitive indicator for schizophrenia. The current DSM explicitly inherits only the latter. It should be emphasized that Schneider's definition of schizophrenia was constructed on the body of psychoses, and it may be a flaw of the DSM that it hardly considers any discussion of psychoses. On the other hand, the missing diagnosis of psychoses is, as was shown by the above-mentioned study, actually used by clinicians, and it is to this that the notion of insight belongs.

This means that the notion of insight still plays an important role in clinical practice and that this notion is worth intensive research.

Actually, insight has been eagerly investigated in the past decade by some outstanding researchers, such as David [1] and Amador [2]. The common premise is that insight should be regarded multidimensionally. The classical notion held by Jaspers, that insight is something like a choice between the two, either the presence and absence, or the psychoses or the nonpsychoses, has been replaced by a more classical and comprehensive viewpoint.

To push this trend of investigation of insight further, we examined the pathway of insight formation that starts from the vague perception of a pathological experience and extends through its recognition to the communication. The three steps require the ability of self-monitoring, medical knowledge, and reliance towards others, respectively. Their distorted form may be hallucination, delusion, and social withdrawal.

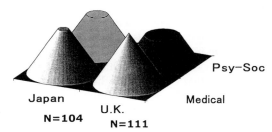

FIG. 1. The view of insight as the definition of schizophrenia

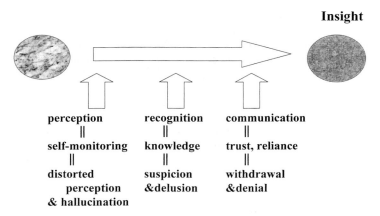

FIG. 2. The process of insight formation

Insight and Subjective Experience

To confirm this schema of insight formation, we investigated the existence of the perception of the pathological experience, regardless of whether it is expressed in an ordinary medical form of knowledge. This step needs to be confirmed, because if there is not any perception of the pathological experience at all, the following steps will lose their significance: it would be just a house of cards.

First, we examined how varieties of the subjective experience of schizophrenia can be categorized [3]. This was necessary because the ordinary symptomatology of schizophrenia consists of objective judgments of the patient's experience and lacks the pure description of subjective symptoms. In addition, it is difficult to categorize various amorphous forms of complaints according to the ordinary symptomatology. Therefore, we developed a self-report questionnaire consisting of 150 items of the subjective complaints derived from a number of case records and administered it to 237 Japanese schizophrenic inpatients. The results were analyzed by a multivariate method to produce the two largest and significant factors. The first factor represents loss of focus and adequacy of thoughts, behavior, and interpersonal perception; it resembles negative symptoms and coincides with the basic symptoms of schizophrenia reported by anthropological psychiatrists. The second factor represents automatic and excessive thoughts and affective loading, and it overlaps "the tremble" of Conrad and the mental automatism of de Clerambault.

Next, we investigated the correlation of these two types of subjective experience and ordinary symptoms, such as positive, negative, and depressive symptoms [4]. It was shown that each type of the subjective experience was significantly correlated with positive and negative symptoms.

Therefore, it is concluded that patients with schizophrenia have at least two types of perception of their experience, and these forms of perception seem to be robust, because they have a significant correlation with objective symptoms. Also, it is impor-

FIG. 3. Awareness of one's pathological state

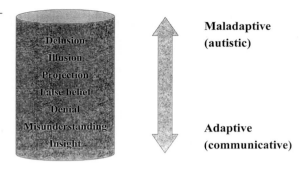

Maladaptive
(autistic)

Adaptive
(communicative)

tant to note that this perception is not distorted by the existence of positive or negative symptoms. This perception can presumably be the core on which patients with schizophrenia can build up insight into their illness.

Last, to expand our understanding of insight further, we would like to add that insight should be viewed from the wide perspective of the awareness of the illness, which may shift from the maladaptive to the adaptive form. Insight represents the adaptive form of awareness, especially from the medical viewpoint. The extreme pole of the maladaptive form may be delusion. In the intermediate forms, there are illusion, projection, false belief, denial, and misunderstanding. It should be pointed out that the patients always try to have an awareness of their illness, but only the extent to which it is adaptive varies.

Conclusions

Schizophrenic patients have an awareness of their own psychopathological changes, but this does not always lead to insight into their illness. As appropriate conceptual framework is needed, not only for patients but also for doctors. Each component and step of insight formation should be investigated individually.

References

1. David A (1990) Insight and psychosis. Br J Psychiat 156:798–808
2. Amador X, Flaum M, Andreasen N, et al (1994) Awareness of illness in schizophrenia and schizoaffective and mood disorders. Arch Gen Psychiat 51:826–836
3. Kim Y, Takemoto K, Mayahara K, et al (1994) An analysis of the subjective experience of schizophrenia. Compr Psychiat 35:430–436
4. Kim Y, Sakamoto K, Kamo T, et al (1997) Subjective experience and related symptoms in schizophrenia. Compr Psychiat 38:49–55

Insight: Theory and Practice

ANTHONY S. DAVID

Summary. The topic of insight in people with psychosis has recently attracted attention from psychiatric researchers. This has been facilitated by operational definitions of poor insight and the publication of number of rating scales. The author has proposed that insight has three overlapping dimensions: awareness that one is suffering from an illness, the ability to relabel certain experiences as abnormal, and acceptance of treatment. Insight is best viewed as a bio-psycho-social construct. It is affected by the presence of psychosis, disturbances in mood, intelligence, personality variables, and family and cultural beliefs. As well as being of theoretical importance, poor insight has a number of prognostic implications. This is mediated by acceptance of treatment or compliance. We have devised a brief and pragmatic cognitive-behavioral intervention (Compliance Therapy), which aims to improve insight and compliance. The results show that insight and compliance improve following the intervention, and that this improvement is maintained throughout the follow-up period. The combination of cognitive-behavioral interventions, patient education, and effective pharmacotherapy offers the best hope for patients with severe mental illness.

Key words. Insight, Psychosis, Compliance, Schizophrenia, Awareness

Introduction

The insight that patients with psychosis have into their mental pathology is no longer considered an all-or-none phenomenon, but rather a dimensional one, so that subjects can have different levels of awareness into their illness. This suggestion was first mooted by Aubrey Lewis [1] in his seminal work on insight. Conceptual exploration of insight has been activated in the last decade and is proceeding in parallel with research into its cognitive, biological, social, and cultural basis.

Institute of Psychiatry and GKT School of Medicine, Denmark Hill, London SE5 8AF, UK

Concepts and Scales

It is generally accepted that insight is, at its simplest, a dimension and probably a complex series of partially overlapping dimensions. Rather than committing to a single definition, researchers and clinicians have devised scales which they hope would capture the essence of the construct. One approach [2] has been to distinguish three main aspects: the awareness that one is suffering, in some general way, from a mental (as opposed to a physical) disturbance, which could be an illness; the more specific awareness that certain experiences, including beliefs and perceptions, may not be veridical and further that they too could be part of an illness; the acknowledgment of the medical implications of the above, a concrete token of which is informed acceptance of treatment.

Some workers in the field have expanded upon these dimensions, proposing a separation of the processes underlying awareness and those of attribution [3]. Kemp and David [4] suggested that awareness of change was also a prerequisite of insight, which could fall short of a medical attribution of illness. Furthermore, there has been much interest in the specificity of insight for certain features of mental disorder, such as positive versus negative symptoms and mood disorder versus abnormal perceptions. There are now a number of psychometric instruments and scales to assess insight [2,3,5–8]. It should be emphasized, however, that there is a large correspondence between most scales in covering such aspects as acceptance of the illness "label," perceived need for treatment, etc. [9,10].

A single-item insight assessment of the traditional mental state examination provides the investigator with little information about the quality or quantity of insight. Which aspects of the therapist's formulation does the patient accept? Does this vary from moment to moment or as the illness evolves? How fixed is it? Does illness awareness lead inevitably to treatment adherence, or is there no connection? Do the patient's actions indicate some awareness of his or her illness, as opposed to the patient's overt statements? Detailed longitudinal monitoring in clinical settings and psychopathology research requires more structured measurement of insight, which is the feature of the scales described above.

Insight and Psychopathology

Schizophrenia

Impairment of insight was the most common and discriminating symptom of schizophrenia in the World Health Organization's International Pilot Study of Schizophrenia [11]. More recent work using more complex (nontautological) definitions of insight [12] found that lack of insight was common in schizophrenia (and psychotic bipolar disorder), but less so in other affective and schizoaffective disorders diagnosed as part of the DSM-IV field trials.

There are a number of recent studies exploring the association of insight and psychopathological symptoms in patients with schizophrenia. McEvoy et al. [13] found a moderately significant association between insight and Brief Psychiatric Rating Scale scores (BPRS) [14], which became less significant by the time of discharge. Thus, as the psychopathology of the schizophrenic episode showed changes toward improvement, lack of insight remained a more stable variable. David et al. [15] revealed moderate though significant (−0.31) correlation between Present State Examination (PSE) [8] total scores and a composite score of the Schedule for Assessment of Insight. This study did not find significant differences in insight scores between patients with schizophrenia and other patients with paranoid and affective psychoses. Several other investigators [12,16] have found significant correlations between insight and psychopathological state, although the range of variance explained by this correlation was generally low (less than 50%). It has been suggested [17,18] that insight might be more strongly related to the subjective experiences of patients, as opposed to observer-rated "behavioral" measures. Kim and coauthors constructed an interview exploring subjective components of psychotic symptoms from standardized rating scales. The study revealed a moderate inverse correlation between observer-rated positive symptoms and insight measures (as assessed by the BPRS and David's scale, respectively). However, the subjective experiences of psychosis did not correlate with the measure of insight, contrary to the authors' hypothesis. It is of course possible that observer ratings of psychopathology contaminated observer ratings of insight.

A few studies have examined insight and symptoms longitudinally. David and colleagues [19] showed that poor insight mediated negative symptoms, disability, and unemployment four years later. Rossi et al. [20] recently found an association between awareness of mental disorder and a measure of global functioning.

Insight in Mood Disorders

Assessment of insight could shed some light on the clinical evaluation of affective and post-affective states. Patients with bipolar disorders investigated by the Insight and Treatment Attitudes Questionnaire (ITAQ) showed that insight was severely impaired in mania (comparable to that in schizophrenia) and less impaired in depressive states [16,21]. These studies also reported different results regarding changes in insight over time compared to schizophrenia. The first study found improvement of insight after recovery from a manic state, and the second found that there was no improvement. Similarly, Peralta and Cuesta [22] showed that patients with mania on admission had greater impairment of insight than those with depression, and at discharge some impairment was still observed in the manic patients, particularly those with mood-incongruent psychotic symptoms. The relationship between "recovery" and insight is again, prone to circularity. Amador and Seckinger [9] argued on pragmatic grounds that there is no need for patients to overtly accept a diagnosis of mental disorder so long as they are able to benefit from treatment.

Focusing on depressive disorders, Ghaemi et al. [21,23] found that patients with Seasonal Affective Disorder (SAD) possessed a moderate amount of insight (as measured by Amador's Scale to Assess Unawareness of Mental Disorder (SUMD) into depressive symptoms that did not change after recovery. Increased severity of illness in SAD was associated with increased insight into depressive symptoms. A positive correlation between insight and depressive states was also found by Sanz et al. [10]. These findings are consistent with the concept of depressive realism [24], which implies that in some cases, depression may result from excessive insight into unfavorable life circumstances. Recently, Ghaemi et al. [25] showed that insight had a strong association with improved global functioning in bipolar depression.

Lay Models of Illness

Can unawareness of illness be caused by lack of knowledge? However plausible this explanation may seem, supporting evidence is lacking. Startup [26] discovered a close to normal ability of patients to recognize the symptoms of mental illness in others (as tested using case vignettes), but this was in stark contrast to their impaired awareness of illness in themselves (as inferred from ITAQ scores). McEvoy et al. [27] had earlier shown that schizophrenia patients admitted to more (or were more aware of) negative symptoms than positive ones [12]. At the same time, patients considered negative features as least typical of mental illness (cf. positive symptoms). Moreover, the study revealed selectivity of (un)awareness towards those negative symptoms which could be construed as most pejorative (e.g., loss of motivation). This is in line with work by Swanson et al. [28], in which patients with schizophrenia and mania were shown the vignettes describing the examples of positive, negative, and manic psychopathology. On admission, schizophrenia patients rated themselves as significantly less similar to the positive-symptom vignettes than psychiatrists rated them, although the patients correctly labeled the presented signs as pathological. Patients with mania did not differ from the psychiatrists' rating of their similarity to the vignettes, but they strongly denied that the vignettes reflected mental illness. It is likely that in at least some cases, apparent lack of insight might be determined by the reluctance of the patients to admit having socially undesirable characteristics.

Insight and Neuropsychological Performance

Studies of the neuropsychological substrate of insight fall into two camps: one which maintains that there are specific neuroanatomical sites, such as the frontal lobes, that are responsible for the impairment of insight in schizophrenia, and the other which claims that if insight is related to cognitive impairment, it results from a global cognitive deficit.

Two research groups [29,30] have shown and replicated a correlation between poor insight, measured by the SUMD, and executive deficits, measured by the Wisconsin Card Sorting Test (WCST) [31]. Other groups [10,32,33] failed to find a significant relationship between insight and frontal task (WCST) performance. David et al. [19] suggested that insight is related not to specifically frontal function, but more to measures of general intelligence, although these relationships were found to be nonlinear.

The WCST is problematic as a measure of executive or "frontal" dysfunction because it is dependent on general cognitive abilities [34,35]. Of much interest is the study of Startup [36], who found that the relationships between neuropsychological performance and insight in schizophrenia are of a complex curvilinear nature. He suggested that besides cognitive deficits, motivational forces could be implicated in the development of insight impairment (particularly in those of above average intelligence).

To conclude, intellectual abilities—whether specific frontal lobe functions or more general abilities—may be meaningfully associated, not just with general scores of insight, but also with more specific tasks, requiring cognitively demanding introspection into particular domains of mental life.

Cultural Influences on Insight

There are at least two simple ways in which external influences may shape insight measures. First, as hinted above in the discussion of "motivational accounts" of illness unawareness, patients may consciously or unconsciously avoid admitting to their clinicians that they are suffering from pathological symptoms, because of unwillingness to bear the stigma of mental illness. On the other hand, the patient may differ from the clinician in terms of educational or cultural background, as well as on a theoretical continuum of conformity, and subsequently in their explanations of the experience of mental disorder. The vignette studies do not support this notion, but it cannot yet be dismissed. In this respect, several investigators [37–39] have argued that patients may have their own explanations of their disturbances (e.g., religious, physical, or interpersonal) that may not coincide with the Western "medical model" of mental disease. The situation can be even more complicated if one tries directly to impose the models of insight on patients from non-Western cultures. Referring to his experience in Singapore, Tan [40] warns that allowances should be made when assessing components of insight. For example, treatment compliance might be applied to either traditional remedies or "modern" treatments. The extent to which the ability to distance oneself from unusual experiences is dependent on cultural norms and is a topic for future multidisciplinary research. Beck-Sander [41] criticizes the concept of insight as being restrictive and internally inconsistent (but see David [42]). As an alternative, an individual explanatory model is proposed, which is grounded on the patient's explanation of his or her illness. Nevertheless, there are benefits to the patient in embracing the "medical model," provided it does not imply lack of autonomy and incurability. In many cases, individual explanations and insight are not mutually exclusive but complementary. Medical professionals should be aware, however, of the patient's use of terms referring to his or her mental state.

McNally and Goldberg [43] avoided terms like "illness" and "symptom" when interviewing schizophrenia patients about their subjective experiences and natural coping strategies. The patients, scoring medium to high on the positive symptoms scale of the Positive and Negative Syndrome Scale (PANSS) [44], reported such coping strategies as "trying to stand outside of one's experience and see it from the perspective of another," "reality checks," etc. Although these descriptions of self-developed strategies would not coincide literally with items on insight scales, they demonstrated an implicit awareness of having a mental disorder. Indeed, insight positively correlated with the number of natural coping strategies employed by the patients with auditory hallucinations [45].

Regarding the influence of culture on coping mechanisms, Wahass and Kent [46] showed that patients with an Islamic background were more inclined towards religious activities to cope with their "voices," whereas native British patients engaged in "physiological" methods, such as sport, using alcohol, and taking medication.

Considering these findings from an insight viewpoint, we should mention that not all of these coping strategies reflect the presence of good insight. Thus, Sanz et al. [10] demonstrated that the use of alcohol and illicit drugs correlated negatively with insight, which subsequently might hinder the adherence to medication. Again, activation of religious practices may be helpful for patients belonging to Islamic culture but may be inappropriate in different settings. In a recent study from inner London, Kirov et al. [47] found that religious affiliations in a group of patients recovering from psychotic relapse were not correlated with insight.

Treatment

The relevance of the concept of insight to therapeutic intervention is increasing. Given the changes in mental health care policy towards a community-based system, the patient is regarded as a participant in (and no longer a mere recipient of) the treatment program. The success of this approach depends to a large extent on the patient's insight and attitudes towards therapy. The association between insight and adherence to medication has been demonstrated in a number of studies [48–50]. Insight has also been found to be associated with social functioning [51].

Despite the most liberal attitudes, sanctioning involuntary treatment under the Mental Health Act is a fact of life for most British psychiatrists. Studies from the United States [13] and the United Kingdom [15] confirm the rather obvious idea that poor insight is a particular feature of involuntary patients, and that it is rather stable in the face of clinical remission. Nevertheless, in some cases (over 50% of the patients in the study of Kemp et al. [52]), enforced compliance may be the first step towards voluntary treatment adherence [53,54].

Psychoeducation has been used to improve the knowledge base of patients and their families about the nature of mental illness and the benefits of medication. However, studies tend to show short-lived benefits at best [55–57]. An 18-month follow-up of a randomized, controlled trial study by Kemp et al. [52] showed that "compliance therapy" had a better outcome in terms of social functioning and community tenure (i.e., longer time before relapse) than a control intervention consisting of nonspecific counseling. This therapy combines interactive, cognitive, and behavioral approaches and promotes clinical improvement via attitudes toward treatment and the increase of insight into existing psychotic symptoms (see also Kemp et al. [58]).

Conclusions

There is good evidence that insight into psychosis is a multidimensional process, unfolding with time. It is domain specific and influenced by a host of factors (cognitive, emotional, social, and cultural), which interact. The concept of insight is far from being fully understood. There are many uncertainties regarding the association of insight with psychopathology and neuropsychological performance. Some of these uncertainties reflect the dynamic nature of insight [59], which implies a certain malleability and opens the door for therapeutic intervention. In conclusion, I have stressed the clinical implications of the insight concept, the meaningfulness of subjective attitudes of patients, and the fact that the quality of patients' lives might be improved by targeting insight and attitudes to treatment.

References

1. Lewis A (1934) The psychopathology of insight. Br J Med Psychol 14:332–348
2. David AS (1990) Insight and psychosis. Br J Psychiatry 156:798–809
3. Amador XF, Strauss DH (1990) The scale to assess unawareness of mental disorder (SUMD). Columbia University and New York State Psychiatric Institute, New York
4. Kemp R, David A (1997) Insight and compliance. In: Blackwell B (ed) Treatment compliance and the treatment alliance in serious mental illness. Harwood Academic Publishers, The Netherlands, pp 61–86
5. McEvoy JP, Apperson LJ, Appelbaum PS, et al (1989) Insight in schizophrenia: its relationship to acute psychopathology. J Nerv Ment Dis 177:43–47
6. Birchwood M, Smith J, Drury V, et al (1994) A self-report insight scale for psychosis—reliability, validity and sensitivity to change. Acta Psychiatr Scand 89:62–67
7. Markova IS, Berrios GE (1992) The assessment of insight in clinical psychiatry: a new scale. Acta Psychiatr Scand 86:159–164
8. Wing JK, Cooper JE, Sartorius N (1974) The description and classification of psychiatric symptoms: an instruction manual for PSE and category system. Cambridge University Press, London
9. Amador XF, Seckinger BA (1997) The assessment of insight: a methodological review. Psychiatr Ann 27:798–805
10. Sanz M, Constable G, Lopez-Ibor I, et al (1998) A comparative study of insight scales and their relationship to psychopathological and clinical variables. Psychol Med 28:437–446
11. World Health Organization (1973) Report of the international pilot study of schizophrenia. World Health Organization, Geneva
12. Amador XF, Flaum M, Andreasen NC, et al (1994) Awareness of illness in schizophrenia, schizoaffective and mood disorders. Arch Gen Psychiatry 51:826–836
13. McEvoy JP, Appelbaum PS, Geller JL, et al (1989) Why must some schizophrenic patients be involuntarily committed? The role of insight. Comp Psychiatry 30:13–17
14. Overall J, Gorham D (1962) The Brief Psychiatric Rating Scale. Psychol Rep 10:799–812
15. David AS, Buchanan A, Reed A, et al (1992) The assessment of insight in psychosis. Br J Psychiatry 161:599–602
16. Michalakeas A, Skoutas C, Charalambous A, et al (1994) Insight in schizophrenia and mood disorders and its relation to psychopathology. Acta Psychiatr Scand 90:46–49
17. Kim Y, Sakamoto K, Kamo T, et al (1997) Insight and clinical correlates in schizophrenia. Comp Psychiatry 38:117–123
18. Kim Y, Sakamoto K, Sakamura Y (1997) Subjective experience and related symptoms in schizophrenia. Comp Psychiatry 38:49–55
19. David A, van Os J, Harvey I, et al (1995) Insight and psychotic illness. Br J Psychiatry 167:621–628
20. Rossi A, Arduini L, Prosperini P, et al (2000) Awareness of illness and outcome in schizophrenia. Eur Arch Psychiatr Clin Neurosci 250:73–75
21. Ghaemi SN, Stoll AL, Pope H (1995) Lack of insight in bipolar disorder—the acute manic episode. J Nerv Ment Dis 183:464–467
22. Peralta V, Cuesta MJ (1998) Lack of insight in mood disorders. J Affec Dis 49:55–58
23. Ghaemi SN, Sachs GS, Baldassano CF, et al (1997) Insight in seasonal affective disorder. Comp Psychiatry 38:345–348

24. Alloy LB, Abramson LY (1988) Depressive realism: four theoretical perspectives. In: Alloy LB (ed) Cognitive processes in depression. Guilford Press, New York, pp 223–265

25. Ghaemi SN, Boiman E, Goodwin FK (2000) Insight and outcome in bipolar, unipolar, and anxiety disorders. Comp Psychiatry 41:167–171

26. Startup M (1997) Awareness of own and others' schizophrenic illness. Schizophr Res 26:203–211

27. McEvoy JP, Schooler NJ, Friedman E, et al (1993) Use of psychopathology vignettes by patients with schizophrenia or schizoaffective disorder and by mental health professionals to judge patients' insight. Am J Psychiatry 150:1649–1653

28. Swanson CL, Freudenreich O, McEvoy JP, et al (1995) Insight in schizophrenia and mania. J Nerv Ment Dis 183:752–755

29. Lysaker PH, Bell MD, Bryson G, et al (1998) Neurocognitive function and insight in schizophrenia: support for an association with impairments in executive function but not with impairments in global function. Acta Psychiatr Scand 97:297–301

30. Young DA, Zakzanis KK, Bailey C, et al (1998) Further parameters of insight and neuropsychological deficit in schizophrenia and other chronic mental disease. J Nerv Ment Dis 186:44–50

31. Heaton RK (1981) Wisconsin Card Sorting Test Manual. Psychological Assessment Resources, Odessa, FL, USA

32. Collins AA, Remington GJ, Coulter K, et al (1997) Insight, neurocognitive function and symptom clusters in chronic schizophrenia. Schizophr Res 27:37–44

33. Cuesta MJ, Peralta V, Caro F, et al (1995) Is poor insight in psychotic disorders associated with poor performance on the Wisconsin Card Sorting Test? Am J Psychiatry 152:1380–1382

34. Dieci M, Vita A, Silenzi C, et al (1997) Non-selective impairment of Wisconsin Card Sorting Test performance in patients with schizophrenia. Schizophr Res 25:33–42

35. Laws KR (2000) A meta-analytic review of Wisconsin Card sort studies in schizophrenia: a general intellectual deficit in disguise. Cogn Neuropsychiatry (in press)

36. Startup M (1996) Insight and cognitive deficits in schizophrenia: evidence for a curvilinear relationship. Psychol Med 26:1277–1281

37. Johnson S, Orrell M (1995) Insight and psychosis—a social perspective. Psychol Med 25:515–520

38. Johnson S, Orrell M (1996) Insight, psychosis and ethnicity—a case-note study. Psychol Med 26:1081–1084

39. Perkins R, Moodley P (1993) The arrogance of insight? Psychiatr Bull 17:233–234

40. Tan T (1993) Assessment of insight in Singapore. Br J Psychiatry 162:565–566

41. Beck-Sander A (1998) Is insight into psychosis meaningful? J Ment Health 7:25–34

42. David AS (1998) The clinical importance of insight. In: Amador XF, David AS (eds) Insight and psychosis. Oxford University Press, New York, pp 332–351

43. McNally SE, Goldberg JO (1997) Natural cognitive coping strategies in schizophrenia. Br J Med Psychol 70:159–167

44. Kay S, Fiszbein A, Opler L (1987) The Positive and Negative Syndrome Scale (PANSS) for schizophrenia. Schizophr Bull 13:261–276

45. Nayani TH, David AS (1996) The auditory hallucination—a phenomenological survey. Psychol Med 26:177–189

46. Wahass S, Kent G (1997) Coping with auditory hallucinations: a cross-cultural comparison between Western (British) and Non-Western (Saudi Arabian) patients. J Nerv Ment Dis 185:664–668

47. Kirov G, Kemp R, Kirov K, et al (1998) Religious faith after psychotic illness. Psychopathology 31:234–245

48. Buchanan A (1992) A two-year prospective study of treatment compliance in patients with schizophrenia. Psychol Med 22:787–797

49. Chan DW (1984) Medication compliance in a Chinese psychiatric out-patient setting. Br J Med Psychol 57:81–89
50. McEvoy JP (1998) The relationship between insight in psychosis and compliance with medications. In: Amador XF, David AS (eds) Insight and psychosis. Oxford University Press, New York, pp 289–306
51. Lysaker PH, Bell MD, Bryson GJ, et al (1998) Insight and interpersonal function in schizophrenia. J Nerv Ment Dis 186:432–436
52. Kemp R, Kirov G, Everitt B, et al (1998) Randomised controlled trial of compliance therapy—18-month follow-up. Br J Psychiatr 172:413–419
53. Kane JM, Quitkin F, Rifkin A, et al (1983) Attitudinal changes of involuntarily committed patients following treatment. Arch Gen Psychiatry 40:374–377
54. Kjellin L, Andersson K, Candefjord IL, et al (1997) Ethical benefits and costs of coercion in short-term inpatient psychiatric care. Psychiatr Serv 48:1567–1570
55. Boczkowski JA, Zeichner A, DeSanto N (1985) Neuroleptic compliance among chronic schizophrenic outpatients: an intervention outcome report. J Consult Clin Psychol 53:666–671
56. Hayward P, Kemp R, David A (2000) Compliance therapy: a collaborative approach to psychiatric medication. In: Martindale B, Bateman A, Crowe M, Margison F (eds) Psychosis: psychological approaches and their effectiveness. Putting psychotherapies at the centre of treatment. Gaskell (Royal College of Psychiatrists), London, pp 50–67
57. MacPherson R, Jerrom B, Hughes A (1996) A controlled study of education about drug treatment in schizophrenia. Br J Psychiatry 168:709–717
58. Kemp R, Hayward P, David A (1997) Compliance therapy manual. Gardiner-Caldwell Communications, London
59. Jorgensen P (1995) Recovery and insight in schizophrenia. Acta Psychiatr Scand 92:436–440

Part 5
Pharmacotherapy

Factors Affecting Drug Compliance Among Patients in Japan with Schizophrenia

KOICHIRO WATANABE, MASAFUMI MIZUNO, GOHEI YAGI, and
HARUO KASHIMA

Summary. Factors affecting Japanese patients with schizophrenia in terms of their drug compliance were investigated. Subjects were patients with schizophrenia who were discharged from a psychiatric hospital for he first time. The target period was 24 months after discharge. Positive and Negative Symptoms Scale (PANSS), Clinical Global Impression (CGI), Global Assessment of Functioning (GAF), Drug Attitude Inventory (DAI), and The Schedule for Assessment of Insight (SAI) were adopted as rating scales. To define drug noncompliance, patients satisfying either of two criteria were chosen: an indication of "not taking medications appropriately" entered in the medical record, or inconsistency in the periods of prescription and visiting the out-patient clinic. There were 58 subjects (48.3% male), of whom 51.7% were fully compliant for 24 months after discharge. Significant factors among the good compliance group were found to be "lack of spontaneity and flow of conversation," "depression," and "emotional withdrawal" at discharge on PANSS subscales; a diagnosis of hebephrenic and residual schizophrenia, longer hospitalization and longer time from first treatment to admission, and positive attitde toward antipsychotics on the DAI scale; and "insight for treatment and drug compliance" on the SAI scale. Factors for noncompliance, on the other hand, were "uncooperativeness" and "lack of judgment and insight" in PANSS subscales at discharge, as well as gastrointestinal symptoms and drowsiness as side-effects, and less complete education.

Key words. Schizophrenia, Drug compliance, Antipsychotics, Insight, Hospitalization

It is well known that drug compliance is a crucial problem that reduces the relapse rate of patients with schizophrenia, but there are some obstacles to drug compliance of patients with schizophrenia in Japan. There are six unique characteristics of Japanese psychopharmacotherapy for schizophrenia, which are unfavorable compared to other countries.

The first is polypharmacy: an average of 2.6 kinds of antipsychotics are given to every patient in Japan [1]. Second, depots should become an indication for drug non-compliant patients. There are three kinds of depots, but they are not widely used yet.

Department of Neuropsychiatry, School of Medicine, Keio University, 35 Shinanomachi, Shinjuku-ku, Tokyo 160-8582, Japan

Compared with other antipsychotics, the ratio of depots is less than 4%. Third, atypical antipsychotics, such as serotonin-dopamine antagonists (SDA) and multi-acting receptor-targeted antipsychotics (MARTA), are well known for having fewer side effects, including extrapyramidal signs, but are effective in treating psychotic symptoms. Unfortunately, at the end of the year 2000, there was only one SDA on the market: risperidone. Other long-awaited atypical antipsychotics are coming on the market on 2001: olanzapine, quetiapine, and perospirone. Clozapine, an antipsychotic well known for treatment-resistant schizophrenia, is not yet available in Japan. Thus, the classical and typical antipsychotics are still prevalent on the market; they have more extrapyramidal signs, making psychiatrists tend to use more antiparkinsonian drugs. Finally, there are many four-times-a-day prescriptions, which require taking medications after every meal and before sleep. This type of multimedication approach is the conventional manner in Japan, despite evidence-based psychiatry. All these factors are thought to have an undesirable influence on drug compliance.

These circumstances exert at least some effect on the attitude of patients with schizophrenia toward antipsychotics in Japan. In the present study, we investigated factors affecting patients with schizophrenia in terms of their drug compliance.

Subjects

The subjects were patients diagnosed as schizophrenic by ICD-10, F20s [2], who discharged from a psychiatric hospital for the first time between August 1996 and January 1998, and who were willing to continue to have consultation at the outpatient clinic of the same hospital after discharge. The hospital, with 380 beds, is located in suburban Tokyo. Informed consent was obtained from all subjects.

Methods

The target period was 24 months after discharge. We used the Positive and Negative Symptoms Scale (PANSS) [3] and the Clinical Global Impression (CGI) [4] to assess psychiatric symptoms and their severity. Global Assessment of Functioning (GAF) [5] was used to assess social functioning, the Drug Attitude Inventory (DAI) [6,7] to assess image and attitude toward antipsychotics, and the Schedule for Assessment of Insight (SAI) [8,9] to rate insight. The data were obtained from medical records and interviews.

To define drug noncompliance, we chose patients satisfying either of two criteria: an indication of "not taking medications appropriately" entered in the medical record, or inconsistency of the periods of prescription and of visiting the outpatient clinic.

The Drug Attitude Inventory (DAI) is a self-rating scale consisting of 30 items that indicate the patient's attitude toward antipsychotics and psychopharmacotherapy. On this scale, a correct answer to a given item is scored as plus one and an incorrect answer as minus one. The sum total of the pluses and minuses gives the final score. A final positive total score means a positive attitude, and a negative total score means a negative attitude.

The Schedule for Assessment of Insight (SAI) consists of three subscales: Compliance, Recognition of Illness, and Relabeling of Psychosis. Besides these three, a subscale Hypothetical Contradiction was added as a supplement. The total of these four scores indicates the grand total insight score. A maximum score of 20 indicates full insight.

Results

The background of the target group is shown in Table 1. There were 58 subjects; 48.3% were male. Of the target group, 51.7% were fully compliant, which means complete drug compliance for 24 months after discharge.

Table 2 shows the statistical differences between the drug-compliant group and the noncompliant group in the following factors. First, during hospitalization, the compliant group remained significantly longer. There were three patients who were hospitalized continuously for more than 1000 days in the compliant group, and after exclusion of those three patients from the compliant group, a significant difference was still found between the two groups. The period from first treatment to admission was also significantly longer in the compliant group. Furthermore, the compliant

TABLE 1. Background of the target group

Characteristic	Value
Sex	
Male	28 (48.3%)
Female	30 (51.7%)
Age at onset (yr)	27.8 ± 10.8
Age at discharge (yr)	34.3 ± 12.0
Diagnosis	
F20.0	37 (63.8%)
20.1	4 (6.9%)
20.2	4 (6.9%)
20.3	2 (3.4%)
20.5	9 (15.5%)
20.6	1 (1.7%)
20.9	1 (1.7%)
Marital status	
Single	35 (60.3%)
Married	15 (22.4%)
Separated	8 (15.5%)
Work situation	
Working	25 (43.1%)
Unemployed/invalid	33 (56.9%)
Type of cohabitation	
Family	45 (77.6%)
Alone	13 (22.4%)
Type of admission	
Voluntary admission	27 (46.6%)
Admission for medical care and custody	22 (37.4%)
Involuntary admission	9 (15.5%)
Mean admission period (days)	343.4 ± 1127.2
Duration of untreated psychosis (mos)	17.8 ± 35.1
Total amount of neuroleptics—chlorpromazine equivalent (mg/day) at discharge	856.1 ± 581.9

TABLE 2. Compliant group vs. noncompliant group

Characteristic	Compliant	Noncompliant
Admission period (days)	595.6 ± 1535.0	73.1 ± 72.8**
Admission period excluding 3 patients (days)[a]	165.4 ± 191.8*	
From the first treatment until admission (mo)	48.9 ± 60.8	18.2 ± 42.7*
Education (yr)	13.4 ± 2.0	12.2 ± 2.4***
DAI	10.1 ± 10.6	3.9 ± 9.0*
SAI compliance	4.9 ± 1.4	4.4 ± 1.1***
Subscales of PANSS at discharge		
Emotional withdrawal	3.4 ± 1.1	2.9 ± 1.0***
Lack of spontaneity and flow of conversation	3.2 ± 1.1	2.6 ± 0.9*
Depression	2.3 ± 1.2	1.8 ± 1.0*
Uncooperativeness	2.0 ± 1.0	2.5 ± 0.9*
Lack of judgment and insight	3.0 ± 1.2	3.6 ± 1.3***

[a] Three patients had been admitted for over 10 years, and therefore we excluded these three subjects

DAI, Drug Attitude Inventory; SAI, Schedule for Assessment of Insight; PANSS, Positive and Negative Symptoms Scale

** $P < 0.01$, * $P < 0.05$, *** $P < 0.1$; Mann-Whitney U test

group tended to have a higher education. Thirteen years of education in Japan is equivalent to completion of high school and at least a year of college.

In the diagnosis, there was a significant difference between the two groups according to the chi-square test. The compliant group had more hebephrenic and residual schizophrenia, whereas in the noncompliant group, there was more paranoid schizophrenia ($P = 0.025$).

The compliant group scored significantly higher in the DAI, reflecting a more positive attitude to antipsychotics and psychopharmacotherapy. The compliant group also tended to score higher on one subscale of SAI, "compliance to treatment and medicine."

In the CGI, "severity of illness" at one year after discharge, the compliant group scored 3.1 and tended to show a better condition. In "global improvement" of CGI, the compliant group was significantly improved compared with the noncompliant group at 1 year and $1\frac{1}{2}$ year after discharge.

As for psychotic symptoms, the results of the subscales of PANSS revealed that the compliant group scored significantly higher in "lack of spontaneity and flow of conversation" and "depression" at discharge; the group also scored higher in "emotional withdrawal." The noncompliant group scored significantly higher in the subscale "uncooperativeness" at discharge and tended to score higher also in "lack of judgment and insight" at discharge. Thus, the noncompliant group had less judgment and insight at discharge than the compliant group. We found no difference in PANSS 2 years after discharge and in GAF at every stage.

Side effects, such as gastrointestinal symptoms ($P = 0.048$), were frequently observed in the noncompliant group, and drowsiness ($P = 0.067$) was also evident in the group.

Finally, the compliant group had a tendency to participate in day hospitals and sheltered workshops and to have more nursery visits ($P = 0.073$).

Using a stepwise multiple regression analysis, we examined the factors that explain the drug compliance. With an R value of 0.725, variables such as length of hospital

TABLE 3. Variables predicting drug compliance

Variable	B
Admission period	0.38*
Lack of spontaneity and flow of conversation	−0.43**
Uncooperativeness	0.29***
Education period	−0.33*
Gastrointestinal symptoms	−0.32*
Drowsiness	−1.95***

** $P < 0.01$, * $P < 0.05$, *** $P < 0.1$; stepwise multiple regression analysis. $R = 0.725$

stay, "lack of spontaneity and flow of conversation," "uncooperativeness," and education period, along with side effects, such as gastrointestinal symptoms and drowsiness, predicted compliance (Table 3).

There was no significant difference in sex, age at onset and discharge, marital status, jobs, type of admission, duration of untreated psychosis, total amount of antipsychotics administered, and other scales of PANSS, such as positive symptoms and social functioning according to GAF.

Discussion

We found the factors for good compliance to be as follows. At discharge, subscales of PANSS including "lack of spontaneity and flow of conversation," "depression," and "emotional withdrawal," diagnosis of hebephrenic and residual schizophrenia, longer hospitalization and longer time from the first treatment until admission, positive attitude toward antipsychotics in DAI, and "insight for treatment and drug compliance" in SAI.

From the results on which traits are preferable for good compliance, psychiatric symptoms, including a passive attitude or behavior, seem advantageous. Van Putten [10], Marder [11], and Kelly [12] cited insight and attitude as factors related to compliance, so measuring these two factors by DAI and SAI would be very useful. McEvoy [13] found that patients who readily take their neuroleptics may have more chronic depression and anxiety. In a Japanese study, Waseda [14] compared compliant and poorly compliant Japanese patients in their characteristics and described compliant patients as depressive, poor in volition, and dependent. Tsumura [15] indicated that compliant patients were hebephrenic and had a passive attitude in common. Thus, the present results are quite similar to those of previous research on Japanese compliant patients.

The factors for noncompliance, on the other hand, were as follows: at discharge, subscales of PANSS, including "uncooperativeness" and "lack of judgment and insight," gastrointestinal symptoms, and drowsiness as side effects and less formed education.

Bartko [16] pointed out that in the noncompliant group, lack of feeling ill and lack of insight into illness were frequently seen, and Marder [11] described the noncompliant group as uncooperative and lacking insight. Therefore, appropriate judgment and insight, along with cooperativeness, would be necessary for good compliance.

Regarding side effects, Van Putten [10] and Buchanan [17] described akathisia, and Kemp [18] described extrapyramidal signs related to poor compliance. Against expectations, gastrointestinal symptoms and drowsiness led to poor compliance in this research. Thus, from the viewpoint of drug compliance, it would be preferable to prescribe antipsychotics with fewer side effects, such as gastrointestinal symptoms and drowsiness. It is no wonder, then, that fewer medications would be better for compliance.

The result that longer hospitalization led to good compliance would suggest that good information on drugs would easily be supplied if the patient received longer treatment or was in a hospital setting longer. Generally, the same doctor who sees inpatients in this hospital continues to see them when they become outpatients after discharge. At the time when the subjects were hospitalized, in 1996 and 1997, drug information service was not yet performed systematically in this hospital, so there might be a possibility that a longer time in the hospital would make a good and tight relationship between the patient and the doctor or nurses that would lead to a positive drug attitude and good compliance.

In Western countries, such as the United States, England, and Germany, the number of beds decreased in the 1970s. But at that time in Japan, the number of beds was increasing, and that trend continued up to 1990. The number of beds in Japan finally decreased in the 1990s. In comparison with other Asian countries, South Korea and China are similar, but the number of beds in Japan is much higher [19].

The mean length of hospitalization of this target group, 343 days, is lower than the average for all psychiatric patients in Japan. The length of hospitalization declined from the mid 1980s in virtually every psychiatric hospital in Japan [19]. However, the target group was longer in comparison with the whole admission period of the same hospital, because, as mentioned before, this group had long-time-admitted patients. As of 1998, 43.2% of all patients in this hospital had stayed for more than 3 years.

In this research, we used patient and family interviews, along with medical records. Other means to determine drug compliance include monitoring of blood levels, urine [20–24], and hair, and, of course, pill counts [25].

The results show that certain scales at the time of discharge predict future drug noncompliance. Kemp pointed out that improvements in insight have been linked to improved medication compliance [18], so if the results of these rating scales were poor upon admission, psychoeducation should be performed simply and individually, and intensive follow-up systems would be necessary to achieve better compliance and thus a better outcome.

References

1. Yamauchi K, Baba K, Ikegami N, Miyaoka H, Kamijima K (1998) A survey of drug utilization in psychiatric hospitals in Japan: the basic analysis of the current status of prescription patterns. Seishin Shinkeigaku Zasshi 100:51–68
2. World Health Organization (1992) The ICD-10 classification of mental and behavioral disorders: clinical descriptions and diagnostic guidelines. World Health Organization, Geneva
3. Kay SR, Opler LA, Fiszbein A (1991) Positive and Negative Syndrome Scale (PANSS) rating manual. Multi-Health System, Toronto
4. Guy W (1976) ECDEU Assessment Manual for Psychopharmacology. Department of Health, Education and Welfare, Washington, DC, pp 217–222

5. American Psychiatric Association (1994) Quick reference to the diagnostic criteria from DSM-IV. American Psychiatric Association, Washington, DC
6. Hogan TP, Awad AG, Eastwood R (1983) A self-report scale predictive of drug compliance in schizophrenics: reliability and discriminative validity. Psychol Med 13:177–183
7. Miyata R, Fujii Y, Inagaki A (1996) Psychopharmacotherapy and quality of life of patients with schizophrenia part 1 by using drug attitude inventory Japanese version. Seishinshinkeishi 98:1045–1046
8. David A (1990) Insight and psychosis. Br J Psychiatry 156:798–808
9. Sakai Y, Kim Y, Akiyama T, Tachimori H, Kurita H (2000) Reliability and validity of the Japanese version of the Schedule for Assessment of Insight (SAI-J). Rinsyoseishinigaku 29:177–183
10. Van Putten T (1974) Why do schizophrenic patients refuse to take their drugs? Arch Gen Psychiatry 31:67–72
11. Marder SR, Mebane A, Chien CP, Winslade WJ, Swann E, Van Putten T (1983) A comparison of patients who refuse and consent to neuroleptic treatment. Am J Psychiatry 140:470–472
12. Kelly GR, Mamon JA, Scott JE (1987) Utility of the health belief model in examining medication compliance among psychiatric outpatients. Soc Sci Med 11:1205–1211
13. McEvoy JP, Apperson LJ, Appelbaum PS, Ortlip P, Brecosky J, Hammill K, Geller JL, Roth L (1989) Insight in schizophrenia: its relationship to acute psychopathology. J Nerv Ment Dis 177:43–47
14. Waseda T, Kawatani D, Nishizono M (1999) The psychology of schizophrenic and mood disorder's patients on taking medicine. Rinsyoseishinigaku 28:603–608
15. Tsumura T, Nishino H, Fujita K, Tsutsumi T, Chiba H (1991) A statistical study of schizophrenic patients; Part 2: Types of medicational course and outcome during 8 years (1982–1989). Seishinigaku 33:71–78
16. Bartko G, Herczeg I, Zador G (1988) Clinical symptomatology and drug compliance in schizophrenic patients. Acta Psychiatr Scand 77:74–76
17. Buchanan A (1992) A two-year prospective study of treatment compliance in patients with schizophrenia. Psychol Med 22:787–797
18. Kemp R, Hayward P, Applewhite G, Everitt B, David A (1996) Compliance therapy in psychotic patients: randomised controlled trial. BMJ 312:345–349
19. Seishinhokenfukushi kenkyuukai (1999) Handbook of mental health and welfare, pp 165–173
20. Carman JS, Wyatt ES, Feck R, Martin D, Gold M (1984) Neuroleptic compliance in schizophrenic outpatients. Psychiatr Hosp 15:173–178
21. McClellan TA, Cowan G (1970) Use of antipsychotic and antidepressant drugs by chronically ill patients. Am J Psychiatry 126:1771–1773
22. Willcox DRC, Gillan R, Hare EH (1965) Do psychiatric outpatients take their drugs? BMJ 2:790–792
23. Parkes CM, Brown GW, Monck EM (1962) The general practitioner and the schizophrenic patient. BMJ 1:972–976
24. Mason AS, Forrest IS, Forrest FW, Butler H (1963) Adherence to maintenance therapy and rehospitalization. Dis Nerv Syst 24:103–104
25. Falloon I, Watt DC, Shepherd M (1978) A comparative controlled trial of pimozide and fluphenazine decanoate in the continuation therapy of schizophrenia. Psychol Med 8:59–70

Long-Term Olanzapine Treatment in Schizophrenic Outpatients: Its Effects on Their Quality of Life and Clinical Outcome

Yasuo Fujii[1], Ryoji Miyata[1], Mitsukuni Murasaki[2], Kunitoshi Kamijima[3], and Gohei Yagi[4]

Summary. This multicenter, open-label study was designed to evaluate the long-term effects of olanzapine on the quality of life (QOL) of persons with schizophrenia. A total of 29 outpatients diagnosed with schizophrenia, schizotypal disorder, or schizoaffective disorder, including 18 day-care patients, were enrolled in 10 treatment facilities. The study period lasted 24 weeks and was extended to 48 to 52 weeks where possible. The patients' QOL was assessed with the Quality of Life Scale (QLS) established by Heinrichs et al. The Mean change from baseline to endpoint showed significant improvement in the total score and in all subscales of the QLS ($P \leq 0.005$). Some patients also showed improvement in real world psychosocial functioning domains. In addition, there was a noticeable decrease in hospitalization rates. Significant improvement from baseline to 24 weeks was observed in the Brief Psychiatric Rating Scale (BPRS) total and all BPRS subscores ($P \leq 0.028$) except hostility. According to the Final Global Improvement Rating (FGIR), 22 patients (75.9%) were assessed as slightly improved or better, with moderate or remarkable improvement observed in 13 patients (44.8%). In terms of extrapyramidal symptoms, significant improvement from baseline to 48/52 weeks was observed for Drug-Induced Extra-Pyramidal Symptoms Scale (DIEPSS) total, overall severity, parkinsonism, and akathisia ($P \leq 0.008$). The results of this study suggest that long-term treatment with olanzapine has beneficial effects not only in the clinical domain, but also on functional status and QOL for Japanese patients with schizophrenia living in the community.

Key words. Olanzapine, Quality of Life (QOL), Quality of Life Scale (QLS), Atypical antipsychotics, Open-label study

[1]Yamanashi Prefectural Kita Hospital, 3314-13 Kamijominamiwari, Asahimachi, Nirasaki, Yamanashi 407-0046, Japan
[2]Department of Psychiatry, School of Medicine, Kitasato University, 2-1-1 Asamizodai, Sagamihara, Kanagawa 228-8520, Japan
[3]Department of Psychiatry, School of Medicine, Showa University, 1-5-8 Hatanodai, Shinagawa-ku, Tokyo 142-8666, Japan
[4]Department of Neuropsychiatry, School of Medicine, Keio University, 35 Shinanomachi, Shinjuku-ku, Tokyo 160-8582, Japan

Introduction

Conventional antipsychotics are very helpful in alleviating the positive symptoms of schizophrenia. They also reduce the risk of relapse [1–4]. However, the use of these drugs can be accompanied by undesirable residual symptoms and serious side effects, which often interfere with a patient's ability to function in society [5–10].

Risperidone, olanzapine, and quetiapine were introduced in the United States following the reintroduction of clozapine in the late 1980s [11]. These new-generation drugs, with their low incidence of extrapyramidal symptoms (EPS) and their beneficial effects on negative symptoms, offer the possibility of improving not only the psychotic symptoms but also the patient's Quality of Life (QOL) and overall functioning [12–16].

In this Japanese clinical phase III study of olanzapine, the research was directed at studying QOL of patients, hospitalization rates, and psychosocial functions. This is the first QOL assessment study using the Quality of Life Scale (QLS) in a clinical trial involving antipsychotics and targeting outpatients, including day-care patients, in Japan.

Methods

Study Design

This study was designed as a multicenter, open-label study conducted by 16 investigators in 10 institutes from January 1996 to September 1997, under consultation by Associate Professor Yagi of Keio University. The study protocol was approved by each site's institutional or ethical review board, and signed, informed consent was obtained from all eligible patients after the procedures and possible adverse events had been explained. The patients started olanzapine therapy at 5 or 7.5 mg/day once daily. Thereafter, investigators could adjust the daily olanzapine dosage upward or downward by 2.5 mg/day every 7 days (range, 5–15 mg/day). The study period was 24 weeks and was extended to 48 to 52 weeks where possible. Concomitant medications were not allowed during the study, with the exception of limited hypnotics and anticholinergic-type antiparkinson drugs as rescue therapy.

Subjects

The patients included men or women between the ages of 18 and 64 who met the ICD-10 criteria for schizophrenia, schizotypal disorders, or schizoaffective disorders, with intelligence within the normal range. Patients could begin the study as day-care patients or as outpatients who could be examined by scheduled laboratory tests. However, a short period of hospitalization during a dose-finding period (four weeks) after the start of administration was permissible. Pregnant or lactating women or patients with serious medical illnesses were excluded. Patients with previous olanzapine medication were also excluded. In addition, patients were excluded of they had abnormal liver function test values more than twice the upper limit of the reference range, tested positive for HBs antigens or HBc antibodies, or had a history of jaundice.

Assessment

The patients' QOL was assessed with the Quality of Life Scale (QLS). The QLS was established by Heinrichs et al. at the Maryland Psychiatric Research Center [17]. The QLS was developed to evaluate the deficit syndrome in schizophrenic outpatients. The deficit syndrome is associated with impaired functioning and reduced reintegration into society [18]. The QLS was suitable for the clinical examination of the drug targeted at the effects on negative symptoms. It contains 21 items rated on a seven-point scale (scored 0 to 6) based on the interviewer's judgement of the patient's functioning. Although self-rated QOL is preferable, it would be difficult in schizophrenic patients with cognitive dysfunction. A total QLS and four subscale scores were calculated, with higher scores indicating less impairment. The four subscale scores are interpersonal relations, instrumental role category, intrapsychic foundations, and common objects and activities. The QLS ratings were obtained through semistructured interviews, conducted by trained raters, of the patient and family members. A training videotape was utilized to ensure interrater reliability. The Japanese version of the QLS and the handling manual were published by Miyata and Fujii [19], and their reliability was confirmed [20]. In addition, psychosocial functions (occupational status and heterosexual relationships in unmarried patients) and hospitalization rates were also studied.

The efficacy measures included the Brief Psychiatric Rating Scale (BPRS) [21,22], which consists of 18 items scored from 1 to 7, and the Final Global Improvement Rating (FGIR). The FGIR is a scale used to evaluate symptom progress after administration of study drug in comparison with the state of progress at the initiation of the study. The change was rated in the following seven categories: remarkable improvement, moderate improvement, slight improvement, unchanged, slight aggravation, moderate aggravation, and remarkable aggravation. When evaluation was impossible because of lack of information or confounding effects, the patient was assessed as unratable. If the improvement with the study drug was equivalent to that with the previous antipsychotic medication, the evaluation was not be changed. However, the results from the use of the previous medication were considered as an improvement with study drug.

Adverse events were observed by clinical evaluation and spontaneous reports at each visit. Hematological tests, blood biochemical tests, and a urinalysis test were also conducted and vital signs, including body weight, were measured at each visit.

Extrapyramidal Symptoms were assessed with the Drug-Induced Extra-Pyramidal Symptoms Scale (DIEPSS) [23], which is scored from 0 to 4 (higher rating represents severe symptoms), and the use of antiparkinsonian medication was also recorded. All medications, including the study drug, were recorded in the case report, and compliance was evaluated by the investigator's observation at every visit.

Statistical Methods

The primary intent of this study was to assess the efficacy, safety, and impact on QOL of olanzapine in the treatment of schizophrenic patients. The primary QOL analysis was the mean change analysis of QLS; the primary efficacy analysis was the analysis of FGIR. Because the extension period after 24 weeks was optional, 24 weeks was set as the endpoint of efficacy and QOL measurement. All obtained data were used for analysis of safety.

All endpoint analysis used a last observation carried forward (LOCF) algorithm; that is, the last available visit within the evaluated period served as the endpoint. When the mean change from baseline to the LOCF endpoint was assessed, patients were included in the analyses only if they had a baseline and a post-baseline measure. Unless otherwise defined, a baseline measure was the week 0 observation; if it was missing, then the baseline measure was the week 1 observation. The significance of the mean change was evaluated by Student's paired t-tests, and 95% confidence intervals were used for the estimation of the mean change.

Results

Baseline Characteristics

Demographic and illness characteristics are summarized in Table 1. A total of 29 out-patients (23 men and 6 women), including 18 day-care patients, were enrolled in the study. The mean age of the patients was 37.6 ± 12.0 years, with a mean age at onset of illness of 23.1 ± 6.4 years. The majority of the patients suffered from schizophrenia, but one had schizoaffective disorder and one had schizotypal disorder. Most patients (65.5%) were living with family members and had never married (89.7%). Eleven patients (37.9%) received a pension for the handicapped, and 6 patients (20.7%) received a livelihood protection pension.

All 29 patients were taking at least one antipsychotic medication prior to study entry. The most frequently used antipsychotic was haloperidol (51.7%). The mean

TABLE 1. Patient background

Item	Analysis Set ($N = 29$)
Age (yr)	37.6 ± 12.0
Onset age (yr)	23.1 ± 6.4
Duration of illness (yr)	15.0 ± 9.9
Sex	
Female	6 (20.7%)
Male	23 (79.3%)
ICD-10 Classification	
Schizophrenia (F20)	27 (93.1%)
Schizotypal disorder (F21)	1 (3.4%)
Schizoaffective disorders (F25)	1 (3.4%)
Living conditions	
Live solitarily	8 (27.6%)
Live with family	19 (65.5%)
Group home, protected home, other	2 (6.9%)
Marital history	
Never married	26 (89.7%)
Had married but unmarried now (lost spouse, divorced)	2 (6.9%)
Married	1 (3.4%)

dosage of previous antipsychotics, as measured in haloperidol equivalents, was 11.24 ± 12.00 mg/day. Antiparkinsonian medication was used by 26 patients (89.7%), and hypnotic medication was used by 14 patients (48.3%) prior to initiation of olanzapine treatment.

Patient Disposition

A total of 18 patients (62.1%) completed the study. Eleven patients (37.9%) were discontinued from the study: 5 because of acute aggravation of psychiatric symptoms (not caused by the study drug), 3 because of the physician's judgment, 2 because of adverse events or abnormal laboratory test values, and 1 because of dropout. The discontinuations due to aggravation of psychiatric symptoms were observed at 3, 6, 9, 15, and 44 weeks and were not concentrated on the time period immediately after the switch from pretreatment drugs.

Medication Use and Compliance with Study Drug

The exposure of patients to olanzapine according to modal dose is summarized in Table 2. The modal dose was defined as the dose that patients received for the greater number of days. The majority of patients (69.0%) were treated for 37 weeks or more. The most common modal dose was 10.0 mg/day (37.9% of patients). The mean modal dose of olanzapine was 10.3 ± 3.7 mg/day.

Compliance with olanzapine during the study was excellent, with the exception of one patient who was discontinued at 40 weeks because he failed to take his medication more than half the time during weeks 37 to 40.

Efficacy

The mean change in QLS from baseline to endpoint (24 weeks, LOCF) showed significant improvement in total score and in all subscales (Table 3). An improvement in QLS total score of 20 percent or more was observed for at least half of the patients at 12, 24, and 48 to 52 weeks (Table 4).

With regard to psychosocial functions, three patients had improved occupational status at 24 weeks and four had improved occupational status, whereas only one patient had reduced occupational status at 48 to 52 weeks. The patient who had reduction in occupational status could not work because of closure of his place of

TABLE 2. Patient exposure to olanzapine therapy

Duration (wk)		Modal dose (mg/day)						Total	
		2.5	5.0	7.5	10.0	12.5	15.0	n	%
1–8			2	1		1	1	5	17.2
9–16				1	2			3	10.3
17–24							1	1	3.4
37–48/52		1	2	1	9	1	6	20	69.0
Total	n	1	4	3	11	2	8	29	
	%	3.4	13.8	10.3	37.9	6.9	27.6		100

TABLE 3. QLS scores (week 24, LOCF)

OLS[a] score	N[b]	Baseline		Change		t statistic[c]	95% CI		P[d]
		Mean	SD	Mean	SD		Lower	Upper	
Total	24	38.96	17.11	13.79	13.86	4.87	7.94	19.65	<.001
Interpersonal relations	24	12.79	7.42	3.38	4.44	3.72	1.50	5.25	0.001
Instrumental role category	24	5.33	5.37	2.96	4.32	3.36	1.13	4.78	0.003
Intrapsychic foundations	24	14.67	6.68	6.46	7.28	4.34	3.38	9.53	<.001
Common objects and activities	24	6.17	2.06	1.00	1.59	3.09	0.33	1.67	0.005

QLS, Quality of Life Scale; LOCF, last observation carried forward; N, total number of patients with a baseline and at least one postbaseline score; SD, standard deviation; CI, confidence interval
[a] Items scored on a scale of 0 to 6
[b] Three patients did not have a postbaseline score; 2 patients had all postbaseline assessments excluded because of concomitant medication violation
[c] Degrees of freedom = 23
[d] Within-treatment-group mean change is tested with Student's t-test

TABLE 4. QLS total score response rates (20% or greater QLS improvement)

Week	N	Patients responding		95% CI	
		n	%	Lower	Upper
12	22	11	50.0	28.2	71.8
24	24	14	58.3	36.6	76.6
48/52	24	14	58.3	36.6	76.6

OLS, Quality of Life Scale; N, total number of patients with a baseline and a postbaseline score; CI, confidence interval

employment rather than his own volition. Furthermore, two patients improved their dating status at 24 weeks, and three improved it at 48 to 52 weeks.

Hospitalization rates in the year of this study were significantly lower than those in the year prior to the study. Three hospitalizations occurred during the study period, compared with 15 during the previous 12 months (Fig. 1). Among the 10 patients who continued olanzapine treatment for 12 months, there was only 1 re-hospitalization during the study period, compared with 10 hospitalizations during the previous 12 months.

Significant improvement from baseline to 24 weeks was observed in BPRS total and all BPRS factor total scores ($P \leq 0.028$) except hostility ($P = 0.442$) (Table 5). In FGIR (24 weeks, LOCF), 22 patients (75.9%) were assessed as slightly improved or better, with moderate or remarkable improvement observed in 13 (44.8%) patients. Three patients (10.3%) were assessed as having slight to remarkable aggravation (Table 6).

Safety

Of the 29 patients enrolled in the study, 27 (93.1%) had at least one treatment-emergent adverse event while receiving olanzapine (Table 7). The most commonly

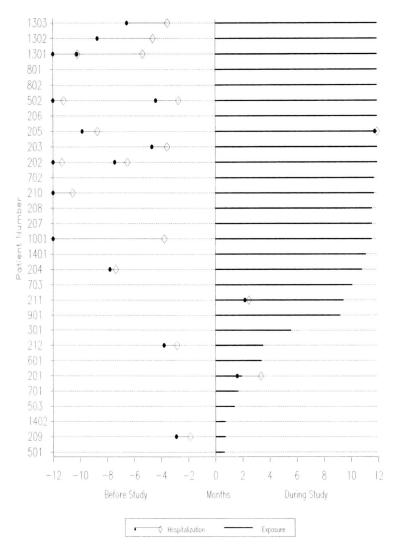

FIG. 1. Hospitalization one year before and during the study

reported treatment-emergent adverse events (≧10% incidence) were insomnia, appetite increase, weight increase, sleepiness, malaise, excitement, depressed state, nasal obstruction, dizziness, blood pressure decrease, diarrhea, anxiety, weight decrease, weakness, akathisia, nausea, vomiting, constipation, and common cold syndrome. The majority of the events were of mild severity. Adverse events such as excitement, insomnia, and anxiety may represent symptoms of schizophrenia.

Six patients (20.7%) had a serious adverse event. Three of these patients were hospitalized for worsening of schizophrenia, and one patient was hospitalized post-study

TABLE 5. BPRS scores (week 24, LOCF)

BPRS[a] score	N[b]	Baseline Mean	SD	Change Mean	SD	t statistic[c]	95% CI Lower	Upper	P[d]
Total	26	41.19	9.94	−9.23	8.06	−5.84	−12.49	−5.97	<.001
Anxiety depression	26	9.19	3.50	−3.08	3.46	−4.53	−4.48	−1.68	<.001
Anergia	26	12.81	3.95	−4.12	2.85	−7.37	−5.27	−2.97	<.001
Activation	26	5.73	1.76	−0.85	1.52	−2.85	−1.46	−0.23	0.009
Thought disturbances	26	8.46	3.75	−0.96	2.11	−2.33	−1.81	−0.11	0.028
Hostility	26	5.00	2.21	−0.23	1.50	−0.78	−0.84	−0.38	0.442

BPRS, Brief Psychiatric Rating Scale; LOCF, last observation carried forward; N, total number of patients with a baseline and at least one postbaseline score; SD, standard deviation; CI, confidence interval

[a] Items scored on a scale of 1 to 7

[b] One patient did not have a postbaseline score; 2 patients had all postbaseline assessments excluded because of concomitant medication violation

[c] Degrees of freedom = 25

[d] Within-treatment-group mean change was tested with Student's t-test

TABLE 6. FGIR scores (week 24, LOCF)

+++	++	+	+/−	-	--	---	Unratable	n (%) Total
3 (10.3)	10 (34.5)	9 (31.0)	1 (3.4)	0 (0.0)	3 (10.3)	0 (0.0)	3 (10.3)	29

13 (44.8)
(95% CI = 26.5, 64.3)

22 (75.9)
(95% CI = 57.7, 89.7)

3 (10.3)
(95% CI = 2.9, 26.5)

+++ Remarkable improvement, ++ Moderate improvement, + Slight improvement, +/− Unchanged, - Slight aggravation, -- Moderate aggravation, --- Remarkable aggravation. CI, confidence interval; FGIR, Final Global Improvement Rating; LOCF, last obstruction carried forward

for dysphagia. One patient died, possibly by suicide, during the study. One patient was discontinued from the study after experiencing suicidal ideation, and was presumed to have committed suicide post-study.

In terms of extrapyramidal symptoms, significant improvement from baseline to 48 to 52 weeks was observed for DIEPSS total, overall severity, parkinsonism, and akathisia ($P \leq 0.008$) (Table 8). Use of antiparkinsonian medication was greatly reduced from 89.7% prior to olanzapine treatment to 34.5% during the treatment period. Seventeen patients (58.6%) used hypnotic medication during the study.

Abnormalities in laboratory analytes that were most commonly identified ($\geq 10\%$ incidence) as adverse drug reactions were increased aspartate aminotransferase/

TABLE   7. Treatment-emergent   adverse events

Event	Analysis set[a] (N = 29)	
	n	%
Insomnia	10	34.5
Appetite increase	9	31.0
Weight increase	8	27.6
Sleepiness	7	24.1
Malaise	6	20.7
Excitement	6	20.7
Depressed state	6	20.7
Nasal obstruction	5	17.2
Dizziness	4	13.8
Blood pressure decrease	4	13.8
Diarrhea	4	13.8
Anxiety	4	13.8
Weight decrease	3	10.3
Weakness	3	10.3
Akathisia	3	10.3
Nausea	3	10.3
Vomiting	3	10.3
Constipation	3	10.3
Common cold syndrome	3	10.3

[a] 27 of 29 (93.1%) patients had at least one treatment-emergent adverse event

TABLE 8. DIEPSS scores (week 24, LOCF)

DIEPSS score	N[a]	Baseline			Change			P[b]
		Median	Mean	SD	Median	Mean	SD	
Total (items 1–8)	28	3.5	4.4	4.4	−2.0	−3.5	4.1	<.001
Parkinsonism (items 1–5)	28	2.5	2.9	2.8	−2.0	−2.3	2.5	<.001
Akathisia (item 6)	28	0.0	0.9	1.2	0.0	−0.7	1.2	0.008
Dystonia (item 7)	28	0.0	0.3	0.8	0.0	−0.2	0.7	0.188
Dyskinesia (item 8)	28	0.0	0.3	0.9	0.0	−0.3	0.8	0.188
Overall severity (item 9)	28	1.0	1.4	1.1	−1.0	−0.9	1.0	<.001

DIEPSS, Drug-Induced Extra-Pyramidal Symptoms Scale; LOCF, last observation carried forward; N, total number of patients with a baseline and at least one postbaseline score; SD, standard deviation
[a] One patients' date were excluded because of concomitant antipsychotic medication
[b] Within-treatment-group change was tested with Wilcoxon signed rank test

serum glutamic oxaloacetic transaminase (AST/SGOT) (14.3%), increased alanine aminotransferase/serum glutamic pymvic transaminase (ALT/SGPT) (25.0%), increased gamma GTP (21.4%), and increased creatine phosphokinase (11.1%). The serum prolactin level was decreased to 39.02 ± 23.07% URL (upper reference limit) from 142.77 ± 160.65% URL at baseline.

Treatment-emergent weight increase as an adverse event was reported for eight patients (27.6%). Overall, weight increase was not of concern. Weight increase ≧10%

was observed in four (14.8%) patients at any point in time during olanzapine treatment and in two (7.4%) at the endpoint. The mean change in body weight from baseline to endpoint was 1.50 ± 4.18kg, not a statistically significant change ($P = 0.074$).

Discussion

When considering the clinical significance of new drugs in general, it is important to examine the therapeutic outcomes of each drug independently. Whereas therapeutic outcomes in patients with schizophrenia should be evaluated from many aspects, social function and QOL of patients, well-being of their family, public safety, and health-care costs have recently become increasingly important, as well as the improvement of psychopathology and prevention of relapse [14,24–26]. However, these kinds of investigations are in their infancy and are extremely rare in Japan. Although this study had a small sample size and no control arm, it was meaningful to examine the effects of this new drug on QOL in patients with chronic schizophrenia in the development process as a phase III clinical trial of olanzapine in Japan.

It is also important to note that more than two-thirds of the included patients were under day care. Schizophrenic patients are treated mainly in psychiatric hospitals in Japan, and thus it is suggested that psychiatric rehabilitation is still insufficient. In spite of this situation, day care has been administered over the last 10 years in many hospitals as a core rehabilitation program for chronic schizophrenia. More positive psychosocial rehabilitation is being used with day care patients than with other patients. Consequently, these treatments give day-care patients opportunities to participate in social activities at a higher level. On the other hand, positive and negative symptoms are found in day-care patients, and hence they should be hospitalized once symptoms are aggravated.

Some reports mention the treatment effects of atypical antipsychotics using QLS. In an open-label, six-month clozapine study of 38 patients with treatment-resistant schizophrenia, the QLS was indicated a favorable response [27]. The mean QLS total score was 36.9 ± 26.9 at baseline and 59 ± 21.4 six months after starting clozapine treatment, an increase of approximately 20 points. Breier et al. performed the same kind of study, including chronic schizophrenic outpatients who had a history of residual positive and negative symptoms after trials of conventional neuroleptics [28]. The mean QLS total score in this study was 44.5 ± 19 at baseline, which was higher than the above, 47.6 ± 23 at 6 months and 54.2 ± 28 at 12 months after starting clozapine treatment. Although the QLS total score increased gradually, no statistically significant differences in QLS between baseline and both endpoints were observed. In these two studies, there was significant improvement in BPRS total score, and the duration of hospitalization was reduced. These results clearly mean that clozapine was effective in improving psychotic symptoms. Therefore, it should be discussed whether improvement of psychopathology would effect QLS evaluation, and how long it would take until such an improvement impacted the scale. It should be considered that some factors other than psychotic symptoms affect the evaluation from QLS. If QLS score decreased due to adverse events and/or movement disabilities caused by conventional antipsychotics, it might be possible to increase the score in a shorter time by switching to atypicals. It might take longer for conventional antipsychotics to improve social functions of patients, and consequently those improvements might affect the QLS score.

With regard to olanzapine, QOL of schizophrenic patients was researched using QLS in the double-blind, randomized, multicenter trials with haloperidol. A total of 828 outpatients diagnosed with schizophrenia, schizotypal disorder, or schizoaffective disorder participated in the global double-blind study and evaluated their quality of life with the QLS [29]. In the study, the baseline QLS total score was 51.6 ± 20.9, and the mean changes were 6.5 ± 14.9 at 6 weeks and 13.2 ± 19.0 at 52 weeks. A total of 335 schizophrenic patients participated in the North American study, which had three olanzapine dosage arms, and they were also evaluated on their QOL by QLS [30]. The mean change in QLS total score from baseline to 24 weeks was 6.7 ± 26.4 in the group receiving 5 ± 2.5 mg/day, 24.6 ± 26.2 in the group receiving 10 ± 2.5 mg/day, and 15.5 ± 21.5 in the group receiving 15 ± 2.5 mg/day. Olanzapine at doses of 10 ± 2.5 mg/day and 15 ± 2.5 mg/day significantly improved QLS total score as compared with baseline ($P \leq .004$).

In the current study, the baseline QLS total score (38.96 ± 17.11) was similar to the results of Meltzer's clozapine study; the patients whose QOL was more severe than that in Revicki's study seemed to be enrolled in this study. For such severe patients, olanzapine increased the QLS total score at 24 weeks by 13.79 ± 13.86 points from baseline. This result suggests that olanzapine has efficacy on QOL in Japanese patients with schizophrenia. Furthermore, according to analysis of responders (defined by 20% or more improvement in QLS total score), 50% of the patients responded at 12 weeks and 58.3% responded at 24 weeks and 48 to 52 weeks. In Hamilton's study, the responder rates were 32.7% at 6 weeks, 44.1% at 14 weeks, 49.7% at 22 weeks, and 55.7% at 52 weeks. Although the time course of QLS improvement should be studied to obtain longer-term data, these results suggest that improvement of QLS total score may be observed at comparative stages and may plateau at approximately six months.

In addition to QLS evaluation, occupational status and heterosexual relationships in unmarried patients were studied, and improvements in these functions were observed in some patients. Although other factors besides medical treatment might influence the change in these psychosocial functions, it is important to study this area in the future.

It is known that atypical antipsychotics such as risperidone can reduce the frequency and duration of hospitalization compared with typical antipsychotics [31–35]. The cumulative relapse rate under olanzapine treatment for outpatients was not compared with haloperidol [36], and the duration of hospitalization with olanzapine treatment was less than that with haloperidol treatment [25]. Olanzapine also reduced the frequency of hospitalization in Japanese schizophrenic patients, which corresponds to the international findings.

Some reports demonstrate that olanzapine has antipsychotic effects equal to or greater than those of haloperidol and fewer extrapyramidal symptoms [37–39]. The efficacy and safety of olanzapine were also confirmed in Japanese patients in this study from the improvements in BPRS, FGIR, and DIEPSS score.

One patient in this study fell from the seventh-story balcony of a building, suffering general contusions and death, after receiving olanzapine for 19 days. Another patient discontinued olanzapine treatment because of suicidal ideation occurring 286 days after the beginning of treatment. Suicidal thoughts and suicidal attempts are often observed in schizophrenic patients, and the risk of death by suicide is 10 times higher than in the general population [40]. It is a complex issue to discuss the relationship between drug treatment and suicidal attempts, because there can be many causes. Patients switched from typical antipsychotics to atypical antipsychotics often experience an improvement of extrapyramidal symptoms, and preliminary data suggest that atypical antipsychotics may have a favorable effect on cognitive functioning. Some problems, such as confusion, suicide attempts, and deviant behavior, occur following these changes [41–43]. In our previous study, suicidal attempts and hyperactivity appeared during the period of switching to risperidone in some patients [44]. On the other hand, clozapine reduced the risk of suicide in treatment-resistant schizophrenic patients [45]. It is inconclusive whether the patient had committed suicide or suffered an accidental fall, but the possibility of suicide is not excluded. It is therefore important to monitor a patient's condition closely when switching from a conventional to an atypical antipsychotic drug, and psychosocial supports corresponding to the change in the patient's condition are essential.

Weight increase is a commonly observed adverse event during treatment with antipsychotic medications, particularly atypical antipsychotics, including clozapine and olanzapine [46,47]. In this study, increased body weight was observed, but it was not statistically significant. Further long-term research on this matter is needed.

Elevation of prolactin levels is clinically important because it is related to adverse effects such as amenorrhea and impotence. In this study, mean prolactin levels declined substantially during olanzapine treatment, and no patients taking olanzapine had increased prolactin levels. It has been demonstrated that the incidence of elevated prolactin levels with olanzapine treatment is lower than that with haloperidol treatment and the value is smaller [48]. Such clinical characteristics of olanzapine demonstrate its superiority to typical antipsychotics and risperidone.

Conclusions

The results of this study suggest that long-term treatment with olanzapine has beneficial effects not only in the clinical domain, but also on functional status and quality of life for Japanese patients with schizophrenia living in society.

References

1. Carpenter WTJ (1996) Maintenance therapy of persons with schizophrenia. J Clin Psychiatry 57(Suppl 9):10–18
2. Hogarty GE, Goldberg SC, Schooler NR, et al (1974) Drug and sociotherapy in the aftercare of schizophrenic patients. Arch Gen Psychiatry 31:603–608
3. Kane JM, Rifkin A, Woerner M (1983) Low-dose neuroleptic treatment of outpatient schizophrenics I. Preliminary results for relapse rates. Arch Gen Psychiatry 40:893–896
4. Kissling W (1992) Ideal and reality of neuroleptic relapse prevention. Br J Psychiatry 161(Suppl 18):133–139
5. Awad AG (1994) Subjective response to neuroleptics and the quality of life: implications for treatment outcome. Acta Psychiatr Scand 89(Suppl 380):27–32

6. Awad AG, Hogan TP, Voruganti LNP, et al (1995) Patients' subjective experiences on antipsychotic medications: implications for outcome and quality of life. Int Clin Psychopharmacol 10(Suppl 3):123–132
7. Kane JM (1994) Clozapine: negative symptoms and extrapyramidal side effects. J Clin Psychiatry 55(Suppl B):74–77
8. Lewander T (1994) Neuroleptics and the neuroleptic-induced deficit syndrome. Acta Psychiatr Scand 89(Suppl 380):8–13
9. Van Putten T, May PRA (1978) "Akinetic depression" in schizophrenia. Arch Gen Psychiatry 35:1101–1107
10. Van Putten T, Marder SR (1987) Behavioral toxicity of antipsychotic drugs. J Clin Psychiatry 48(suppl):13–19
11. Kane JM, Honigfeld G, Singer J, et al (1988) Clozapine for the treatment-resistant schizophrenic. Arch Gen Psychiatry 45:789–796
12. Franz M, Lis S, Pluddemann K, et al (1997) Conventional versus atypical neuroleptics: subjective quality of life in schizophrenic patients. Br J Psychiatry 170:422–425
13. Green MF (1996) What are the functional consequences of neurocognitive deficits in schizophrenia? Am J Psychiatry 153:321–330
14. Meltzer HY (1992) Dimensions of outcome with clozapine Brit J Psychiatry 160(suppl 17):46–53
15. Meltzer HY, Thompson PA, Lee MA, et al (1996) Neuropsychological deficits in schizophrenia: relation to social function and effect of antipsychotic drug treatment. Neuropsychopharmacoly 14(Suppl 3):27S–33S
16. Sullivan G, Wells KB, Leake B (1992) Clinical factors associated with better quality of life in a seriously mentally ill population. Hosp Commun Psychiatry 43:794–798
17. Heinrichs DW, Hanlon TE, Carpenter WT Jr (1984) The quality of life scale: an instrument for rating the schizophrenic deficit syndrome. Schizophr Bull 10:388–398
18. Kirkpatrick B, Buchanan RW, Mckenney PD, et al (1989) The schedule for the deficit syndrome: an instrument for research in schizophrenia. Psychiatr Res 30:119–123
19. Miyata R, Fujii Y (1995) Quality of Life Scale (QLS): guide to its usage. Seiwa Shoten, Tokyo
20. Miyata R, Fujii Y, Inagaki A, et al (1995) Reliability of the Japanese version of Quality of Life Scale (QLS). 91st Annual Meeting of the Japanese Society of Psychiatry and Neurology, Nagasaki
21. Overall LE, Gorham DR (1962) The Brief Psychiatric Rating Scale. Psychol Rep 10:799–812
22. Miyata R, Fujii Y, Inagaki A, et al (1995) Reliability of the Japanese version of Brief Psychiatric Rating Scale (BPRS). Clin Eval 23:357–367
23. Inada T (1996) Evaluation and diagnosis of drug-induced extrapyramidal symptoms: commentary on DIEPSS and guide to its usage. Seiwa Shoten, Tokyo
24. Foster RH, Goa KL (1998) Risperidone: a pharmacoeconomic review of its use in schizophrenia. Pharmacoeconomics 14:97–133
25. Hamilton SH, Revicki DA, Edgell ET, et al (1999) Clinical and economic outcomes of olanzapine compared with haloperidol for schizophrenia. Results of a randomized clinical trial. Pharmacoeconomics 15:469–480
26. Lehman AF (1996) Evaluating outcomes of treatments for persons with psychotic disorders. J Clin Psychiatry 57(Suppl 11):61–67
27. Meltzer HY, Burnett S, Bastani B, et al (1990) Effects of six months of clozapine treatment on the quality of life of chronic schizophrenic patients. Hosp Commun Psychiatry 41:892–897
28. Breier A, Buchanan RW, Irish D, et al (1993) Clozapine treatment of outpatients with schizophrenia: outcome and long-term response patterns. Hosp Commun Psychiatry 44:1145–1149

29. Revicki DA, Genduso LA, Hamilton SH, et al (1999) Olanzapine versus haloperidol in the treatment of schizophrenia and other psychotic disorders: Quality of life and clinical outcomes of a randomized clinical trial. Qual Life Res 8:417–426

30. Hamilton SH, Revicki DA, Genduso LA, et al (1998) Olanzapine versus placebo and haloperidol: Quality of life and efficacy results of the North American double-blind trial. Neuropsychopharmacology 18:41–49

31. Addington DE, Jones B, Bloom D, et al (1993) Reduction of hospital days in chronic schizophrenic patients treated with risperidone: a retrospective study. Clin Therapeut 15:917–926

32. Albright PS, Livingstone S, Keegan D, et al (1996) Reduction of healthcare resouce utilisation and costs following the use of risperidone for patients with schizophrenia previously treated with standard antipsychotic therapy. Clin Drug Invest 11:289–299

33. Csernansky J, Okamoto A, Brecher M (1999) Risperidone vs haloperidol for prevention of relapse in schizophrenia and schizoaffective disorders: a long-term double-blind comparison. Biological Psychiatry Annual Meeting, Washington, DC

34. Lindstrom LH, Eriksson B, Hellgren A, et al (1995) Efficacy and safety of risperidone in the long-term treatment of patients with schizophrenia. Clin Ther 151:825–835

35. Viale G, Mechling L, Durkin M, et al (1997) Impact of risperidone on the use of mental health care resources. Psychiatr Serv 48:1153–1159

36. Tran PV, Dellva MA, Tollefson GD, et al (1998) Oral olanzapine versus oral haloperidol in the maintenance treatment of schizophrenia and related psychosis. Br J Psychiatry 172:499–505

37. Beasley CMJ, Tollefson GD, Tran PV (1997) Efficacy of olanzapine: an overview of pivotal clinical trials. J Clin Psychiatry 58(Suppl 10):7–12

38. Beasley CMJ, Tollefson GD, Tran PV (1997) Safety of olanzapine. J Clin Psychiatry 58(Suppl 10):13–17

39. Fulton B, Goa KL (1997) Olanzapine: a review of its pharmacological properties and therapeutic efficacy in the management of schizophrenia and related psychoses. Drugs 53:281–298

40. Allebeck P (1989) Schizophrenia: a life shortening disease. Schizophr Bull 15:81–89

41. Cooper H, Klewe J (1995) Insight and acceptance of the need for medication. Primary Care Psychiatry 2(Suppl 1):1–3

42. Larsen P, Ashleigh EA (1996) Response to risperidone: a two edged sword? J Calif Alliance Mentally Ill 7:17–18

43. Weiden P, Aquila R, Standard J (1996) Atypical antipsychotic drugs and long-term outcome in schizophrenia. J Clin Psychiatry 57(Suppl 11):53–60

44. Fujii Y, Hayama T, Inagaki A, et al (1998) Switching from conventional antipsychotics to risperidone for schizophrenic patients and one year follow-up. Jpn J Psychopharmacol 1:527–541

45. Meltzer HY, Okayli G (1995) Reduction of suicidality during clozapine treatment of neuroleptic-resistant schizophrenia: impact on risk-benefit assessment. Am J Psychiatry 152:183–190

46. Allison DB, Mentore JL, Heo M, et al (1998) Weight gain associated with conventional and newer antipsychotics: a meta-analysis. 21th CINP, Glasgow

47. Wirshing DA, Wirshing WC, Kysar L, et al (1999) Novel antipsychotics: comparison of weight gain liabilities. J Clin Psychiatry 60:358–363

48. Crawford AMK, Beasley CMJ, Tollefson GD (1997) The acute and long-term effect of olanzapine compared with placebo and haloperidol on serum prolactin concentrations. Schizophr Res 26:41–54

Keynote Lecture: The Integration of Innovative Biomedical and Psychosocial Strategies into Clinical Practice

Ian R.H. Falloon[1], Rita Roncone[2], Patrizia Giosiu[2], Chiara Mela[2], Tilo Held[3], John Coverdale[1], and the Optimal Treatment Project Collaborators

Summary. In recent years, advances in neurobehavioral research have begun to contribute to the development of more effective therapeutic interventions. It is now evident that the vulnerability to schizophrenic disorders is complex, and includes combinations of factors such as genetics, brain injury, and endogenous and exogenous toxins. However, as with most major illnesses, the biomedical factors are only part of the equation, and psychosocial stressors appear to play an important role in determining the onset and long-term course of the disorder. Comprehensive treatment that integrates the strategies designed to modify the biomedical factors with those designed to modify the social and psychological factors appears to lead to substantial improvements in the rates of recovery from the impairment, disability, and handicaps associated with these disorders. The application of these integrated treatment strategies requires a teamwork approach that ensures that optimal treatment is individualized, targeted to recovery of functioning, and provided throughout the entire course of the disorder. Such an approach has been demonstrated as feasible in centers throughout the world. However, only a tiny proportion of cases are receiving the benefits of such an approach. The challenge for the new century is to ensure that every person with a schizophrenic disorder receives the optimal treatment, until they have all made a full and lasting recovery.

Key words. Schizophrenia, Integrated, Biomedical, Psychosocial, Evidence-based treatments

Background

Schizophrenia is a medical disorder with one of the largest socioeconomic burdens on sufferers, carers, and the community [1]. Until recently, the recovery rate from

Advanced Research Institute for Effective Treatment and Education: ARIETE Perugia, Italy
[1] Department of Psychiatry & Bahavioural Science, School of Medicine, University of Auckland, Private Bag 92019, Auckland, New Zealand
[2] Dipartmento di Medicina Sperimentale, Universita L'Aquila, Coppito, Blocoo 11, 67100 L'Aquila, Italy
[3] Wilhelm Levison Str. 23, 53115 Bonn, Germany

schizophrenia had not changed from the 13% reported by Kraepelin almost a century ago [2]. This has led to the view that palliative care was the best that could be offered people who were considered to be suffering a slowly degenerative brain disease. At best, treatment could only control the behavioral excesses of the disorder [3]. Social care and support of a "hospice" variety took precedence over effective treatment and restoration of functioning until research and political pressure suggested that our hospital care was possibly contributing to the handicaps of patients and, moreover, was a major public expense. Care in the community became the slogan for closing hospitals, but not for curing disorders.

Forty years have passed since the pioneers of home-based care initiated a revolution in housing and social support for people with schizophrenia. During that time several major advances in treatment strategies have been developed and refined. These have included drug strategies, psychoeducation, stress management strategies, skills-based rehabilitation training, and specific cognitive-behavioral strategies. It is our point of view that the refinement of these approaches, supported by well-designed controlled research trials, has achieved a level where they should be readily available for every person with a schizophrenic disorder. Recent authoritative reviews have drawn similar conclusions with remarkable consensus on those strategies that should be provided in standard clinical practice [4–7]. This paper will outline a theoretical base for integrating biomedical, social, and psychological strategies and describe an international initiative to assist in the development of optimal services.

The Vulnerability/Stress Model

Advances in the treatment of schizophrenia have been derived largely from a research-based model of its pathogenesis. Although the precise causes of schizophrenic disorders remain unclear, several factors that appear to increase the risk of the characteristic psychotic episodes have been elucidated. The hypothesis that has the clearest support is that psychotic episodes result from a disturbance of brain chemistry that is triggered by stress. Risk factors for the chemical imbalance include hereditary, prenatal developmental anomalies, some of which may be caused by in-utero viral infections, birth injury or later serious brain injury, endogenous and exogenous toxins (such as fevers, encephalitis, hallucinogenic and stimulant drugs), and withdrawal from alcohol and other sedative drugs [8,9]. Of course some toxic factors are readily reversed, at least theoretically if not in practice, and tend to contribute to brief psychotic disorders, which recur only if the toxic state recurs. The precise abnormalities and areas of the brain that are affected may be clarified as technological innovations allow greater refinement in studies of brain anatomy and physiology. This may help the clinician to target medication to the specific deficits of specific individuals. Control of neuroviruses, improved obstetric care, reductions in severe head injuries, and less substance abuse may all contribute to a reduced vulnerability to schizophrenic disorders. Lower incidence of some of these factors may account for the observed reduced incidence of schizophrenia in countries with effective public health services [10–13].

Stress factors have been associated with the onset and exacerbation of psychotic episodes. Studies of ambient stress have found a consistent association between exacerbations and high levels of interpersonal stress in the social environment [14]. Almost all these studies have used the Camberwell Family Interview and the Expressed Emotion Index that is derived from this. Where one or more people living in, or in frequent contact, with the person who has had one or more episodes of schizophrenia express critical or overinvolved attitudes towards that person, the risk of further major episodes is increased three to four times. A similar increase in risk of exacerbation is seen when the individual has a life event that is experienced as highly stressful [15]. Fewer studies have been conducted on life events stress, and the results are less consistent [16]. Very few studies have examined all types of stress impinging on the vulnerable individual at any one time, or the cumulative effects of continued stresses. However, on the strength of the current data, it seems reasonable to conclude that when a person who is biologically vulnerable to schizophrenia experiences high levels of stress in the social environment there is a risk of developing psychotic episodes. Thus, it has been concluded that strategies that lead to a reduction in stress, or enhance a person's ability to cope with stresses, would improve the course of the disorder. Unfortunately, few studies of stress factors have explored these issues. There is evidence that the presence of a supportive relationship in the person's immediate social network may counter the stress of a coexisting stressful home environment [17]. Further, effective coping behaviour has been shown to modify the pathogenic effects of life events stress [18]. Further research that examines all forms of stress in a prospective, longitudinal way may elucidate this important factor and may lead to greater specificity in psychosocial strategies.

Comprehensive Assessment Strategies: Case Management

Key to effective case management is assessment of all the specific biomedical vulnerability and life stresses of each patient. This enables specific treatment strategies to be chosen that are targeted to resolve those individual problems. This process is aided by standardized rating procedures, including straightforward measures of outcome, particularly the achievement of the personal life goals of each person. The vulnerability/stress model provides a clear rationale for a comprehensive assessment that includes medical and psychiatric history; pattern of symptoms and diagnosis; comprehensive medical screening; family history; social factors—current stresses in social support system and major life stressors, including problems of housing, finances, and basic support; social and coping skills; and side effects and stresses associated with medication and psychosocial treatment currently provided, including the benefits and stresses associated with the treatment process. In the traditional hospital setting, these assessments were conducted in a somewhat piecemeal fashion by referral to the different disciplines within the team, e.g., medical, nursing, psychology, social work, and occupational therapy. Community-based assessments have integrated this process to enable all members of the team to conduct comprehensive assessments, at least at a basic screening level. However, it is important that all key aspects of the assessment be completed in all patients, and that assessments be closely supervised by the professional representatives of each discipline, who are readily available to provide more specialized assessment when indicated. For example, nurses and other key workers can be trained to conduct standardized psychiatric histories and mental status examinations, aided by instruments such as the CPS-50, SCID, Brief Psychiatric Rating Scale (BPRS), or Positive and Negative Syndrome Scale (PANSS). However, each assessment should be reviewed with a team psychiatrist, who may decide to conduct further assessment on some aspects that are not clear. The same key worker may complete an assessment of the patient's interpersonal support network, which should be reviewed by the team social worker. In most cases such reviews can be conducted in group meetings similar to the hospital ward round, with more detailed review and supervision arranged individually. In summary, it is crucial that the same rigor applied in good hospitals is replicated in all mental health services in the community.

Until recently psychiatry has focused extensively on the initial diagnostic assessment and formulation, and much less on assessing the beneficial outcomes of comprehensive treatment plans. The development of global measures of clinical and social outcomes has facilitated this process. Helping patients set concrete goals for their treatment and rehabilitation helps focus on the problems that they see as most critical to overcome and empowers them and their support network to become actively involved in the teamwork needed to achieve such goals [19]. In most situations, the first step to achieving personal goals is to control disabling aspects of the disorder, but not always to eliminate all symptoms, particularly if some of the unwanted effects of the treatment are more disabling than the symptoms themselves [20]. The necessity to maximize the benefits while minimizing the unwanted effects of our treatment strategies is clearly recognized when both of these aspects are assessed on a continuing basis, with the opinion of the patient given top priority.

Medication Strategies

The pharmacological management of schizophrenic disorders ranks among the greatest advances of medical science of the past century. Medications are able to induce a significant reduction in psychotic symptoms in 75% of patients. The benefits are greatest for acute hallucinations and delusions, and less beneficial for blunted affect, cognitive deficits, and autistic features [21]. An added problem is the side effects, which often contribute to the deficit states or negative syndromes, as well as adding to the overall stress that the patient must cope with from day to day [22].

Low dose continuation of medication after recovery from an acute episode has been highly effective in reducing the risk of further episodes from around 70% to 30%–40% [23]. But this long-term preventive use of drugs requires strategies to develop and maintain adherence to an adequate dosage regimen. Efforts do this have been relatively unsophisticated, usually relying on depot drugs with frequent monitoring, and the use of coercion by mental health legislation. However, educational and cognitive-behavioral strategies employed in other branches of medicine may be equally effective in psychiatry. These include patient education; involving carers; self-monitoring of benefits and unwanted effects; dosage variation within a prescribed range; titrating to the minimal effective dosage, aided by plasma assays; regular assessment of all side effects and assertive responses to them; detecting early warning signals; and rewarding good adherence behaviour, while immediately problem-solving and watching for signs of unauthorized reduced adherence [24].

It is important to recognize that even with optimal adherence to medication, not all patients respond, and not all recurrences can be prevented. If the pathophysiological reaction has been triggered by a clear increase or persistence of high stress, the most effective strategy is resolution of the stress, not an increase in the dose of medication, provided this is already within the therapeutic range [25,26]. This simple integration of biomedical and psychosocial strategies that appear to have synergistic effects may over time lead to full and lasting remissions for many people [27].

To date, well-controlled research studies have shown similar beneficial effects for all antipsychotic drugs. Recent studies of some new atypical drugs have suggested an added benefit for cases in which the response to other drugs has been minimal [6]. It is worth noting that earlier studies of new drugs with fewer sedative side effects showed similar benefits [28,29]. However, it has been suggested that any pharmacological advantages are maximized when optimal drug treatment is integrated with optimal psychosocial treatment programmes [30]. A series of reviews of clinical cohorts has suggested that depot drugs confer an advantage over oral preparations in long-term prevention of exacerbations [31]. These findings were not seen in controlled studies that compared the two types of preparations under identical conditions. It is possible that the regular nursing monitoring and added support provided by administering depot injections may be the critical variable, and could be replicated with the strategies used for the administration of oral drugs. Furthermore, these reviewers have failed to note that any marginal clinical benefits seen in controlled trials of depot drugs were often outweighed by greater side effects and greater social disability [32,33]. It is concluded that the specific indications for depot drugs should be for those cases in which oral self-administration is contraindicated by malabsorption problems or rapid metabolism, resulting in minimal plasma levels despite excellent adherence, or for people who choose this strategy after education about the clinical and social risks and benefits.

Psychoeducation

Educational strategies that were pioneered by Professor Robert Liberman in the early 1970s to give patients and their informal carers a clear understanding of the nature of their disorders and a rationale for treatment strategies have finally been accepted as a standard part of clinical practice. The specific benefits of education are in helping encourage patients and their carers to become actively engaged in comprehensive clinical management programmes and to enhance their self-efficacy with medication and stress management strategies [34–36]. Effective long-term treatment requires a shared care approach based on a shared framework of understanding. This can be achieved through good education. Such education is not merely the brief dissemination of factual information, but a process of helping people to make sense of their experiences with the disorders and with the treatments. Those people with persisting cognitive deficits will find this process may be slow and arduous, and they may need repeated brief interventions over months and years.

Carer-Based Stress Management Training

A major advance in the treatment of schizophrenia has been the reduction in major episodes when patients and their immediate carers receive training in stress management strategies that enhance the efficiency of their coping efforts. This benefit is in addition to that obtained by optimal drug therapy and reduces the risk of major exacerbations by two to three times. The most efficacious stress management programs include psychoeducation, strategies to improve interpersonal communication about personal goals and problems, and training in structured problem-solving strategies that enable everyday stresses as well as major life crises to be resolved efficiently [31,37–39]. Most of these approaches use skill training methods that help participants to actively seek and implement their own solutions to their own problems. This educative approach is contrasted to the traditional psychosocial approaches, such as the mental asylums, sheltered rehabilitation units or day centers that provide a relatively narrow range of solutions, mainly based upon *reducing* rather than *managing* stress. Undoubtedly there will are some individuals with very high biological vulnerability who will need a very gentle rehabilitation approach. But catering only for the needs of this minority may obscure the benefits of empowering the majority of sufferers to achieve their more ambitious personal life goals. The stress management training approach is not limited to natural family groups and can be applied in all forms of household or social support groups, such as hostels, schools, group homes or even in acute hospital wards. The aim of this goal-oriented strategy is not to prevent recurrences, but to enhance life quality. Just as medication needs to be titrated to maximize benefits and minimize side effects, stress levels can be balanced to maximize pleasant experiences and to minimize the effects of unpleasant events. Patients are encouraged to learn to recognize not merely the early symptoms of a major episode, but also their individual stress responses. In this way they can be alerted to the everyday experiences of excessive stress and develop a range of coping mechanisms to enable them to gradually manage to lead a full and active life. Minimally effective doses of medication may enable patients to maintain their sensitivity to the psychological and physiological effects of stress, whereas higher doses may tend to obscure them [40]. The process of learning to manage stress may lead to frequent minor exacerbations initially, which can be readily nipped in the bud by using stress reduction strategies and possibly brief increases of medication (within the therapeutic windows). This is rather similar to the management of diabetes, where patients learn to covary drugs and lifestyle to maximize their functioning [41].

Like drug treatment, there is growing evidence that a minimum amount of psychosocial treatment is needed to obtain maximum benefits. Interventions that only provide information or that last less than six months show few effects. Those continuing for at least two years have more lasting clinical and social benefits [38]. As expected, withdrawal of psychosocial treatment leads to a similar reduction of benefits to that seen when medication is withdrawn [42]. However, it seems likely that psychological treatment can be tapered off to a "low-dosage" regimen after the first three to six months of care, once there is evidence that patients and carers have acquired efficient stress management skills [43]. Boosters of greater intensity may be needed to support people through periods of major life stress, changes in biological vulnerability, or times when the early signs of symptom exacerbation may emerge. The long-term management of combinations of drug and psychosocial stress management strategies requires further sophisticated research studies to provide guidelines for optimal "dosage" regimens [23].

Social and Work Skills Training

Skills training using a cognitive–behavioral approach has not been evaluated as extensively as the psychoeducational and stress management approaches [39]. The excessive concern of research to focus on simplistic clinical outcomes such as "relapse" and hospital readmission may account for the relative lack of studies to demonstrate the value of this and other strategies that aim primarily to enhance social functioning and achievement of personal life goals [39,44,45]. Where living skills training has been integrated with carer-based stress management there is evidence that social functioning is improved, and substantial reductions in clinical morbidity are achieved [38,44,46]. It is worth noting that in these programs family members and friends are assisted in achieving their own personal goals, and are given training to assist them to improve the quality of their own lives, especially when they are providing continuing care for a chronically disabled person. Remarkably, despite the focus on improving social functioning, relatively few studies of social skills training in schizophrenia have reported benefits in this area. Part of the problem appears to be that many inventories of social functioning measure higher-order work and relationship functions that are not the targets of skills training of more disabled people. In addition, many of the studies are of relatively short duration that does not permit the achievement of major changes in social and interpersonal goals. A series of excellent long-term studies of combinations of optimal pharmacotherapy strategies with social living skills training have shown significant social improvements, with clinical stability [47–50].

Skills training strategies include role rehearsal, constructive coaching with positive feedback, and real-life practice. The best results occur when skills training is targeted to each person's chosen goals. Areas of training frequently include issues of self-care, occupational, leisure and recreation, friendship, and intimacy skills. An important part of living skills training is the development of local community resources that actively support people with disabilities associated with mental disorders [51,52]. Comprehensive integration with the full range of vocational, educational, recreational, and business resources available in the community necessitates specific communiy education and liaison strategies to minimize discrimination and to maximize citizenship for all disabled people. This reduces the need for provision of housing, work, and recreational resources by psychiatric services and allows such specialized resources to focus on those few patients who require such specialized services and cannot currently be integrated into existing community facilities. An excellent application of these principles has been the supported employment model of Professor Robert Drake that has show that many people with serious mental disabilities can be integrated into normal work environments in the community [53].

Specific Drug and Cognitive-Behavioral Strategies

When all the strategies outlined above have been applied competently, a small but significant proportion of patients continue to have residual symptoms and disability. In the past, most of these unfortunate people were considered untreatable and left in the care of long-suffering families or long-term hospitals. In recent years, strategies for treating these residual problems have been developed. These include pharmacological and psychological strategies for depressive and anxiety symptoms, sleep disorders, eating dysfunction, persistent psychotic symptoms, anger and aggression, sexual dysfunction, substance abuse, underactivity and deficit symptoms, or negative thought patterns. The criterion for general application of such strategies is that they have been tested under replicated random controlled trial conditions [54]. Unfortunately, few of these adjunctive strategies have been tested in people with schizophrenic disorders. Exceptions to this are the atypical medications and cognitive behavioral strategies for persistent psychosis [55–57], and the addition of antidepressant, anxiolytic and lithium drugs to neuroleptics for specific mood disturbances [58].

Although the long-term benefits of pharmacotherapy approaches remain unclear, a series of controlled studies of cognitive-behavioral therapy as an adjunct to optimal drug treatment shows promising results. Eight studies have now been published that show added and lasting benefits of cognitive-behavioral therapy in terms of reduction in the severity of psychotic and deficit symptoms [59–67]. However, when these specific strategies have been compared with control psychosocial treatments that involve similar time in contact with and support from therapists, the benefits have been less striking than comparisons with optimal medication alone. Indeed, the effect sizes of some of these supportive control treatments have been similar to those found in many of the early clozapine studies.

One possible conclusion from this body of research is that people with schizophrenic disorders remain highly sensitive to the positive attitudes of professional caregivers, and that all enthusiastic biomedical or psychosocial efforts to help them in a way that they clearly believe to be beneficial may assist them to deal with the stress of persisting unpleasant symptoms, and may even lead to lasting reductions in the intensity of those symptoms. The need for a collaborative educational and caring approach in the delivery of both the new drug and the psychological strategies may account for a substantial part of their benefits. Further sophisticated research may help elucidate the specific optimal components and integration of both.

The problems of comorbid mood disturbance, suicide risk, anxiety symptoms, violence, and substance abuse remain major impediments for many people with a diagnosis of a schizophrenic disorder. Early efforts to apply evidence-based cognitive-behavioral therapy strategies appear helpful, but more research is needed to establish the most effective approaches [68,69].

Training to Improve Cognitive Deficits

A limiting factor for psychosocial strategies that require learning of complex skills is the cognitive ability of the student. A notable feature of schizophrenic disorders is the discrete impairment of information-processing functions, such as sustained attention, iconic and short-term recall memory, and executive problem-solving functions [70]. Most approaches to skills training have attempted to remedy these deficits through specific teaching strategies, such as simplifying instructions, error-free learning, repetition, positive feedback, and shaping [71]. More recently, efforts have begun to focus on direct remediation of the information-processing deficits [72]. These studies remain essentially laboratory-based, although there have been some promising indications that when improvements of cognitive ability can be achieved with training, they may be associated with gains in social functioning and psychological well-being [73,74]. Preliminary results from a study of family stress management aimed at enhancing interpersonal communication and problem-solving skills have shown substantial improvements in cognitive deficits [75]. In addition, one benefit of atypical medication may be a similar amelioration of information processing [76]. All these findings require further well-controlled trials in clinical settings to demonstrate the specific benefits in terms of assisting patients to recover from the impairments of schizophrenia and the associated disabilities so that they can more readily achieve their personal life goals.

Community-Based Intensive Treatment

A series of controlled studies of alternatives to hospital admission shows that approximately 80% of crisis management can be provided effectively in locations other than the psychiatric hospital [77]. The provision of well-trained ambulatory multidisciplinary teams enables most of the intensive care functions of the hospital to be replicated in the settings most conducive to full and rapid recovery of function. The home environment is the location preferred by most patients. Mobile services enable skilled nursing strategies to be provided in almost any location in the community, including jails and general medical wards, nursing homes, hostels, boarding houses, and motels.

This process of home-based crisis management is aided by early detection of exacerbations and by training patients and their carers in basic clinical management strategies. This enables intensive care to start at the earliest phase of an exacerbation before a major crisis has developed, and then to continue well beyond traditional hospital and day hospital crisis management. When personal safety issues are of concern, it should be evident that it is the provision of *skilled nursing strategies* that is the key to effective clinical management of such problems, *not the physical settings* in which such care is provided [78]. Just as the quality of treatment provided by an inpatient unit will vary according to the availability of adequate numbers of skilled nurses, home-based crisis management is effective only when this key resource is available. Services should be discouraged from attempting to provide intensive care in any setting with insufficient staff, or with staff who are not trained to competently administer the strategies needed.

Results of Integrated Biomedical and Psychosocial Treatment Strategies

Continued minimal-dose medication has well established benefits and is used routinely in clinical practice. In contrast, the added benefits of psychosocial strategies have been less well promoted. More than 70 studies that meet high standards of controlled research design have been completed, with results consistently supporting the benefits of combined drug and psychosocial strategies in reducing the long-term morbidity of schizophrenic disorders [7,39,79]. Furthermore, it is clear that the addition of increasingly complex strategies, such as social skills training and cognitive-behavioral therapy for residual symptoms, provides even more benefits. It is tempting to consider providing all these strategies to all patients with schizophrenia. However, the preferred approach is one in which patients receive the particular strategies that they find most beneficial for the achievement of their current life goals in a targeted manner. These goals and the key problems will change over time, so it is essential to review progress regularly and to modify the treatment program accordingly.

One major area of concern is the need to train mental health professionals in the competent application of all effective strategies. In their landmark review of evidence-based treatment strategies for schizophrenia, Lehman and his colleagues [7] highlighted the problem of the untrained mental health workforce. They concluded that "Practitioners must ask themselves whether they are trained to offer the interventions that have demonstrated efficacy, including the various pharmacotherapies, family interventions, and assertive community treatment, and those for which efficacy data are growing, including social skills training and supportive employment." In a follow-up assessment of routine clinical practice in the United States [80,81], they noted that very few patients with schizophrenic disorders were receiving optimal treatment and that even basic drug strategies were poorly implemented in services. The clarion call had been largely ignored by service providers and planners.

The pharmaceutical industry provides substantial funding for the implementation of effective new products. On the other hand, public health services provide minimal funding for the implementation of effective new psychosocial strategies, which require considerably more skill than the prescribing of medication. So it is understandable that the penetration of evidence-based psychosocial strategies is a slow and poorly rewarded process, dependent mainly on the altruism of its pioneers.

A further concern that has been expressed by service providers is that the addition of effective psychosocial strategies to optimal drug therapy requires more professional time than is presently available in community-based services. However, research shows that over the course of a year, a substantial amount of professional time is actually *saved* when effective strategies are used [63,82–84]. Of course, most of this saving results from a reduction in crisis management and hospital care. In services in which hospital and community units function independently, the savings from one may be at the expense of the other. But even when this is the case, the difference between traditional supportive case management and implementation of all the strategies outlined above is relatively small. In a field trial with community nurses, Brooker and colleagues [85] showed that the weekly time spent per case was 33 minutes for the nonspecific approach and 47 minutes for the comprehensive psychosocial approach. The latter resulted in a 10-fold reduction in time spent in the hospital. The implications of this small investment in skilled community resources are clear, and would appear to answer many of the current concerns about improving mental health services while containing costs.

There can be no reasonable excuses for not implementing effective and efficient mental health strategies. The only problem for services is to choose the precise approaches to implement, to provide training of all staff, and to review the quality of application of the methods to improve and maintain competence. Manuals, workbooks and in-service training courses are readily available [38,85–87].

Optimal Treatment Project: An International Programme for Service Development and Evaluation

The Optimal Treatment Project (OTP) is a field trial of the benefits and costs of applying optimal biomedical and psychosocial strategies for schizophrenic and other nonaffective psychotic disorders over a five-year period. Multidisciplinary teams of integrated hospital and community services are trained to administer the effective treatment strategies in a competent manner, with continuous audits of their quality, and further supervision and annual updates. Independent assessments of clinical, social, carer, and economic benefits are made every three months throughout the programme. The study aims to provide optimal treatment to patients as soon after onset as possible, and hypothesizes that this will be the single best predictor of long-term recovery. However, in order to test this hypothesis, it is essential to include a wider range of patients than those experiencing their first psychotic episodes. Thus, centers are including all patients up to 10 years from onset of the initial signs of a mental disorder.

Workbooks, manuals, and consumer guidebooks have been developed and translated to enhance the consistency of treatment. More than 70 teams have been trained to competence in 18 countries. Continuous reviews are conducted to examine the fidelity of applications of these strategies and to provide continuing enhancement of the clinical skills of the treatment team. The integration of biomedical, psychological, social, and nursing strategies requires considerable teamwork. The manner in which teams work together is being assessed throughout the project.

A battery of global outcome measures has been devised that can be applied readily in clinical practice. These have been derived from existing scales. They include modified versions of the Clinical Global Impressions Scale [88], Charing Cross Disability and Distress Scales [89], Global Carer Stress Scale [90], and the Community Resource Inventory [82]. Research centers are encouraged to add biological, clinical, neuropsychological, and social measures and to employ randomized control methodology where selection of cases into the project is not representative of all cases in the community. A straightforward database using World Health Organization EPI-INFO software (supplied at no cost) has been developed for use at each center. The collaborative data are being managed at the University of Auckland, where it is anticipated that outcome data on more than 1000 cases will be available for analysis. Detailed background data, including delays until initial and comprehensive treatment, family history, premorbid social functioning, and substance use will enable predictive analyses to be conducted with power seldom available in smaller studies. Funding for each center is provided by local grants, with a small contribution to the collaborative costs. As well as providing a systematic and comprehensive approach to service development, it is hoped that the OTP will provide a model for further large-scale field trials in psychiatry.

Preliminary results have demonstrated that the full range of evidence-based strategies can be applied in routine clinical practice, and that the outcomes seem similar to those found in more rigorous randomized, controlled trials [91]. Clinical research of this kind should not be undervalued. It holds similar promise of finding new ways to facilitate recovery from major mental disorders as the important laboratory research on brain functioning. We hope that this project will be a small step to integrate both in the search for more effective cures for schizophrenic disorders.

References

1. Andrews G (1991) The cost of schizophrenia revisited. Schizophr Bull 17:389–394
2. Kraepelin E (1919) Dementia praecox and paraphrenia. Livingstone, Edinburgh
3. Shepherd M, Watt D, Falloon I, et al (1989) The natural history of schizophrenia. Psychol Med Monograph 16. Cambridge University Press, Cambridge
4. Quality Assurance Project (1984) Treatment outlines for the management of schizophrenia. Aust N Z J Psychiatry 18:19–38
5. World Health Organization (1991) Evaluation of methods for the treatment of mental disorders. WHO Technical Report Series 812, Geneva
6. Kane JM, McGlashan TH (1995) Treatment of schizophrenia. Lancet 346:820–825
7. Lehman AF, Carpenter WT, Goldman HH, et al (1995) Treatment outcomes in schizophrenia: Implications for practice, policy and research. Schizophr Bull 21:669–675
8. McGlashan TH, Johannessen JO (1996) Early detection and intervention with schizophrenia: rationale. Schizophr Bull 22:201–222
9. McGorry PD, Singh BS (1995) Schizophrenia: risk and possibility. In: Raphael B, Burrows G (eds) Handbook of studies on preventive psychiatry. Elsevier, Amsterdam, pp 491–513
10. Der G, Gupta G, Murray RM (1990) Is schizophrenia disappearing? Lancet 335:513–516
11. Eagles JM, Whalley LJ (1985) Decline in the diagnosis of schizophrenia among first admissions to Scottish mental hospitals from 1969–1978. Br J Psychiatry 146: 151–154
12. Joyce PR (1987) Changing trends in first admissions and readmissions for mania and schizophrenia in New Zealand. Aust N Z J Psychiatry 21:82–86
13. Munk-Jorgensen P (1986) Decreasing first admission rates of schizophrenia among males in Denmark from 1970 to 1984: changing diagnostic patterns? Acta Psychiatr Scand 73:645–650
14. Kavanagh DJ (1992) Recent developments in expressed emotion and schizophrenia. Br J Psychiatry 160:601–620
15. Ventura J, Nuechterlein KH, Lukoff D, et al (1989) A prospective study of stressful life events and schizophrenic relapse. J Abnorm Psychol 98:407–411
16. Hirsch SR, Bowen J, Emami J, et al (1995) A one-year prospective study of the effect of life events and medication in the aetiology of schizophrenic relapse. Br J Psychiatry 168:49–56

17. Falloon IRH (1988) Expressed emotion: current status. Psychol Med, 18:269–274
18. Hardesty JP, Falloon IRH, Shirin K (1985) The inpact of life events, stress and coping on the morbidity of schizophrenia. In: Falloon IRH (ed) Family management of schizophrenia. Johns Hopkins University Press, Baltimore
19. Falloon IRH, Talbot RE (1982) Achieving the goals of day treatment. J Nerv Ment Dis 170:279–285
20. Coverdale JH, Falloon IRH (1993) Home or hospital-based emergency care for chronic psychiatric patients? N Z Med J 106:218–219
21. Goldberg SC, Klerman GL, Cole JO (1965) Changes in schizophrenic psychopathology and ward behaviour as a function of phenothiazine treatment. Br J Psychiatry 111: 120–133
22. Wing JK (1978) Social influence on the course of schizophrenia. In: Wynne LC et al (eds) The nature of schizophrenia. Wiley, New York
23. Schooler NR (1991) Maintenance medication for schizophrenia: strategies for dose reduction. Schizophr Bull 17:311–324
24. Falloon IRH (1984) Developing and maintaining adherence to long-term drug-taking regimens: a behavioral analysis. Schizophr Bull 10:412–417
25. VanPutten T, Marder SR, Wirsching WC, et al (1991) Neuroleptic plasma levels. Schizophr Bull 17:197–216
26. McEvoy JP, Hogarty GE, Steingard S (1991) Optimal dose of neuroleptic in acute schizophrenia. A controlled study of neuroleptic threshold and higher haloperidol dose. Arch Gen Psychiatry 48:739–745
27. Falloon IRH, Liberman RP (1983) Interactions between drug and psychological therapy in schizophrenia. Schizophr Bull 9:543–554
28. Falloon IRH, Watt DC, Shepherd M (1978) A comparative controlled trial of pimozide and fluphenazine decanoate in the continuation therapy of schizophrenia. Psychol Med 7:59–70
29. Falloon IRH, Watt DC, Shepherd M (1978) The social outcome of patients in a trial of long-term continuation therapy in schizophrenia: pimozide vs fluphenazine. Psychol Med 8:265–274
30. Meltzer HY (1992) Dimensions of outcome with clozapine. Br J Psychiatry Suppl 17:46–53
31. Dixon LB, Lehman AF, Levine J (1995) Conventional antipsychotic medications for schizophrenia. Schizophr Bull 21:567–577
32. Hogarty GE, Schooler NS, Ulrich RF, et al (1977) Fluphenazine and social therapy in the after care of schizophrenic patients. Arch Gen Psychiatry 36:1283–1294
33. Schooler NR, Severe JB (1984) Efficacy of drug treatment for chronic schizophrenic patients. In: Mirabi M (ed) The chronically mentally ill: research and services. Spectrum, New York
34. Macpherson R, Jerrom B, Hughes A (1996) A controlled study of education about drug treatment in schizophrenia. Br J Psychiatry 168:709–717
35. Solomon P, Draine J, Mannion E, et al (1996) Impact of brief family psychoeducation on self-efficacy. Schizophr Bull 22:41–50
36. Atkinson JM, Coia DA, et al (1996) The impact of education groups for people with schizophrenia on social functioning and quality of life. Br J Psychiatry 168: 199–204
37. Mari JDJ, Streiner DL (1994) An overview of family interventions and relapse of schizophrenia: meta-analysis of research findings. Psychol Med 24:565–578
38. Falloon IRH, Graham-Hole V, Fadden G, et al (1996) Integrated mental health care: a programme of training in clinical management of mental disorders using effective, efficient intervention strategies within a multidisciplinary team. University of Auckland, Auckland, New Zealand
39. Penn DL, Mueser KT (1996) Research update on the psychosocial treatment of schizophrenia. Am J Psychiatry 153:607–617

40. Gruzelier J, Thornton S, Staniforth D, et al (1980) Active and passive avoidance learning in controls and schizophrenic patients on racemic propanolol and neuroleptics. Br J Psychiatry 137:131–137
41. Falloon IRH, OTP Collaborators (1997) Integrated mental health care: a guidebook for consumers and professionals. ARIETE, Perugia, Italy
42. Tarrier N, Barrowclough C, Porceddu K, et al (1994) The Salford Family Intervention Project: relapse of schizophrenia after five and eight years. Br J Psychiatry 165:829–832
43. Doane JA, Goldstein MJ, Miklowitz DJ, et al (1986) The impact of individual and family treatment on the affective climate of families of schizophrenics. Br J Psychiatry 148:279–287
44. Hogarty GE, Anderson CM, Reiss DJ, et al (1991) Family psychoeducation, social skills training, and maintenance chemotherapy in the aftercare treatment of schizophrenia. II. Two-year effects of a controlled study on relapse and adjustment. Arch Gen Psychiatry 48:340–347
45. Scott JE, Dixon LB (1995) Psychological interventions for schizophrenia. Schizophr Bull 21:621–630
46. Wallace CJ, Liberman RP (1985) Social skills training for patients with schizophrenia: a controlled clinical trial. Psychiatry Res 15:239–247
47. Hogarty GE, Kornblith SJ, Greenwald D, et al (1997) Three-year trials of personal therapy among schizophrenic patients living with or independent of family. I: Description of study and effects on relapse rates. Am J Psychiatry 154:1504–1513
48. Hogarty GE, Greenwald D, Ulrich RF, et al (1997) Three-year trials of personal therapy among schizophrenic patients living with or independent of family. II: Effects on adjustment of patients. Am J Psychiatry 154:1514–1524
49. Liberman RP, Wallace CJ, Blackwell G, et al (1998) Skills training versus psychosocial occupational therapy for persons with persistent schizophrenia. Am J Psychiatry 155:1087–1091
50. Marder SR, Wirsching WC, Mintz J, et al (1996) Behavioral skills training versus group psychotherapy for outpatients with schizophrenia: two-year outcome. Am J Psychiatry 153:1585–1593
51. Falloon IRH, Fadden G (1993) Integrated mental health care. Cambridge University Press, Cambridge
52. Lehman AF (1995) Vocational rehabilitation for schizophrenia. Schizophr Bull 21:645–656
53. Drake RE, Becker DR, Clark RE, et al (1999) Research on the individual placement and support model of supported employment. Psychiat Q 70:289–301
54. Andrews G (1996) Talk that works: the rise of cognitive behaviour therapy. Br Med J 313:1501–1502
55. Buchanan RW (1995) Clozapine: efficacy and safety. Schizophr Bull 21:579–591
56. Birchwood M (1999) Psychological and social treatments: course and outcome. Curr Opin Psychiatry 12:61–66
57. Jones C, Cormac I, Mota J, et al (1999) Cognitive behaviour therapy for schizophrenia (Cochrane Review on CD-ROM). Cochrane Library, Oxford
58. Kane JM, Marder SR (1993) Psychopharmacologic treatment of schizophrenia. Schizophr Bull 19:287–302
59. Drury V, Birchwood M, Cochrane R, et al (1996) Cognitive therapy and recovery from acute psychosis: a controlled trial. Br J Psychiatry 169:593–601
60. Haddock G, Tarrier N, Morrison AP, et al (1998) A pilot study evaluating the effectiveness of individual inpatient cognitive-behavioural therapy in early psychosis. Soc Psychiatry Psychiatr Epidemiol 34:254–258
61. Jackson H, McGorry P, Edwards J, et al (1998) Cognitively-oriented psychotherapy for early psychosis (COPE): preliminary results. Br J Psychiatry 172 (Suppl 33):93–100

62. Kuipers E, Garety P, Fowler D, et al (1997) London-East Anglia randomised controlled trial of cognitive-behavioural therapy for psychosis. I: Effects of the treatment phase. Br J Psychiatry 171:319–327
63. Kuipers E, Fowler D, Garety P, et al (1998) London-East Anglia randomised controlled trial of cognitive-behavioural therapy for psychosis. III: Follow-up and economic evaluation at 18 months. Br J Psychiatry 173:61–68
64. Pinto A, La Pia S, Mennella R, et al (1999) Cognitive-behavioral therapy and clozapine for clients with treatment-refractory schizophrenia. Psychiatr Serv 50:901–904
65. Sensky T, Turkington D, Kingdon D, et al (2000) Arch Gen Psychiatry 57:165–172
66. Tarrier N, Beckett R, Harwood S, et al (1994) A trial of two cognitive behavioural methods of treating drug-resistant residual psychotic symptoms in schizophrenic patients: I. Outcome. Br J Psychiatry 162:524–532
67. Tarrier N, Yusupoff L, Kinney C, et al (1998) Randomised controlled trial of intensive cognitive behaviour therapy for patients with chronic schizophrenia. Br Med J 317:303–307
68. Falloon IRH, Morosini PL, Roncone R, et al (1998) Cognitive-behavioral strategies for the treatment of schizophrenic disorders. In: Sanavio E (ed) Behavior and cognitive therapy today: essays in honor of Hans J. Eysenck. Elsevier Science, Oxford
69. Hafner RJ, Crago A, Christensen D, et al (1996) Training case managers in cognitive-behaviour therapy. Aust N Z J Men Health Nursing 5:163–170
70. Green M (1996) What are the functional consequences of neurocognitive deficits in schizophrenia? Am J Psychiatry 153:321–330
71. Bowen L, Wallace C, Glynn S, et al (1994) Schizophrenics' cognitive functioning and performance in interpersonal interactions and skills training procedures. J Psychiatry Res 28:289–301
72. Brenner HD, Hodel B, Roder V, et al (1992) Treatment of cognitive dysfunctions and behavioral deficits in schizophrenia. Schizophr Bull 18:21–26
73. Spaulding WD, Reed D, Sullivan M, et al (1999) Effects of cognitive treatment in psychiatric rehabilitation. Schizophr Bull 25:657–676
74. Wykes T, Reeder C, Corner J, et al (1999) The effects of neurocognitive remediation in executive processing in patients with schizophrenia. Schizophr Bull 25:291–307
75. Mazza M, DeRisio A, Pirro R, et al (2000) Psychosocial treatments: effects on cognitive functions. WAPR World Congress, Paris, 9 May 2000
76. Green M, Marswhall B, Wirshing W, et al (1997) Does risperidone improve verbal working memory in treatment-resistant schizophrenia? Am J Psychiatry 154:799–804
77. Scott JE, Dixon LB (1995) Assertive community treatment and case management for schizophrenia. Schizophr Bull 21:657–668
78. Holloway F (2000) Mental health policy, fashion and evidence-based practice. Psychiatr Bull 24:161–162
79. Falloon IRH, Held T, Coverdale JH, et al (1999) Psychosocial interventions for schizophrenia: a review of long-term benefits of international studies. Psychiatr Rehabil Skills 3:268–290
80. Lehman AF, Steinwachs DM (1998) Patterns of usual care for schizophrenia. Initial results from the Schizophrenia Patient Outcomes Research Team (PORT) client survey. Schizophr Bull 24:11–20
81. Lehman AF, Steinwachs DM (1998) Translating research into practice. The Schizophrenia Patient Outcomes Research Team (PORT) treatment recommendations. Schizophr Bull 24:1–10
82. Cardin VA, McGill CW, Falloon IRH (1985) An economic analysis: costs, benefits and effectiveness. In: Falloon IRH (ed) Family Management of Schizophrenia. Johns Hopkins University Press, Baltimore
83. Tarrier N, Lowson K, Barrowclough C (1991) Some aspects of family interventions in schizophrenia. II. Financial considerations. Br J Psychiatry 159:481–484

84. Held T (1995) Schizophreniebehandlung in der Familie. Eine kontrollierte Studie zur Wirsamkeit familiärer Verhaltenstherapie bei der Rückfallprophylaxe schizophrener Erkrankungen. Peter Lang, Frankfurt am Main

85. Brooker C, Falloon I, Butterworth A, et al (1994) The outcome of training community psychiatric nurses to deliver psychosocial intervention. Br J Psychiatry 165:222–230

86. Liberman RP and associates (1986–89) Modules for training social and independent living skills. Psychiatric Rehabilitation Consultants, Camarillo/UCLA Research Center, Box A, Camarillo, CA 93011, USA

87. McGorry P, Edwards J (1997) Early psychosis training pack. Gardiner-Caldwell Communications, Cheshire, UK

88. Guy W (1976) E.C.D.E.U. assessment manual for psychopharmacology. US Department of Health, Education, and Welfare, Washington, DC

89. Rosser RM, Kind P (1978) A scale of valuations of states of illness: Is there a social consensus? Int J Epidemiol 7:347–358

90. Falloon IRH (1985) Family management of schizophrenia. Johns Hopkins University Press, Baltimore

91. Falloon IRH, and The Optimal Treatment Project Collaborators (1999) Optimal treatment for psychosis in an International Multisite Demonstration Project. Psychiatr Serv 50:615–618

Part 6
Consumer Collaboration

What Can the Family Do as a Consumer Collaborator?

Kazuyo Nakai

Summary. These days, thanks to many professionals and nonprofessionals, family education seems to have prevailed to some extent in Japan, and family education is now changing to family empowerment. On the other hand, I wonder if families come within the psychiatrists' field of vision adequately. Generally, most doctors do not regard families as educable people or possible good collaborators. Why have we come to this circumstance? I will try to suggest a better direction for collaboration between families and professionals, especially doctors.

Key words. Zenkaren, Consumers, Family education, Psychoeducation, Informed consent

Introduction

Zenkaren (National Federation of Families of the Mentally Ill) was founded in 1965 as the sole nationwide Japanese self-help organization for families with members who are mentally ill. It now has approximately 120 000 family members belonging to 1500 branches all over the country. I am a mother of a schizophrenic daughter, and for 10 years I have worked as a counsellor in our organization. My presentation is based not on my personal experience or scientific theories, but on the voices of consumers (patients and families) I have heard during everyday consultation.

The Relationship Between Doctors and Consumers

The subject of my presentation is how consumers can collaborate with professionals, especially with psychiatrists, to achieve better treatment. The following questions is very important: Why do most psychiatrists not listen to families' voices? Why do consumers find it difficult to communicate with doctors? The main excuses from the doctors are that (1) they are always busy (too many patients and limited hours); (2) it is best to make out a prescription with silence (silence is golden in mental treat-

Zenkaren, 1-4-5 Shitaya, Taito-ku, Tokyo 110-0004, Japan

ment); and (3) they do not think family consultation is necessary (families do not come in sight of the doctors).

The main excuses from the consumers are that (1) they hesitate to ask doctors because they seem busy; (2) doctors do not respond to questions adequately (lack of suitable explanation or answer from doctors); and (3) doctors seem to get angry or irritated if consumers ask a question (doctors have high Emotional Expression).

Consumers seem to be like sheep that obey their sheepdogs. Under these conditions, doctors and consumers are far from partners or collaborators. If the sheepdogs were excellent and reliable and guided a flock of sheep in an appropriate or better direction, the consumers could remain silent sheep with no complaint. However, we found that professionals are not always professional or reliable.

An Appeal to Doctors from Consumers

Although it may sound rude or frank, I must appeal to doctors, as this symposium is a rare and precious opportunity to send consumers' messages. The following is an appeal to doctors from consumers.

A Dull Sheepdog will Remain Behind Empowered Sheep

If doctors cling to their license without brushing up their arts and knowledge, they will be behind the times and even behind consumers. Our organization provides up-to-date information by monthly newsletters and various opportunities, and especially during the last 10 years, inspired by WFSAD (World Fellowship for Schizophrenia and Allied Disorders, formerly WSF) and the World Health Organization (WHO), Zenkaren has been successful in family education. I must stress that the family education is the result of collaboration with understanding professionals and consumers.

Thanks to family education, we have learned what mental illness is, how to cope with patients, what new medicines are on the market, and, as an important and practical matter, how to communicate with doctors without making them angry or irritated. We have found that not all doctors know how to manage patients, what Expressed Emotion (EE) is, and that many doctors are reluctant to try atypical antipsychotics in our country.

For example, when a family member asks a question about how to manage a patient, some doctors are very open-minded and say, "We do not know exactly. We just consult with a patient once or twice a month, but you, as a family member, spend a lot of time with the patient. So you must know how to cope with him much better than doctors." They are very honest. Still, is it an adequate response to a family in need? We do not recognize these doctors as professionals.

Do Not Drive Sheep to the Edge of a Cliff

Although it is incredible, every year our organization must cope with the anxiety of families who ask about electroconvulsive therapy (ECT). Most of them are told to decide whether the patient should try ECT or not and to answer the doctor in a few days. Needless to say, this is a vital question for families. Nevertheless, families are not informed about ECT, except that the therapy might be somewhat effective and it is not so dangerous today. That is the information, and there is no detailed explanation about how it is administered, what kind of side effects it has, to what degree a patient is expected to recover, and so on. How can consumers decide whether or not to accept ECT under these poor conditions?

This is far from "informed consent." Doctors seem to be satisfied by just going through the procedure for the sake of form. Doctors should not throw consumers into the sea suddenly with no lifejacket.

A Sheepdog in High EE Sometimes Kills Sheep

Research on EE seems to be one of the main topics of this symposium, and family members have learned how important it is to keep EE low to reduce the relapse rate of patients. Still, I dare say that the EE theory should be highlighted not only in the patient–family relationship but also in the consumer–doctor relationship. In Japan it is as difficult to meet an understanding and supportive doctor as to find a diamond in the sand. We go to the hospital to be treated and healed, but not a few consumers become worse after visiting the hospital because of the critical comments of doctors with high EE. We strongly recommend that psychoeducation be carried out among psychiatrists to their EE low, at least during mental treatment.

Conclusion

I have stated boldly what we want mental doctors to be. If consumers are well informed and empowered, they will become good collaborators to achieve better treatment. For this purpose, consumers must continue to learn and understand the situation that we are in. Through this effort, consumers will change from obedient, silent sheep to empowered howling dogs. Aiming at the new century when consumers and professionals become real collaborators, we hope that doctors will accept and understand the appeal I have just made, having made up my mind to be frowned at by many psychiatrists.

Consumers, Carers, and Clinicians in Collaboration: What Does This Mean?

MARGARET LEGGATT

Summary. The puzzling nature of major mental illnesses creates conflict among the key players. This causes family carers, consumers (patients), and clinicians to work in different directions. In order to achieve better results for people with schizophrenia, this paper suggests a three-stage model of treatment and care that utilizes the experiential knowledge of consumers and carers along with the professional knowledge of clinicians in a process of collaboration. This process gradually changes the power dimension from the clinician to the consumer and carer, so that the latter are more able to take control of their situation as then self-esteem and confidence are restored. This further enables family carers and consumers to take on active roles as advocates and advisors in many areas of mental health policy and reform. Underlying these techniques is the basic understanding that carers, consumers, and clinicians are equal partners. Doctors must change their negative attitudes, join with family carers and consumers in an equal partnership, and support consumers and carers to develop their own strengths and resources. Some family carers and consumers are then able to become valuable assets in many aspects of treatment and care.

Key words. Consumers (patients), Family carers, Clinicians, Collaboration, Care

Of all the medical conditions suffered by human beings, it is probably the case that major mental illnesses have the greatest potential to create conflict among those key players who become involved, namely, the consumers, their family carers, and the clinicians.

The primary cause for this has been, and still is, the often puzzling nature of mental illness itself. Many of the symptoms create situations that turn people against each other. For example, paranoid ideation is frequently directed at family members. Consumers blame their families for many of their problems. Families feel ignored by the clinicians' lack of attention to their needs as carers, and insignificant because of the doctors' unwillingness to communicate with them. Doctors are often placed in unrealistic positions by families and consumers, who expect them to have all the answers and to provide a complete cure—an uncomfortable situation for doctors who are aware that major mental illnesses are not necessarily able to be cured, and that

29 Mary Street, North Carlton, 3054, Victoria, Australia

treatments may not always bring about the desired results. Frequently, the end result of these conflicts means that professionals, family carers, and consumers are isolated from each other, striving to achieve resolution of problems but often working in different directions.

Attitudes of Mental Health Professionals

In the last two decades, in Western countries that have undergone a process of transferring the treatment of the mentally ill from psychiatric institutions to community-based mental health facilities, family carer and consumer surveys have reported dissatisfaction with the therapeutic relationship between mental health clinicians and family carers and consumers. For example, two surveys from the Asian region have reported problems with this relationship. Phillips and Gao (personal communication) found that

mental health professionals tend to share community beliefs about the dangerousness and unpredictability of the mentally ill, about the burden the mentally ill place on society, about the advisability of avoiding social contacts with the mentally ill, and about the need to impose restrictions on the social activities of the mentally ill. . . . If they convey these attitudes to their patients (which is likely) they could easily magnify the damaged self-esteem of their patients and, thus, decrease patients' and family members' willingness to seek care and to comply with treatment . . . We must change clinicians' attitudes about the mentally ill, improve their understanding of the negative effects stigma and discrimination have on their patients, and provide them with interventions that they can use to help patients and family members "positively reframe" the illness. Interventions that decrease patients' and family members' loss of self-esteem and that provide hope despite the altered social status of the patient, need to become an integral component of the comprehensive treatment and rehabilitation of all schizophrenic patients.

Kim [1] states that

Among mental health professionals, attitudes towards the mentally ill, especially schizophrenic, can be characterized by . . . a tendency to focus on highly functioning patients, a tendency to have unrealistic expectations for the rehabilitation of this section of the population. There is little success or satisfaction associated with the treatment of these people because of the high refractory rates and negative prognosis and therefore a lack of personal fulfillment in one's work. It is the current consensus among Korean health care professionals that this section of the population is not worth the effort. . . . People with these diseases demonstrate behaviour which makes engagement with them difficult. There has been a general upgrading in both education and autonomy among mental health professionals. This has enabled them to move away from what has been a medically dominated field and to seek opportunities with other more diverse populations.

These negative attitudes of health care professionals towards people with schizophrenia and their families increase their already low self-esteem and loss of confidence. Health care professionals are therefore working against more positive outcomes for these consumer consumers.

How is it possible then, to work in collaboration, to work together in a more equal partnership, in order to produce better outcomes for our consumers and their family carers, and to give better work satisfaction to professionals?

A collaborative model of care can be developed that involves a process of education and training for the key players in the management of mental illness. This model emphasizes the need for clinicians, carers, and consumers to develop greater respect for each other, thus enabling a more fruitful outcome for all concerned. This model is divided into three stages.

Stage 1. Initial Contacts—Engagement

In the beginning of mental illness, families are bewildered and confused, anxious and frightened, particularly if their relative displays a total lack of insight and cannot be reasoned with. Consumers are equally terrified by their experiences. There is often denial. Clinicians need to be in control of the situation in these early stages, hence the diagram places the clinician at the top of the triangle in Fig. 1. It is often in these very early stages, though, that clinicians do not empathize enough with the distress of the patient and the family. There can be many reasons for this, but one of the major ones relates to their professional training, which tends to emphasize the need for "objectivity," often causing clinicians to behave in a cold, formal, and uninvolved manner.

In these early stages, then, it is vital that clinicians openly express greater compassion and understanding of the fears of their patients and their families, combined with a much more positive attitude of hope than they have shown in the past. It is also important for clinicians to tell families that they have not caused this illness, as well as to say that they need the families to help them in the treatment and care of the patient. This process is called "engagement," or "joining with" the carers and consumers [2].

What Is It That Families and Consumers Can Explore with the Clinician in the Engagement and Joining Process in Stage 1?

Exploration of precipitants. What stress has the consumer experienced? People with schizophrenia are sensitive to environmental pressures.

Review of prodromal symptoms and signs. These can be very specific for each individual.

These first two points are aimed at learning how to prevent relapse.

Discussion of the emotional and behavioral reactions of the family and consumer to illness.

Coping strategies. How are they coping?

Social supports. It may be too early, but clinicians should refer family members to family support organizations and consumers to peer support groups. This should be seen by clinicians as a vital part of help for families and consumers; often it is only when family members join family organizations that their emotional distress

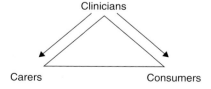

Clinicians

Carers   Consumers

FIG. 1. Stage 1: initial contacts

and then sense of isolation and powerlessness disappears, leaving them with greater energy for positive coping.

Mourning. What are their experiences of grief and loss? How are they managing this?

The last four points are designed to help families develop the best social and emotional environment in which the person with schizophrenia will be able to function most effectively.

Preparation for an education and training program. In the early stages, families and consumers cannot absorb much information. It is therefore important to recognize that education and training is a process that needs to continue for as long as it is needed.

When the doctor involves the family carers in an education and training program, the family feels reassured because they are made aware of the fact that this will be a partnership; they need not fear that they will be abandoned and have to cope by themselves. Meeting these needs through initial positive contacts with families enhances their ongoing relationship with mental health service providers and prevents the occurrence of experiences with professional workers that leave family carers feeling frustrated, angry, depressed, and powerless.

Stage 2. Rehabilitation

The rehabilitation stage is characterized by an awareness that the illness is a long-term one; that the mentally ill person is not going to make a complete recovery or to become the person with the capabilities that he or she once had. It is often a time of sadness and depression for the family as well as the consumer. It is also a time when professionals are often not as available as much as required, nor are there enough services to provide for the rehabilitation needs of consumers.

It is a time when the negative symptoms of schizophrenia become the primary focus. In the past, and still far too often, the negative symptoms were the ones of least concern to clinicians, mainly because, since the discovery of antipsychotic medications, their training emphasizes more the control of positive symptoms; they are not trained in techniques for the improvement of negative symptoms.

It is a time too, when family carers, consumers, and professionals tend to have different priorities. Shepherd et al. [3] carried out a study that revealed a general consensus on the important elements of "packages of care," but some differences in the priorities as seen by each group. The "users" (consumers) gave more emphasis to practical help (housing, finance, and occupation), whereas the professionals emphasized treatment and symptom monitoring. The families felt that everything was important. Given these different emphases, it is vitally important that the partnership among clinicians, families, and consumers does not disappear. This is the time when it is too easy for the three groups to be working in different directions.

The diagrammatic depiction of this stage (Fig. 2) shows family carers, consumers, and clinicians interacting along a straight line. This is to represent the fact that the contributions of each group to treatment and care are all of equal importance.

Carers ◄──────► Clinicians ◄──────► Consumers

FIG. 2. Stage 2: rehabilitation

Experiential Knowledge

By this stage, clinicians need to recognize that family carers and consumers have accumulated a great deal of experience in learning how to live with mental illness on a
day-to-day basis. It is often only through a trial-and-error process that families and
consumers learn the best way of coping with the symptoms and their behavioral consequences. When a consumer is unable to develop insight into his or her condition,
family members are in the best position to know whether or not the medication is
useful; they understand the person's illness better than anyone, because they are in
closer and more regular contact.

Families have many strengths and resources. These include the development of
an optimal emotional and social atmosphere, the provision of information on a very
wide range of issues, protection of their mentally ill relative from adverse community
responses, and personal connections—particularly if they belong to self-help support
groups—which they can use in the person's rehabilitation. There is a need to
work out a plan of action that shares the responsibility of treatment and care with
clinicians.

As well as relying on medication, consumers can learn a variety of psychological
and social techniques for managing the effects of their symptoms. It is important that
they feel free to reveal the nature of many symptoms and problems. Consumers report
that they do not feel free to discuss shameful matters with their clinicians, and that
these problems prevent them from making as good a recovery as possible. They need
to be able to share all of this information about their symptoms with their clinicians,
without fear of being punished or made to feel ashamed.

Problem-Solving and Empowerment

The role of the clinician in this stage of rehabilitation, as well as continuing to monitor
symptoms, is to act as a facilitator for the resolution of problems that arise, and to
help in the determination and implementation of goals that families and consumers
wish to achieve.

Structured problem-solving techniques are well documented in the literature [4].
They are "structured" because the lives of people with mental illnes and their family
carers can often become chaotic, particularly if people are working with different
goals in mind. There is a need to look at problem resolution in a formal and structured way. Problem-solving involves definition of the exact problem, listing possible
solutions to the problem, evaluation of the suggestions, choosing the most practical
solution, careful planning of how to implement the solution, and, later, a review of
progress with the plan.

When family carers and consumers learn these techniques, they become empowered to take control over their own lives; this improves their self-esteem and confidence; it helps them to realize that the illness is manageable; it helps them to realize
that they do not have to be passive victims of this illness. When this stage is success-

fully completed, then families and consumers are able to move into stage three of this model.

Stage 3. Family and Consumer Empowerment

For many family carers and consumers, Stage 3 becomes possible with an acceptance of their situation and a belief that they are able to manage their circumstances in as effective a way as possible. The diagram (Fig. 3) depicts this by placing family carers and consumers in an equal partnership, with clinicians in less of a position of control but available when and as needed. As well as continuing to use Stages 1 and 2, this acceptance can lead to family carers and consumers becoming active as advocates and advisors in a variety of different mental health areas.

Family carers and consumers can become all of the following.

Educators and Trainers of Mental Health Professionals. The experiential knowledge that family carers and consumers accumulate as they learn to live with mental illness is an essential part of mental health training. Without this, professionals tend to see only the symptoms and the need for medication; they see an illness, and not a person. Mental health service consumers wish to be accepted as human beings, not just as symptoms of a particular mental disorder. It is only when professionals learn from and accept the individuality of each patient that they will be able to provide an individualized treatment plan that the consumers and families are able to implement.

Advisors in Policy Development for Mental Health Services. Family and consumer perspectives must inform mental health policies through family and consumer advisory groups that alert governments to mental health issues.

Developers of Pilot Rehabilitation Projects. Because governments have not provided community-based services, non-government family support organizations are among those groups that have developed many pilot rehabilitation programmes.

Advocates for Community Acceptance of Mental Illness. Stigma and discrimination associated with mental ilness can be overcome when family and consumer groups themselves take on the role of community education and awareness. This means that they themselves are no longer ashamed of their illness and are prepared to talk openly about their condition. This is a hard task, and it is not achievable unless family and consumers have successfully gone through Stages 1 and 2 as described and can continue to rely on support from the shared partnership with professionals.

Educators and Trainers of Other Families and Consumers. In many countries throughout the world, family education programs and consumer peer support programs are being developed by carer organizations in which family members educate, train,

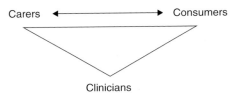

Fig. 3. Stage 3: family and consumer empowerment

and support each other [5,6]. Trained family members have the advantage of personal experience in caregiving, and are particularly appropriate for helping each other come to terms with the distressing emotions that accompany the development of mental illness in a relative. These programs are cost-effective in that families support other families without payment. Consumer groups also support each other—a process that is particularly benefical for overcoming isolation and stigma.

Summary and Conclusions

This paper recommends a three-stage progression of treatment and care for people with schizophrenia. These stages are not mutually exclusive nor do they imply that there is a steady and uncomplicated progression from one stage to the next. The model is designed to help keep in mind the overall goal of helping families and consumers learn the most effective methods of managing mental illness—methods that enable them to move from feeling passive and powerless to feeling they can be active and powerful in achieving positive outcomes.

In order to make this model effective, the greatest changes have to happen in the attitudes of clinicians, who will then need to be educated and trained in a different way of working with families and consumers. This important change must commence at the very first contact with families and consumers. This way of working with families and consumers demands an equal partnership based on mutual respect for each other's expertise. In the beginning of the development of mental illness, unless there is the development of equal partnerships with families and consumers, this model will not work, and opportunities for better outcomes may be lost.

References

1. Kim S (1999) Community-based mental health nursing programme for rehabilitation of long-term psychiatric patients. Final Report. United Nations Development Programme—Supported Project, Seoul, Korea
2. McFarlane W (1994) Families, patients, and clinicians as partners. In: Lefley H, Wasow M (eds) Helping families cope with mental illness. Harwood Academic Publishers, Poststrasse 22, 7000 Switzerland, pp 195–222
3. Shepherd G, Murray A, Muijen M (1995) Perspectives on schizophrenia: a survey of user, family carer and professional views regarding effective care. J Ment Health 4:403–422
4. Andrews G, Hunt CJ, Schmich HJ (1995) The management of mental disorders. Handbook of management skills. World Health Organization Training and Reference Centre for CIDI Fast Books in Print, Sydney, Australia, Vol 1:42–48
5. Alexander K (1991) Understanding and coping with schizophrenia—14 principles for the relatives. Schwartz and Wilkinson, Melbourne, Australia
6. Burland J (1998) Family-to-family: a trauma and recovery model of family education. New Directions for Mental Health Services 77:33–41

Part 7
Putting Effective Settings into Practice

Ensuring Quality and Continuity of Care for Psychiatric Patients Making the Transition from Hospital to Community Care in Japan

Kei Sakuma

Summary. The author introduced strategies employed in his efforts to ensure the quality and continuity of care for psychiatric patients as they make the transition from the hospital to the community in Japan. The number of psychiatric beds per 10000 people in the medical service area of Asaka Hospital is about 40, which is much higher than the average of 28.7 for Japan. Decreasing the number of hospital beds by building up an appropriate support system in the community is the aim of the policies of Asaka Hospital. The key concept in managing health care is "quality assurance," which has three main components: structure, process, and outcome. Among the structured factors, the importance of a wide spectrum of care to support patients from the hospital to the community, the amenity of the hospital unit as a therapeutic milieu, and the information management system were stressed. The Optimal Treatment Project (OTP) was employed for improving quality and continuity of care. From studying OTP as a psychosocial approach, the knowledge and skill of the staff have improved dramatically. OTP as a common language made multidisciplinary teamwork more systematic and extremely consistent for the customer. Finally, an innovative project was introduced to help patients progress from hospital beds to a combination of residential care facilities and day and night care. This project aims eventually to close small hospitals.

Key words. Schizophrenia, Psychosocial approach, Health care management, Quality assurance, Optimal Treatment Project

Introduction

In many Western countries, styles of psychiatric care have changed drastically since the 1980s, moving towards deinstitutionalization. Although many health professionals recognize the importance of such movements, changes in Japan have taken place at a slower pace than expected.

Psychiatric care in Japan is provided mainly by private hospitals. They account for about 90% of all available beds for psychiatric patients in Japan and, since the

Asaka Hospital, 45 Asakamachi, Koriyama, Fukushima 963-0198, Japan public sector does not play a major role in mental health services, must provide the majority of community-based care. Some hospitals have already shifted their style of care from inpatient-centered to outpatient-centered and also provide some degree of successful community care. However, many of them are still struggling with restructuring.

The author introduces strategies employed in his efforts to ensure the quality and continuity of care for psychiatric patients as they make the transition from the hospital to the community.

Circumstances of Asaka Hospital

In Japan 2170000 patients suffer from chronic psychiatric diseases (Table 1). About one-seventh of them are hospitalized, of whom 61% suffer from schizophrenia. In the City of Koriyama, its surrounding medical service area, and indeed throughout Fukushima Prefecture, the proportion of hospitalized patients is much higher than the national average, and there are comparatively few residential care facilities or day-care centers.

Asaka Hospital, with 581 beds, is an ordinary Japanese psychiatric hospital. It is located in a medium-sized city with a population of 330000 people, about 250km north of Tokyo. The medical service area around the hospital is about 40km in diameter, and has about 550000 residents, with more than 2000 beds available for psychiatry. The number of psychiatric beds per 10000 people in this area is about 40, which is much higher than the average of 28.7 for Japan.

Asaka Hospital consists of the 10 units: an acute care unit, a stress care unit, two dementia units, a physical comorbidity unit, a long-term refractory unit, two chronic rehabilitation units, and two units for epilepsy and other diseases (Table 2).

There are also some affiliated facilities. Sasagawa Hospital is a rehabilitation hospital with 102 beds. Kibou 98 is a kind of halfway house with 10 beds (8 single, one double). Patients can stay up to two years for life skills training. Asaka Home Care consists of three divisions: a care management center for geriatrics, a community nurse station for psychiatry and geriatrics, and a day-care center for the elderly with behavioral problems due to severe dementia. A satellite clinic is also located near the Koriyama station.

TABLE 1. Psychiatric patients and social resources; Koriyama City and its surrounding medical service area, Fukushima Prefecture, and Japan

Resource	Koriyama city and surroundings	Fukushima Prefecture	Japan
Population	557850	2132 4910	125570000
Total patients	6748	30296	2170000
Beds for psychiatry	2192	7772	336000
Beds/10000	39.4	39.9	28.7
Mean hospital days	—	524.2	423.7
Residential care facility (beds)	30	50	6728
Day care	4	14	759

TABLE 2. Asaka Hospital and its affiliated facilities

Inpatient service	Sasagawa Hospital
Acute care (1/50)	Rehabilitation hospital
Stress care (1/50)	Kibou '98
Dementia (2/95)	Residential care facility (10 beds)
Physical comorbidity	Satellite clinic
(1/69)	Nearby Koriyama Station
Chronic rehabilitation	Asaka home care
(3/192)	Case management center
Epilepsy, etc. (2/124)	Community nurse station
Outpatient service	Day care for severe dementia
Outpatient	
Day care	

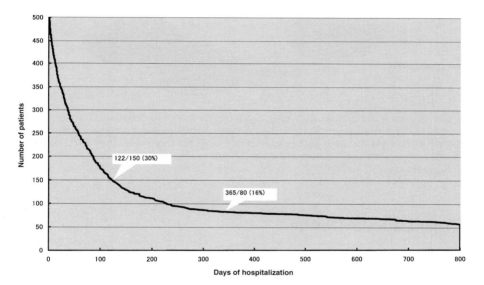

FIG. 1. Among patients admitted to Asaka Hospital in 1996–1997, 70% were discharged within four months and 84% were discharged within one year

Among 500 patients admitted to Asaka Hospital in 1996–1997, 84% were discharged within one year (Fig. 1). The strategies for long-term patients and recently admitted patients should be discussed separately, because many factors distinguish these two groups. Long-term patients often have no relatives who will allow them to live with them, and they have more difficulty in obtaining discharge from hospitals because they tend to suffer from more residual symptoms and often become hospitalized [1]. Therefore, they need a variety of specific services to help them readjust to living in the community.

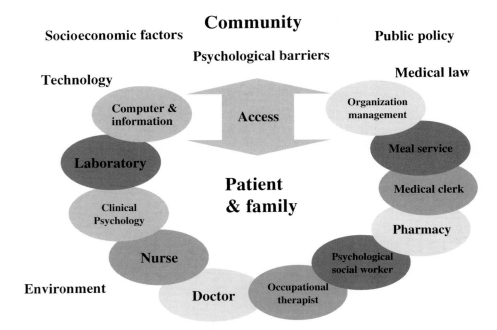

FIG. 2. Schema proposed to hospital staff, suggesting the role of the hospital in the larger community. The main philosophy is centered on the customer (patient and his or her family), with the hospital serving the needs of the customer and his or her community. Psychiatric hospitals should be open for the community and should be able to adapt to medical, socioeconomic, and political changes

Organizational Design

The author proposes a schema to hospital staff, suggesting the role of the hospital in the larger community (Fig. 2) [2]. The main philosophy is customer centered, with the hospital serving the needs of the customer and his or her community. Psychiatric hospitals should be open for the community and should be able to adapt to environmental, medical, socioeconomic, and political changes.

In organizational management, the clarification of objectives and goal setting are key strategies for implementing changes, and enable value integration among staff [3]. Assuring the quality and continuity of psychiatric care is the ultimate objective. Decreasing the number of hospital beds by building up a support system in the community is the aim of the policies of Asaka Hospital.

Strategy for Integrated Care System

The crucial concept in managing health care is "quality assurance," which has three main components: structure, process, and outcome (Fig. 3).

FIG. 3. Quality assurance has three main components: structure, process, and outcome. The factors of structure are personnel, spectrum of care, amenity, and information management system. For process, therapeutic guideline, team approach, case management, and software are indispensable. Outcome should be measured by assessment scale, readmission rate, quality of life, customer satisfaction, and cost effectiveness

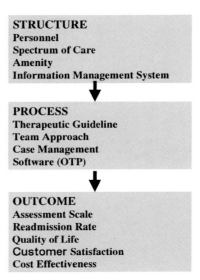

STRUCTURE
Personnel
Spectrum of Care
Amenity
Information Management System

PROCESS
Therapeutic Guideline
Team Approach
Case Management
Software (OTP)

OUTCOME
Assessment Scale
Readmission Rate
Quality of Life
Customer Satisfaction
Cost Effectiveness

Structure

Of course hospitals need good active personnel with appropriate knowledge. A wide spectrum of care to support patients as they move from the hospital to the community is absolutely necessary. With regard to amenity, psychiatric hospitals have traditionally been regarded as dark, dirty, and dangerous places. Amenity is especially important for psychiatric hospitals, because psychiatric units should serve as a therapeutic milieu. In Asaka Hospital, the use of space has been considered anew (Fig. 4). Because it is economically difficult to offer private rooms for all patients due to insufficient government reimbursement for psychiatric care, a special four-bed room has been proposed. Each person has his or her own window and a private space for lying down or sitting in a chair (Fig. 5). Each wing consists of four rooms: a washroom, laundry facilities, a shower room, and a small dining area (Fig. 6). There is a big hall in the center of the care unit. One can choose the privacy of one's own bed and window area, the intimacy of a small group of people in one's room, the company of a small community of 10 to 16 people, or the opportunity to interact with a larger number of people in the big hall.

Information management systems are indispensable for effective team approaches to caring for psychiatric patients. Network systems enable real-time information exchanges and are accessible to all departments and affiliated facilities (Fig. 7). They can provide data on types of medication, results of serological tests, imaging, nursing records in units, reports of community nurses, rehabilitation assessments [4] during occupational therapy or day care, assessment of geriatrics, care plan, etc.

Process

In psychiatry, a team approach and sound case management are the most important factors in the process of administering care [5]. Important to successful team

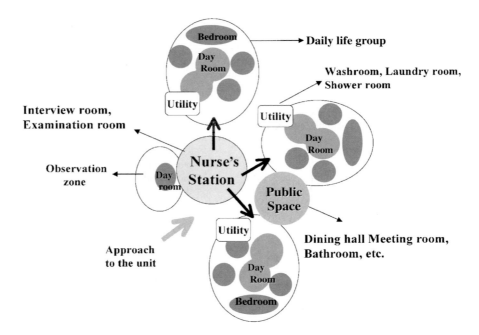

FIG. 4. Cocnept of unit. In Asaka Hospital, the use of space has been reconsidered. A unit consists of four groups, each of which has a day room and utilities, including washroom, shower room, and laundry room

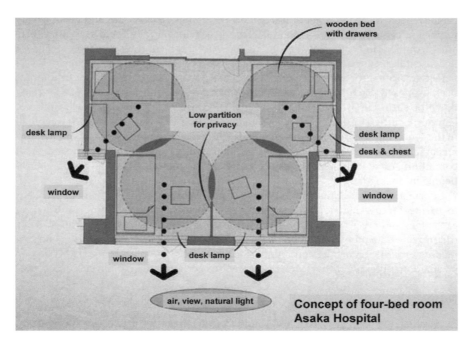

FIG. 5. Proposal for special four-bed room. Each person has his or her own window and also a private space when either lying down or sitting in a chair

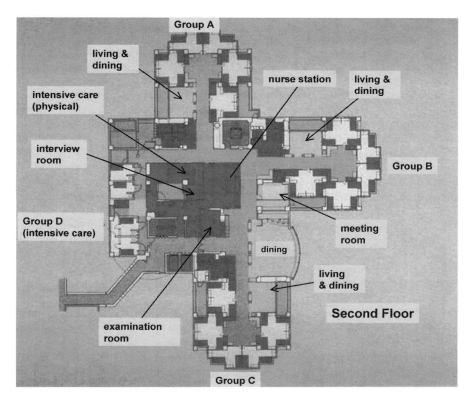

FIG. 6. Floor plan of a unit. Each group consists of four bedrooms, a washroom, laundry facilities, a shower room, and a small dining area. There is a large hall in the center of the care unit

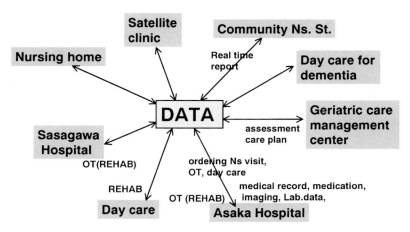

FIG. 7. Information management system. Network systems enable real-time information exchanges and are accessible to all departments and affiliated facilities. They can provide data on types of medication, results of serological tests, imaging, nursing records at units, reports of community nurses, and results of assessment by rehabilitation. *Ns*, nurses; *St.*, station; *OT*, occupational therapy; *REHAB*, rehabilitation

approach is the presence of a common language and value integration among many professionals, that is, "software." The Asaka Hospital was the second in Japan to implement the Optimal Treatment Project (OTP) [6,7].

From studying the psychosocial approaches of OTP, the knowledge and skill of the staff have improved dramatically. OTP as a common language makes multidisciplinary teamwork more systematic and extremely consistent for the customer. It gives staff confidence by providing an explicit standard of care for psychiatric patients rather than relying on a vague, implicit kindness. Furthermore, OTP works quite well in both outpatient and inpatient settings.

At Sasagawa Hospital, an innovative project has recently been designed to help patients progress from hospital beds to a combination of residential care facilities and day and night care. This project aims eventually to close small hospitals. By employing OTP as the software, a variety of clinics, day-care centers, and community nurses are able to integrate their services. Psychoeducation basically starts with a careful, honest explanation of the doctor's diagnosis. Because patients who have been hospitalized for a long time may not have cooperative family members, the hospital staff, friends, other patients, and volunteers will be able to work as the supporters and can act as a community.

Discussion

The outcome has not been assessed yet, because OTP started just a year ago. Decreasing the number of hospital beds by building up a support system in the community is the goal of the Asaka Hospital. In many Western countries, such as Great Britain or Italy, many psychiatric hospitals were closed without sufficient preparation, and later psychiatric community services were established when their importance was recognized. Although Japan is behind those countries in this aspect, it is possible to achieve a smoother shift of the style of care from inpatient-centered to community-based by learning from those countries. The author believes that the innovative Sasagawa project will be a good model of a sound shift from hospital beds to a combination of residential care facilities and other outpatient services, while maintaining quality and continuity of care.

References

1. Hibbard T, Campitelli J, Liberman HJ (1989) Off-unit activities programming for long-stay psychiatric inpatients: clinical and administrative effects. Occupati Ther Ment Health 9:49–61
2. Griffith JR (1990) Foundation of the hospital organization. In: Kovner AR, Neuhauser D (eds) Health service management. Health Administration Press, Ann Arbor, MI, pp 102–120, 196–235
3. Rosenberg NS (1990) Choosing the assessment method that meets your needs. In: Graham NO (ed) Quality assurance in hospitals. Aspen Publishers, Rockville, MD, pp 96–117
4. Baker RD, Hall JN (1983) REHAB: a multipurpose assessment instrument for long-stay patients. Vine Publishing, Aberdeen

5. Moor S (1992) Case management and integration of services: how service delivery system shape case management. Soc Work 37:418–423
6. Falloon IRH, Fadden G (1993) Integrated Mental Health Care: A comprehensive community-based approach. Cambridge University Press
7. Mizuno M, Murakami M, et al (2000) Psychiatric rehabilitation workbook. Chuohouki Tokyo

Training Long-Term Schizophrenic Inpatients in Illness Self-Management: A Randomized Controlled Trial

Nobuo Anzai[1], Shusuke Yoneda[1], Naoki Kumagai[1], Yukako Akaki[1], Emi Ikebuchi[2], and Hajime Kazamatsuri[1]

Summary. Although far behind that of other developed countries, Japanese psychiatry has started shifting from hospital-based to community-based services. For many long-term inpatients, it is necessary not only to provide welfare work but also to strengthen their ability to live outside the hospital. In order to determine whether long-term inpatients with schizophrenia could learn and retain knowledge related to self-management of illness, we conducted a randomized controlled trial. The subjects were 32 inpatients with schizophrenia (ICD-10) who agreed voluntarily to participate in this study. Their mean age was 46.8 years, the mean number of years after onset was 20.5, and the mean duration of current hospitalization was 4.0 years. They were randomly assigned to the training group of the Community Re-Entry Program or to occupational rehabilitation activities. Each program consisted of 18 1-h sessions, twice a week. The results showed that knowledge of self-management of illness was significantly better in the training group than in the control group immediately and 1 year after training. Retention of knowledge 1 year after training was negatively correlated with the number of years after onset of illness. REHAB scores were significantly better in the training group than in the control group after training. Discharge rates 1 year after training were significantly higher in the training group (10/14; 71.4%) than in the control group (3/15; 20.0%). We conclude that improvement of knowledge and the high rate of discharge in the training group suggest the effectiveness of the program. Of the 10 patients in the training group who were discharged after training, 9 lived alone in the community and 8 received home-visit service by psychiatric nurses of the ward from which they were discharged. This suggests that the high discharge rate of patients in the training group was the result of the improvement of relationships between patient and nurses and/or improvement of the patients' attitude to treatment from training in self-monitoring of warning signs.

Key words. Schizophrenia, Insight, Discharge from hospital, Cognitive behavioral therapy, Social skills training

[1] Department of Psychiatry, Tokyo Metropolitan Matsuzawa Hospital, 2-1-1 Kamikitazawa, Setagaya-ku, Tokyo 156-0057, Japan
[2] Department of Psychiatry, Teikyo University, School of Medicine, 2-11-1 Kaga, Itabashi-ku, Tokyo 173-8606, Japan

Objectives

Discharge from psychiatric hospitals may depend on differences in the community mental health systems from country to country. Psychiatric services in Japan are characterized by an overabundance of psychiatric beds. There are 340 000 beds, or 29 beds per 10 000 population. This is two or more times the ratio in the United States or the United Kingdom.

Of the 340 000 psychiatric inpatients in Japan, 65% have schizophrenia. The average hospital stay in Japan is about 400 days, and 46.5% of patients stay in the hospital for more than 5 years. Recently, day care and sheltered workshops have increased in number, but residential care and case management services have only just started. These deficiencies of the rehabilitation resources in the community cause difficulties in discharging many patients from psychiatric hospitals in Japan.

Of the psychiatric beds in Japan, 89% are in private hospitals and only 11% are in public hospitals. The public hospitals are expected to treat more difficult patients. Tokyo Metropolitan Matsuzawa Hospital is the largest and oldest public mental hospital in Japan. Our patients in the rehabilitation wards were transferred from acute or subacute wards in our hospital because of treatment refractoriness to medication. They were characterized by a long history into their illness, persistent psychotic symptoms, and poor insight into their illness. Most of them received little or no support from their families to live in the community.

For planning of discharge of patients in the rehabilitation wards, we use the tentative criteria for discharge from a psychiatric hospital described below. Because community support systems are weak in Japan, 1) patients should have room and/or financial support to live alone or with their relatives; 2) have skills to live independently, such as food preparation and money management, or have relatives who support their daily living; 3) receive medication independently and see a doctor regularly; 4) have the skills to monitor themselves for prodromal signs of relapse and be able to contact staff if the signs occur; 5) overcome the causes of present hospitalization, such as excitement, violence, suicide attempts, illegal drugs or alcohol, etc.; 6) accept outreach support of nurses or public health nurses if needed; 7) and not have severe physical complications.

Thus, Japanese inpatients might require much higher skills to live outside the hospital than patients in other countries with well-established community support systems.

Liberman [1] produced the Community Re-Entry Program for patients who are preparing to be discharged from the hospital, consisting of an educational skills training method based on cognitive-behavioral principles.

Kopelowicz et al. [2] conducted a random assignment study comparing the effects of the Community Re-Entry Program and occupational therapy for their short-term inpatients, and reported that knowledge and performance were significantly improved in patients in the Community Re-Entry Program compared with patients in occupational therapy. They also reported that the Community Re-Entry Program participants were significantly more likely to attend their first aftercare appointments than those in the occupational therapy group. Although their results are encouraging and cause us to expect that the Community Re-Entry Program will also be effective for our patients, there is no evidence of its effectiveness for long-term inpatients in quite different surroundings, such as in Japan.

We introduced this program to help our inpatients meet our criteria for discharge. In order to evaluate the efficacy of the Community Re-Entry Program, we conducted a randomized controlled trial of our inpatients.

Methods

The Community Re-Entry Program consists of 16 sessions, which focus on teaching participants the knowledge and skills to understand their disorder and the medications that control it, determine discharge readiness and community re-entry planning, connect with the community and cope with stress in the community, evaluate the effects of medication and solve medication problems, identify and keep track of warning signs of relapse, and develop an emergency relapse prevention plan. We used the Japanese version developed by Dr. Shimpei Inoue.

The subjects were 32 patients with schizophrenia spectrum disorder who stayed in two rehabilitation wards. All of them agreed voluntarily to participate in this study. Thirty-one patients met the criteria of the *International Classification of Diseases*, 10th revision (ICD-10) diagnosis of schizophrenia (F20.0–F20.9), and one patient had amphetamine psychosis (F15.0) and schizoid personality disorder (F60.1). Their mean age was 46.8 years, the mean time after onset was 20.5 years, and the mean duration of current hospitalization was 4.0 years. They were transferred from acute wards in our hospital to rehabilitation wards because of their treatment refractoriness to medication. They were characterized by a long history of illness, persistent psychotic symptoms, and poor insight into their illness.

The participants were randomly assigned (balanced by sex and age) to either the training group of the Community Re-Entry Program or the control group of the occupational rehabilitation activities. We allocated eight patients to the training group and eight patients to the control group in each ward. Two training groups started at once in the two rehabilitation wards. We added one introduction and one review session to the original 16 sessions, so the training program consisted of 18 sessions. Among about 10 ward nurses in a ward, 2 of the day shift nurses conducted 18 1-hr sessions twice a week in turn.

All of the subjects attended the rehabilitation programs, such as painting, calligraphy, leathercraft, cane work, and gardening, conducted by occupational therapists. The control group attended these activities 2 hr in the morning and 2 hr in the afternoon five times a week, and the training group also attended these activities, except for the hour of the Community Re-Entry Program.

Comparisons between the training and control groups were conducted before and after training, and 1 year after the end of training. The statistical package SPSS for Windows was used for the analysis.

The main characteristics of the patients randomly assigned to the training group and the control group are shown in Table 1. The mean age of patients in the training group and the control group, respectively, was 45.9 and 47.7 years, the mean duration of illness was 17.2 and 23.9 years, the mean number of hospitalizations was 3.5 and 5.1, and the mean duration of current hospitalization was 3.2 and 4.7 years. Although the control patients were slightly older and had a longer duration of illness than the

TABLE 1. Characteristics of patients randomly assigned to training group ($n = 16$) or control group ($n = 16$) (mean ± SD)[a]

Characteristic	Training group	Control group
Age (yr)	45.9 ± 11.5	47.7 ± 10.8
Duration of illness (yr)	17.2 ± 11.4	23.9 ± 11.1
No. of hospitalizations	3.5 ± 3.1	5.1 ± 3.4
Duration of current hospitalization (yr)	3.2 ± 3.0	4.7 ± 5.4
Total REHAB score	31.2 ± 18.2	37.3 ± 25.1

[a] There were no significant differences in clinical indices between the training group and the control group

TABLE 2. Medications before and after the treatment period in both groups (mean ± SD chlorpromazine equivalents)[a]

Group	Before	After
Training	1013.8 ± 715.6	993.0 ± 724.6
Control	1385.4 ± 1191.4	1380.7 ± 1195.1

[a] Although the mean dose of medication was slightly higher in the control group than in the training group, there were no significant differences between the two groups (*t*-test). There were no significant changes in dosage in either group before and after the training period

training patients, there were no significant differences in clinical indices between the training group and the control group.

The medications before and after the treatment period for both groups are shown in Table 2. Although the mean chlorpromazine equivalents of medications were slightly higher in the control group than in the training group, there were no significant differences between the two groups (*t*-test). There were no significant changes in dosage in either group before and after the training period (*t*-test).

Assessments were by the test of knowledge in the manual, a questionnaire of 21 items; the Positive and Negative Symptoms Scale (PANSS); and REHAB to evaluate the behaviors in the ward. We also conducted evaluation the World Health Organization Quality of Life (WHO-QOL) and role-play tests, but neither of these evaluations is reported in this paper.

The test of knowledge was conducted before training, after training, and at 1-year follow-up. Scoring was done by researchers blinded to the group of the subject. The REHAB was scored before and after training by three or four ward nurses who were working on the day of evaluation. The PANSS was evaluated by psychiatrists who were independent of the program and who were blinded to the subject's group.

We treated patients in both groups under the same discharge services from the same ward staff. For both groups, the doctor in charge discharged patients who met the criteria listed above. Follow-up was conducted until 1 year after the training.

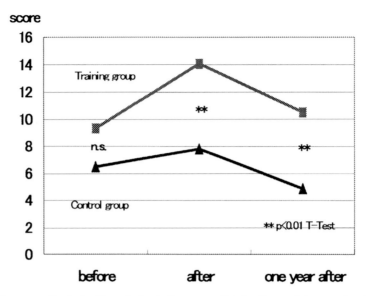

FIG. 1. Scores on the test of knowledge before, immediately after, and 1 year after training. Although the differences in the scores on the test of knowledge between the training and the control groups were significant after training and at 1-year follow-up, a significant decline in the scores occurred during the period from immediately after training to 1-year follow-up in the training group

Results

The results of the test of knowledge are shown in Fig. 1. Before training, there was no significant difference between the training group (9.3 ± 5.7) and the control group (6.5 ± 3.1). After training, the scores of the training group significantly increased from the values before training (from 9.3 to 14.1), and after training, there was a significant difference between the training group (14.1 ± 6.1) and the control group (7.8 ± 4.7) ($p < 0.01$, t-test). At 1 year after training, the scores of the training group (11.0 ± 5.0) were still significantly higher than those of the control group (4.9 ± 3.4) ($p < 0.01$, t-test). Although the differences between the two groups were significant, there was a striking decline in the knowledge test scores from immediately after training (14.1 ± 6.1) to 1 year after training (11.0 ± 5.0) in the training group ($p < 0.05$, t-test).

To study the reason for this decline in the knowledge scores in the training group, we studied the relationship between the knowledge scores and the duration of illness and the number of admissions in the training group. The gain in knowledge was defined as the score in the knowledge test 1 year after the program minus the score before the program in the training group.

The relationship between the gain and the duration of illness is shown in Fig. 2. There was a significant negative correlation ($r = -0.65$) between the gain and the duration of illness. The participants with a shorter history after the onset of illness had a

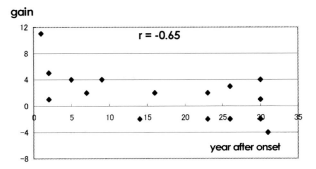

FIG. 2. Duration of illness and gain in scores on the test of knowledge 1 year after minus scores before training in the training group. The gain was defined [score before training] − [score 1 year after training]. The gain was negatively correlated with the year after onset of schizophrenia in training group patients

FIG. 3. Number of admissions and gain in scores of test of knowledge 1 year after minus scores before training in the training group. The gain was negatively correlated with the number of admissions in training group patients

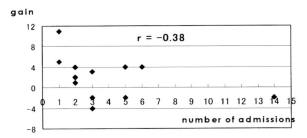

tendency to retain gains of knowledge, whereas the participants with a longer history had a tendency to lose the gains during the follow-up year.

The relationship between the gain and the number of previous admissions is shown in Fig. 3. There was a slight negative correlation between them ($r = -0.38$). This shows that the participants with a smaller number of previous admissions tended to keep their gains, and the participants with more previous admissions tended to lose their gains.

The Positive and Negative Symptoms were evaluated before and after training by the PANSS scale. In both groups, there was no significant difference before and after training (Table 3).

The total scores (CS score) of the REHAB scale are shown in Table 4. Before training, there was no significant difference between the training group and the control group. After training, the scores of the training group significantly improved from 31.2 to 18.2, and there was a significant difference between the training group and the control group (18.2 and 32.5; $p < 0.05$, t-test).

We conducted a follow-up study of both groups up to 1 year after the end of training. After recruitment of the participants and before the start of training, two participants in the training group and one participant in the control group were discharged from the hospital. Although they attended the program, comparison of

TABLE 3. Mean ± SD Positive and Negative Symptoms Scores (PANSS) before and after training[a]

Group	Before training	After training
Training group (*n* = 15)		
Positive symptoms	15.7 ± 5.7	13.5 ± 5.2
Negative symptoms	17.5 ± 4.7	18.7 ± 4.7
General psychopathology	34.4 ± 8.0	34.1 ± 7.8
Control group (*n* = 15)		
Positive symptoms	15.5 ± 4.8	18.3 ± 5.1
Negative symptoms	18.9 ± 4.2	20.8 ± 3.8
General psychopathology	34.9 ± 7.0	37.1 ± 6.3

[a] There were no statistically significant differences between scores before and after training on any group

TABLE 4. Mean ± SD total (CS) scores on the REHAB scale before and after training[a]

Group	Before training	After training
Training (*n* = 16)	31.2 ± 18.2* n.s.	18.2 ± 13.0*
Control (*n* = 16)	37.3 ± 25.1 n.s.	32.5 ± 22.7

[a] The total (CS) scores of the REHAB scale revealed no significant difference before training, and a significant difference after training between the two groups. n.s., Not significant
* $p < 0.05$, t-test

TABLE 5. Discharge rates during the year after the end of training

Group	No.	Rate
Training (*n* = 14)	10/14**	71.4%
Control (*n* = 15)	3/15	20.0%

[a] During the follow-up period, 10 of 14 (71.4%) in the training group and 3 of 15 (20%) in the control group were discharged from the hospital
** $p < 0.007$, Fisher's test

discharge rates was performed excluding these participants. Thus, the number of participants was 14 for the training group and 15 for the control group.

During the follow-up period, 10 of 14 (71.4%) of the patients in the training group, and 3 of 15 (20%) of those in the control group were discharged from the hospital (Table 5). This difference was statistically significant ($p < 0.007$, Fisher's test).

The numbers of days in the community and the relapse rates in each group are shown in Table 6. The mean number of days outside the hospital during the 1-year follow-up period was 139.8 days in the training group and 40.3 days in the control group. The patients in the training group stayed significantly longer than those in the control group ($p < 0.05$, t-test). During the follow-up period, 3 of 10 participants (30%)

TABLE 6. Mean ± SD number of days in the community and readmission rates

Group	Days in community	Readmissions
Training ($n = 14$)	139.8 ± 124.6*	3/10 (30.0%)
Control ($n = 15$)	40.3 ± 106.1	2/3 (66.7%)

[a] The mean number of days outside the hospital during the year after training was significantly greater in the training group than in the control group

*$p < 0.05$, t-test

TABLE 7. Possibility estimation of discharge for long-term inpatients in Japan (Kuroda [3])

Possibility Condition	%
Possible	
Without any conditions	4.0
If the patient can take medication regularly	2.0
If residential and financial support is available	8.7
If both conditions improve	17.7
Impossible	67.5

The subject group consisted of 19,342 inpatients who were staying more than 1 year in a psychiatric ward in Japan. The possibility and conditions of discharge within 6 months were evaluated by the psychiatrist in charge

in the training group and 2 of 3 (67%) in the control group were readmitted to the hospital. Although the readmission rate of the training group was lower than that of the control group, we could not draw a conclusion about the effect of the program on the prevention of readmission because the numbers were too small.

Among the discharged patients during the 1-year follow-up after training, only one patient in the training group lived with parents. Another nine patients in the training group and three patients in the control group discharged to live alone in the community were supported by the home-visit services of the ward nurses.

Discussion

As mentioned above, the deficiency of the community supports tended to require higher expectations to the psychiatric inpatients for their discharge from hospitals in Japan. Kuroda et al. [3] reported the results of a survey of 19342 patients who had inpatient stays of over 1 year in a Japanese psychiatric ward. In this study, the psychiatrist in charge estimated the possibility and conditions of discharge within 6 months for each inpatient. Sixty percent of the inpatients had no home to return to, and 67.5% were considered impossible to discharge within 6 months. It is noteworthy that of the remaining 32.5 %, only 8.7% were considered eligible for discharge if had a home to return to. More than half of the patients who were judged as having a possibility of being discharged within 6 months had problems of residence and compliance with medication to be resolved. These findings reveal the strong need of the population of long-term inpatients to facilitate their understanding of their illness and the importance of their medication.

Fenton et al. [4] reviewed the literature and stated that compliance with medication by patients with schizophrenia might be affected by the severity of illness, insight, medication-related factors, available social support, substance abuse comorbidity, and the quality of the therapeutic alliance. They also mentioned that among educational approaches, several reports providing information about schizophrenia and its treatment failed to improve the patients' knowledge and attitudes about medication compliance. Social skills training in areas related to medication seemed to be more effective than providing factual information.

Our results suggested that the Community Re-Entry Program was effective in improving knowledge of the illness and its treatment for our chronic long-stay inpatients. We will discuss the decline in the knowledge scores during the follow-up period.

Eckman et al. [5] reported that the effects of modularized skills training of schizophrenic outpatients were retained without significant erosion over a 1-year follow-up period. Liberman et al. [6] also reported that the group receiving skills training showed greater independent skills during a 2-year follow-up. What is the difference between these reports and our results?

One reason might be the difference in the duration of illness of the subjects: our subjects were slightly older and had a longer history of illness than their subjects. Another reason might be related to the number of training sessions and the total number of hours of training. The number of sessions in Eckman's study [5] was about 50, and the total duration of training in Liberman's study [6] was 288 hr. There is a possibility that the decline in knowledge in our study was due to the smaller number of sessions. Our findings suggest that the participants with longer histories from the onset of illness and with more hospitalizations may have a tendency to lose gains in knowledge. These patients might need more frequent and repeated learning experiences.

Because all but one of the discharged patients lived alone in the community supported by the home-visit services of ward nurses, the effects of the program on families might be small. Many patients had lost support from their family members because of previous episodes of assault or antisocial behavior, which victimize family members. Home-visit services by ward nurses were provided for 8 of the 10 discharged patients in the training group and 2 of the 3 discharged patients in the control group. The ward nurses repeatedly reported their strong impressions that the home-visit services became easier in the training group when the patients themselves reported the warning signs of relapse. They had been trained to monitor themselves during the sessions in the Community Re-Entry Program. The higher rate of discharge in the training group than in the control group might be related to this facilitated collaboration in the the the management of illness in the training group.

Conclusions

Improvements in the patients' knowledge of their illness and its care and a high rate of discharge in the training group suggest that the program was effective. Because the community support system is not satisfactory in Japan, patients are expected not only to find a place to live but also to understand their illness and the importance of the medication. By attending the Community Re-Entry Program, many participants became sufficiently knowledgeable and skilled to meet the discharge criteria. For some patients with a longer history of illness and many previous admissions, more frequent and repeated learning experiences might be necessary. Although the identification and self-monitoring of the warning signs in this program seem effective to build the coping ability of the patients and facilitate an effective coalition between patients and health care providers, more studies will be needed to confirm the effectiveness of this program for long-term prevention of relapses.

References

1. Liberman RP (1994) Social and independent living skills: the Community Re-Entry Program. Psychiatric Rehabilitation Consultants, Los Angeles
2. Kopelowics A, Wallace CJ, Zarate R (1998) Teaching psychiatric inpatients to re-enter the community: a brief method of improving the community of care. Psychiat Serv 49:1313–1316
3. Kuroda K, Toida S, Kawamuro Y, et al (1999) Estimated possibilities of discharge and the rehabilitation needs among the long-term inpatients in Japan. Psychiat Neurol Japonica 101:762–776 (in Japanese)
4. Fenton WS, Blyler CR, Heinssen RK (1997) Determinants of medication compliance in schizophrenia: empirical and clinical findings. Schizophr Bull 23:637–651
5. Eckman TA, Wirshing WC, Marder SR, et al (1992) Technique for training schizophrenic patients in illness self-management: a controlled trial. Am J Psychiat 149:1549–1555
6. Liberman RP, Wallace CJ, Blackwell G, et al (1998) Skills training versus psychosocial occupational therapy for persons with persistent schizophrenia. Am J Psychiat 155:1087–1091

Need for an Integrated Program of Case Management and Psychoeducation for Long-Stay Psychiatric Patients in Japan

Iwao Oshima[1,2], Junichiro Ito[3], and Naoko Taira[2]

Summary. The need for an integrated program of case management and psychoeducation for people with mental disabilities and their families is discussed in this chapter. Such programs are needed in Japan in order to resolve the problems of long-stay patients and to change the hospital-centered mental health care system into a community-based system. First we present the results of our nationwide research and analysis of governmental statistics, and second we argue the feasibility and effectiveness of such programs.

Key words. Psychoeducation, Case management, Needs assessment, Long-stay patients, Schizophrenia

Introduction

Over the last 10 years, there have been remarkable developments in community mental health in Japan, resulting in a rapid introduction of numerous new programs, such as sheltered workshops and rehabilitation facilities, as well as case management and psychoeducation. However, these programs have not yet effectively treated the most serious mental health problems of long-stay patients in psychiatric hospitals in Japan. Japan still has the highest number of psychiatric beds per person in the world.

We discuss here the need for an integrated program of case management and psychoeducation for people with mental disabilities and their families. Such programs are needed in Japan in order to resolve the problems of long-stay patients and to change the hospital-centered mental health care system into a community-based system. We will present the results of our nationwide research and analysis of governmental statistics, and we will argue the feasibility and effectiveness of such programs.

[1] Department of Mental Health, Graduate School of Medicine, University of Tokyo, 7-3-1 Hongo, Bunkyo-ku, Tokyo 113-0033, Japan
[2] Zenkaren Mental Health and Welfare Institute, 1-4-5 Shitaya, Taito-ku, Tokyo 110-0004, Japan
[3] National Institute of Mental Health, National Center for Neurology and Psychiatry, 1-7-3 Kohnodai, Ichikawa, Chiba 272-0827, Japan

Japanese Mental Health Systems and the Issues of Psychosocial Intervention Programs

In the last two or three decades, while Western countries have gradually decreased their number of psychiatric beds, there has been no similar decrease in Japan. The number of psychiatric beds was on the rise up to a few years ago. The number of psychiatric beds per 100 000 people in 1998 was 287, which was the highest rate in the world.

The characteristics of psychiatric inpatients and psychiatric hospitals are as follows [1]. Of the total number of inpatient beds, 71% are occupied by those who stay for more than one year. There has been a gradual aging of inpatients: 30% are more than 65 years of age. In addition, there is a very restrictive environment in inpatient wards. The percentage of involuntary admission cases is no less than 32%, whereas the percentage of admission to unlocked wards is only 40%. We found in our nationwide survey that the quality of the living environment within psychiatric hospitals is much poorer than those of sheltered accommodations under the Livelihood Protection Law, which was enacted to ensure a minimum level of quality of life in Japan [2,3]. Consequently, we believe that the most important issue facing Japanese mental health care is the problems experienced by long-stay patients in psychiatric hospitals.

On the other hand, progress in community mental health policy has been made from the mid-1980s onwards. Social rehabilitation facilities in line with the new mental health law, amended in 1987, have been established in several districts throughout Japan, and the number of facilities has been increasing rapidly. The number of sheltered workshops founded by family groups has been growing since around 1980, and this has led to the development of community-care programs for persons with mental disabilities. Although advances in housing programs were delayed until recently, the group home program, established in 1992, has made remarkable progress. Nowadays various types of community mental health programs have been put in place, although the provisions allocated for these programs are not yet sufficient.

Nevertheless, such community-care programs have not been effective in solving the problems of long-stay patients in Japan. According to several nationwide surveys, a certain segment of the patient population, ranging from 30% to 40%, have been evaluated by psychiatrists as being capable of living within the community, if community support programs were available (Fig. 1) [4].

Approximately 60% of long-stay patients in several nationwide surveys responded that they wished to be discharged from the psychiatric hospital [4]. We used a self-reporting questionnaire to assess 6417 inpatients staying at 154 psychiatric hospitals for more than one year and found that 55% of inpatients wished to be discharged [2,3]. However, the proportion of those who wanted to use social resources such as group homes and hostels was less than 10%. Many of them hoped to live with their families (39%) or alone (19%) without social resources [2,3].

As an underlying cause of these responses, we found that patients understood very little about the social resources and practical arrangements open to them, and many did not understand how to bring about the conditions necessary for their discharge [2,3]. Although they had some knowledge and demands about economic security, such

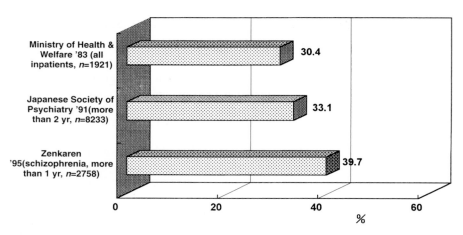

Fig. 1. Proportion of inpatients who were evaluated as capable of living within the community by psychiatrists

as disability benefits, they knew very little about direct personal services, such as group homes and sheltered workshops, aside from day-care services.

We constructed a scale of positive attitudes toward community living (PACL). In terms of determinant factors of PACL, we found that the family environment of long-stay patients was much more significant (Table 1) [5]. On the other hand, the contribution of social resources was less important in determining a positive attitude toward community living. Thus, many inpatients have very little knowledge about social resources for living independently within the community. Such patients wish to be discharged to families who in reality do not have the capacity to take care of their relatives.

If we are to promote a discharge policy for long-stay patients in Japan, we should attempt to enhance the readiness of inpatients to use community support programs, as well as to arrange for appropriately trained personnel to act as advocates for the inpatients after their discharge from the hospital.

Introduction of Nationwide Case Management System and Long-Stay Patients

Case management in Western countries emerged as a means of compensating for the fragmentation and lack of coordination of care services at an early stage of community mental health in the process of deinstitutionalization. In Japan, consideration has eventually swung toward the introduction of a nationwide case management system, where there has been a lack of progress recently in the development of community mental health care. The system is expected to play an important role in solving the problems of long-stay patients in Japan, even though the order of introduction is different from that in Western countries.

TABLE 1. Regression on a scale of positive attitudes toward community living (PACL)

Variable	Equation (1) Beta	Equation (2) Beta
Background variables		
Sex (male)	0.063**	0.063**
Age	−0.090**	0.005
Current admission period	−0.126**	−0.106**
Duration of illness	0.006	−0.019
No. of admissions	0.031	0.019
PACL determinant variables		
Family resources scale		0.042
Family's expectation toward discharge		0.264**
No. of known social resources		0.076**
No. of social resources demanded to be used		−0.045
Dissatisfaction with life in wards		0.113**
No. of activities attended in wards		0.083**
R	0.200	0.381
R^2	0.040	0.145

** $P < 0.001$; * $P < 0.01$

The nationwide case management system was originally introduced for the care of the elderly as a national nursing care insurance program established in April 2000. Introduction of a similar system for people with severe mental illnesses is currently being developed by the Ministry of Health and Welfare (MHW).

The Japan Case Management Guidelines (JCM-GL), published by a professional committee in the MHW, was formulated in 1998 to facilitate introduction of a national case management system in Japan. The nationwide case management trial project has been conducted in every prefecture since 1999 using the JCM-GL.

The guidelines primarily show the fundamental principles and core functions of case management, such as care assessment and planning, as well as linkage to services. In addition, the components of case management, which were proved to be effective by previous studies [6–8], are presented in JCM-GL. As stated in JCM-GL, the case manager provides direct client service, personalized contact, organization of a multidisciplinary team, and continuity of staffing. He or she also works closely with support systems, including informal carers and development of informal care, and is responsible for a number of other services. Models similar to clinical or intensive case management models are considered.

We constructed Fidelity Scales (FS) that were used to measure program implementation based on JCM-GL in a nationwide trial study in 1987. This is a 27-item scale that includes effective components of case management, in addition to the standard case management components, which refer to the fidelity indices of Assertive Community Treatment [9].

The item with the highest implementation rate is "try to assess the comprehensive needs" (99.8%). The rates of items related to procedure implementation from the beginning of intake to care planning ("Client's demands are sufficiently received in the assessment," "Making a care plan based on client's needs," and "Informed consent of the client") were greater than 95%. Furthermore, the rates for items classified as "quality of services" ("Responsible behavior for the protection of the client's privacy," "To have a positive relationship with the client at the initial stage," "Case manager provides services," and "To respect the self-determination of the client") were greater than 90%.

On the other hand, items with low implementation rates were "Development of care services to meet client's needs" (25.7%), "Team approach with well-defined leadership" (31.0%), "To hold case conferences in the service execution" (31.4%), "Work closely with informal support system" (31.9%), "To hold case conferences," and "Work closely with informal support system." These items received particular emphasis in the JCM-GL [10].

We constructed a total fidelity scale (TFS) by summing all of the FS items (Table 2). We generated high-, low-, and intermediate-score groups by dividing TFS into three groups by three-quantiles and compared the outcome variables before and after the trial for about two months in the high and low groups. We used three outcome variables: the Objective Quality of Life Scale (QOLS), the number of categories in the Personal Care Service list (nPCS), and the Life Satisfaction Scale (LSS).

The high-TFS-score group showed significant increases in nPCS, QOLS, and LSS at the end of the trial (paired t-test). In addition, significant increases in the low-score group were observed in nPCS and LSS, whereas no changes were found in QOLS in the low-score group. The high-TFS-score group had significantly higher QOLS scores than the low-score groups (independent samples t-test) after the trial [11].

Our model demonstrated some effective elements (coordinator provides direct client service, in vivo contacts, etc.) that can be added to the standard case management model and showed objective and subjective short-term effectiveness, at least in the beginning stages of its introduction. However, in regard to the low implementation rate of items thought to be important in JCM-GL, such as "To hold case conferences" and "Work closely with informal support system," the study findings demonstrated that many difficulties occurred in the implementation of care services according to the care plan.

Possibility of Integrated Program of Case Management and Psychoeducation

We will return to our original consideration of the problems of long-stay patients. This group is believed to represent the most important target population of case management, given that most people with severe persistent mental illnesses requiring case management in Japan are inpatients in psychiatric hospitals. However, the proportion of enrolled clients in a nationwide research trial in 1987 staying at a hospital for longer than one year was only 9% [12].

To enhance the efficacy of case management for long-stay patients, we need to consider an integrated program of case management and psychoeducation. Psychoeducation for long-stay patients is expected to provide clients with the necessary information about social resources available in the community, as well as to foster within them the self-confidence and incentives needed to live independently within the community. In addition, a psychoeducation program for the family should be integrated to achieve the same goal.

TABLE 2. Comparison of outcome variables before and after the trial in the high and low groups of fidelity scales

Test	Group	nPCS (1)		QOLS (2)		LS (3)		Paired t-test (comparison between)		
		Before	After	Before	After	Before	After	(1)	(2)	(3)
Total fidelity scale	Low (n = 104)	0.64	2.06	2.12	2.19	2.24	2.58	***	ns	**
	High (n = 99)	0.51	2.38	2.10	2.34	2.24	2.79	***	***	***
	t test (High vs Low)	ns	ns	ns	*	ns	ns			
Formation of team and support system scale	Low (n = 93)	0.58	2.02	2.17	2.25	2.29	2.64	***	ns	**
	High (n = 97)	0.52	2.34	1.97	2.23	2.07	2.72	***	***	***
	t test (High vs Low)	ns	ns	**	ns	ns	ns			
Needs-oriented approach scale	Low (n = 82)	0.66	2.16	2.16	2.20	2.38	2.66	***	ns	*
	High (n = 98)	0.54	2.27	2.12	2.36	2.19	2.71	***	***	***
	t test (High vs Low)	ns	ns	ns	*	ns	ns			
Organization of case management system	Low (n = 63)	0.54	2.02	2.07	2.17	2.16	2.70	***	ns	**
	High (n = 94)	0.62	2.22	2.14	2.34	2.17	2.78	***	***	***
	t test (High vs Low)	ns	ns	ns	*	ns	ns			
Total		0.58	2.16	2.11	2.26	2.22	2.68	***	***	***

*P < 0.05; **P < 0.01; ***P < 0.001

We will confirm the goals of a psychoeducation program. According to the responses of a self-reporting questionnaire we administered to 726 persons with mental disabilities being cared for by members of family groups from every district in Japan [13], the issues predicted to be the most important for inpatients of psychiatric hospitals were related to various types of information, such as "Hope to receive an explanation on the effects and side effects of medicines," "Hope to receive an explanation of prognosis."

A nationwide self-reporting mail survey of 1566 members of family groups providing care for inpatients revealed that the issues predicted to be the most important in the psychiatric hospitals agreed with the responses of persons with mental disabilities [14]. These results suggested that sufficient information on psychiatric illnesses and the method of care have not been adequately provided by the staff members of psychiatric hospitals in Japan.

Psychoeducation provides adequate and scientifically sound information to persons with mental disabilities and their families. However, even the patient's diagnosis is left unexplained in Japan, not only to the psychiatric patients themselves, but also sometimes to their families. Thus, there was little expansion of the use of psychoeducational approaches until recently.

Around the year 1990, we at last entered into the age of community care, and as a result, psychoeducation programs for families have seen rapid development over the last 10 years. Currently, 33% of psychiatric hospitals and 69% of public health centers run family psychoeducation programs. We found that an adequate and accurate explanation of the patient's diagnosis was given to the families directly (65.1%) in these recently introduced programs in Japan [13]. However, structured psychoeducation programs for people with mental disabilities themselves are now in the beginning stages.

Conclusions

Several psychosocial intervention programs for people with mental disabilities and their families have been proved effective over the last 20 years. One factor recognized as important is the creation of more effective integrated programs according to the clients' needs. In light of this, we need to take a much greater interest in an integrated program of case management and psychoeducation for long-stay patients in Japan. The problems facing such patients represent the most serious problems to be overcome within the mental health field, and the effectiveness of these programs needs to be established in future research.

Many Japanese mental health workers are now interested in the possible effectiveness of case management and psychoeducation. We believe we are now in a position to introduce integrated programs systematically and to realize community care for long-stay patients.

From an international perspective, the problems facing elderly long-stay patients in psychiatric hospitals are among the most pressing issues throughout the world. We believe our trial will contribute to some extent to solving this problem.

References

1. MWF (1999) Patient Survey 1996. Statistics and information department, Minister's secretariat, MHW (in Japanese)
2. Zenkaren Health and Welfare Research Institute (1994) The needs of care and support of people with mental disorders and their families (III): a nationwide survey of long stay psychiatric patients in Japan. Zenkaren Health and Welfare Institute Monograph No.7. Zenkaren (in Japanese)
3. Oshima I, Yoshizumi A, Inazawa K, et al (1996) The intention of the community living and the idea of the life style after the discharge expressed by long stay patients: an analysis of a nationwide self-rating survey for long stay schizophrenics in about 40 000 psychiatric beds in Japan. Jpn J Hosp Commun Psychiatry 38(4):558–567 (in Japanese)
4. Zenkaren Health and Welfare Research Institute (1998) Research on institutional care for long-term inpatients in Japan. Zenkaren Health and Welfare Institute Monograph No.15. Zenkaren (in Japanese)
5. Oshima I, Yoshizumi A, Inazawa K, et al (1996) The attitude toward the community living and the determinant factors for the long stay patients in Japan: the analysis of a nationwide self-rating survey. Seishinigaku 38(12):1248–1256 (in Japanese)
6. Mueser KT, Bond GR, Drake RE, et al (1998) Models of community care for severe mental illness: A review of research on case management. Schizophr Bull 24:37–74
7. McGrew JH, Bond GR (1995) Critical ingredients of assertive community treatment. J Ment Health Admin 22:113–125
8. Teague GB, Drake RE, Ackerson TH (1995) Evaluating use of continuous treatment teams for persons with mental illness and substance abuse. Psychiatr Serv 43:689–695
9. McGrew JH, et al (1994) Measuring the fidelity of implementation of a mental health program model. J Consult Clin Psychol 62:670–678
10. Cho N, Oshima I, Takahashi K (2000) A study of the guidelines of case management for persons with mental disorders analyzed with fidelity index: the conditions of effective implementation. Jpn J Public Health 47:411–420 (in Japanese)
11. Oshima I, Cho N, Takahashi K (in preparation) Program evaluation of a national case management system for people with severe mental illnesses in Japan: a follow-up study of effective components based on case management guidelines in a nationwide trial
12. JCM-GL Committee (1998) Japan Case Management Guidelines for people with mental disabilities (in Japanese)
13. Zenkaren Health and Welfare Research Institute (1999) Family support programs in hospital setting: current situation and evaluation of trial programs. Zenkaren Health and Welfare Institute Monograph No.23. Zenkaren (in Japanese)
14. Zenkaren Health and Welfare Research Institute (2001) The third national survey of families: members of hospital based family groups. Zenkaren Health and Welfare Institute Monograph. Zenkaren (in Japanese)

Vocational Rehabilitation for Persons with Schizophrenia: Recent Advances in Japan

Naoki Kumagai

Summary. In Japan vocational rehabilitation for persons with mental illness has made gradual advances in social resources and clinical practices for the past decade. In the 1980s, social participation of people with mental illness started to be promoted eagerly, with significant revisions of the related laws. In 1996, a seven-year-plan for normalization was begun, with much emphasis on vocational rehabilitation of persons with mental illness. Social resources are increasing, though not enough. We report the effectiveness of an integrated program support with group activities, individualized care, maintenance medication, and cognitive-behavioral therapy for job finding. At the psychiatric day treatment unit of Tokyo University Hospital, 27 patients with schizophrenia received skills training in job finding from 1991 to 1995. They developed employment readiness through group activity. Most of them acquired targeted skills, reported increased self-efficacy, and generalized in real job interviews. Individual care and peer support of the group seemed effective in overcoming stressful situations. The supportive relationship enabled them to comply with medication. Twenty-two were employed with disclosure of their illness and maintained employment for more than three months. Development of social resources combined with effective support may help persons with schizophrenia work according to their abilities and improve their quality of life.

Key words. Vocational rehabilitation, Schizophrenia, Cognitive-behavioral therapy, Day treatment, Normalization

Introduction

In Japan, vocational rehabilitation for persons with mental illness, including schizophrenia, has made gradual advances over the past decade in the areas of support systems, social resources, and clinical practices, as well as psychosocial techniques. In this paper, I first present the advances in the areas of support systems and service

Department of Psychiatry, Tokyo Metropolitan Matsuzawa Hospital
Current address: Tokyo Metropolitan Comprehensive Mental Health Center—Central District, 2-1-7 Kamikitazawa, Setagaya-ku, Tokyo 156-0057, Japan

provision, and second my clinical experience with an integrated psychosocial approach to utilize resources effectively, the combination and integration of group activities, individual care, maintenance pharmacotherapy, and cognitive-behavioral therapy for skills related to job finding.

Advances in Support Systems

Discrepancy Between Hopes and Conditions

There is still a great discrepancy between the hope of work and the actual vocational condition among persons with mental disablement. According to Zenkaren [1], the national federation of families of the mentally ill in Japan, more than two-thirds of clients with mental disablement who live in the community hoped to work, although only 20% were employed, more than 40% had no job, and about 20% used the community workshop for persons with disablement in the early 1990s. Of course, not every person with mental disablement is able to be employed or even work in a sheltered situation. Moreover, work is not the sole style of social participation. When the hope of work prevails, I consider that vocational rehabilitation is important in satisfying social participation needs and enabling more socially integrated and independent living and enhanced quality of life. How to resolve the above discrepancy is a great issue in comprehensive rehabilitation for persons with schizophrenia.

Barriers to Working: Client Factors and Environmental Factors

People with schizophrenia usually face many barriers when they try to hold jobs. The barriers may be divided into client factors and environmental factors. Client factors are classified as vocational handicap, disability, impairment, and subjective disablement. They involve decreased work ability and deficits in social skills in job finding or in the workplace. Instability of performance causes much trouble. People with schizophrenia are so vulnerable to environmental changes that they have much difficulty in changing tasks, interpersonal environment, staffs, and transition stresses like job finding. They often have inadequate readiness for employment, including appropriate social behavior as well as activities of daily living. Therefore, in vocational rehabilitation for persons with schizophrenia, not only support in work but also support and care in daily living is required. Environmental factors include the stigma of illness

TABLE 1. Disablement in vocational life of persons with schizophrenia

Objective disablement			
Handicap	Disability	Impairment	Subjective disablement
Difficulty in functioning as a worker Difficulty in getting jobs Easily dismissed	Disability in transition Decreased work skills Difficulty in learning Deficit in social skills instable performance	Cognitive deficit Residual symptom instable functioning Relapse vulnerability Lack of motivation Medical side effects	Agony in living Emptiness Loneliness Lost in reverie

and the shortage of work appropriate for people with mental illness. Patients who try to work without disclosing their disability are expected to work more than six hours per day and more than four days per week when they need to continue medication and clinical counseling for support and prevention of relapse. Opportunities for employment with disclosure of disability are fewer, and the wages are not high enough to satisfy daily needs and permit independent living. These problems arise because people with mental illness are not been provided with social and vocational rehabilitation services. Financial and technical support for companies employing people with mental disablement is inadequate. Before the 1980s, only a few charitable companies employed people with mental illness who disclosed their disability. Only after 1990 did supported or sheltered employment have legal ground and public support. Outside the legal care system, private community workshops, of which there are more than 1000 today, have been offering opportunities for unsatisfied needs for work with little public support.

Advances in the Legal System

Since the later 1980s, promotion of rehabilitation and community care has become the mainstream of public mental health policy, and practices in vocational rehabilitation at community settings are increasing gradually, with backup of significant revisions of related laws. After World War II, the new Japanese constitution expressively stated the basic human right to a healthy and cultural life. Accordingly, the policy was adopted that first medical services should be disseminated, especially hospitalization. In 1950s, the great progress in psychopharmacology promoted dissemination of medical care further. On the other hand, persons with mental disablement were long left outside of social rehabilitative services. In later 1980s, the Mental Health Law, a revision of the Mental Hygiene Law, promoted social rehabilitation. The law for promotion of employment of the handicapped did not exclude services for persons with mental disability. In the 1990s, sections for the disabled in public employment security offices, about 500 in Japan, started vocational counseling and placement with disclosure of illness. Companies that employed people with mental disablement through public employment security offices began to be financially supported. Vocational rehabilitation centers were founded in each prefecture, where prevocational training programs were administered. Treaty 159 of the International Labor Organization

TABLE 2. Changes in legal system

1946	New constitution of State of Japan
1950	Mental Hygiene Law
1987	Mental Health Law (the above revised)
	Law for Employment Promotion for the Disabled
1991	Vocational Rehabilitation Center
1992	Financial support for companies to employ mentally disabled or retarded
	ILO Treaty 159, ratified
1993	Fundamental Law for Persons with Disabilities
1995	Mental Health and Welfare Law (revised)
	Seven-Year-Plan for Normalization
1999	Mental Health and Welfare Law (revised)

(ILO), which deals with placement, maintenance, and promotion in the employment of people with handicaps, was ratified in the Diet. Thereafter, sheltered factories and sheltered work institutes were clearly stated in the Mental Health Law. In 1995, a seven-year-plan for normalization, called the Normalization Plan, was established, which has emergent, numerical goals of sheltered rehabilitative services in seven years from 1996.

Normalization Plan: Minimal, Emergent Goal

About half of the limited term of the Normalization Plan has passed, and the progress does not seem to be sufficient. The numerical goal is merely emergent, minimal resource preparation. It seems to be necessary to increase opportunities to work according to ability and enhance social integration and enable support on the job. Employment of mentally disabled people integrated into the competitive work setting is still limited, partly because of lack of numerical goals in the plan. In Japan, by law, at least 1.8% of all employees of companies or public offices must be people with physical disablement or mental retardation, and employers are fined if they do not comply with the rule. But there is no such rule for people with mental disablement. There is little advantage to companies in employing people with mental disablement and no disadvantage in not employing them.

An Innovative Practice in Vocational Rehabilitation

Objective: Supports for Transition from Day Treatment to Work

Psychosocial techniques are necessary for supporting persons with mental disablement to make the transition to work, maintaining the position and enhancing quality of life. They should be administered comprehensively in a needs-oriented way, because the difficulties in placement and maintenance are so pervasive. I introduced the vocational rehabilitation program at the psychiatric day treatment unit (Day Hospital) [2] of Tokyo University Hospital in the 1990s. In this program, cognitive-behavioral therapy for learning job-finding skills is administered combined with group activities, individual care, and maintenance pharmacotherapy. More than 400 clients with schizophrenia have received rehabilitative services in the Day Hospital. Since 1991, a job-finding training group has been conducted as an adjunct program to clients who are almost ready for job finding.

Subject

The subjects of this report include 27 clients with schizophrenic-related disorders who attended this group from 1991 to 1995. There were 12 men and 15 women, with a mean age of 27.2 years. Intelligence assessed with WAIS-R was 98.5 in VIQ, 94.2 in PIQ on average. Fifteen clients had no experience of job finding or work. Five had been continuously employed for more than one year. The mean duration of illness was 7.8 years, and the mean duration of use of the Day Hospital before training was 29.0 months. The mean level of psychiatric symptoms according to the Japanese version of the Psychiatric Rating Scale (PRS) was −11.2. All the subjects hoped to practice job-finding skills and gave consent to videorecording their role plays.

TABLE 3. Disorder

Diagnosis	Males	Females
Schizophrenia	11	13
Schizoaffective disorder	0	1
Schizotypal disorder	1	1
	12	15

Age: 27.2 ± 4.8 yr
Education: 13.0 ± 2.5 yr
WAIS-R: VIQ98.5 ± 16.8; PIQ94.2 ± 16.4
Employment: Never (15), <1 yr (7), ≥1 yr (5)
Illness duration: 7.8 ± 4.4 yr
Day hospital use: 29.0 ± 15.3 mo
Symptom: −11.2 ± 4.5 (PRS)
WAIS-R: Revised Wechsler Adult Intelligence Scale; VIQ: Verbal Intelligence Quotient; PIQ: Performance Intelligence Quotient; PRS: Rsychiatric Rating Scale

TABLE 4. Weekly program of day hospital of Tokyo University Hospital

Time	Mon	Tue	Wed	Thu	Fri
10:00	Doctor interview	Sports	Cooking	Off for clients staff meeting	Game
12:00 13:00	Lunch	Lunch Shopping	Lunch		Lunch
13:30	Easy work	Social skills training	Tea party		Sports
15:00	Meeting	Meeting	Meeting		Meeting
15:15			Job-finding training		

There are about 30 patients, with a staff member in charge of each (8 staff members). Each patient meets weekly with a doctor for interview and prescription. Job-finding training: Adhoc program held from 15:15 to 16:15, for selected patient members almost ready to work

Methods

Group Activity Program of the Day Hospital

About 30 clients with schizophrenia (all under 35 years of age) attended the Day Hospital, cared for by eight staff members. A staff member and a psychiatrist were in charge of each client. The responsibility and roles in managing group activities rested on the clients as much as possible, so that the Day Hospital was a model with social life with self-help and mutual support, with advice from the staff. The staff members and psychiatrists observed and assessed the simulated social behavior in the Day Hospital and utilized the information for individual care, support in group activities, and follow-up.

Support for Job Finding

Most clients who were accepted by and adjusted to the Day Hospital group hoped to work. The staff administered ability examinations, including the WAIS-R, and usually organized a joint meeting with the family and client before job finding. After 1990, most of the patients aimed at employment with disclosure of disability using a public employment security office. With a goal of job finding, the staff member visited the section for the disabled at the office with referral by the psychiatrist in charge. The staff member met the officer there to ask for assistance and search for appropriate situations. The client then visited the section accompanied by the staff member and was interviewed by the officer for registration as a job seeker. After registration, the client researched employment situations with support from the staff member and/or the officer. If the client found an appropriate situation, the client asked the officer for referral. When the employer agreed to an interview, the client visited the workplace and was interviewed by the manager there. When the manager agreed to employ the client and the work was appropriate, the client was placed there. The client started working, and the Day Hospital staff and the officer of the section continued to support both the client and the manager.

Job-Finding Training Group

In the course of job finding, specific skills were required for clients to cope with many kinds of social interactions, including the job interview. The Day Hospital ordinary program was not adequate for them to acquire and develop the skills. Many clients felt anxious in coping with social interactions related to job finding. We started group training in job-finding skills with cognitive-behavioral techniques. This is an adhoc hour-long program held from 15:15 once a week, for selected patient members, who agreed and hoped to find jobs with support by staffs, and were considered by the psychiatirsts to be almost ready to work. The session progressed in a similar manner to the basic training model of social skills training [3], which involved the steps of goal setting and instruction of skills, group discussion about the target skill, demonstrating the skills by role playing or videotape, role playing by clients, positive feedback, and videofeedback, corrective feedback, and homework assignment. The skills taught usually involved interpersonal situations that the client was expected to cope with in the process of job finding. In general, the steps included training in nonverbal behavior in the interview, common easy responses in the interview, registration interview at a public employment security office, job interview at a workplace, coping with stressful questions such as disclosing illness or explaining about a gap in personal history, and skills necessary for initial adjustment in placement such as greeting briefly, following instructions and questioning, and making a positive request to the manager.

Assessment and Evaluation

Before and after the training, the staff member in charge of the client assessed the client in terms of motivation for work, self-efficacy, and nonverbal, paralinguistic, and verbal behavior. When the client had a interview for registration or a job accompanied by the staff member, the staff member assessed how he or she performed in the real interview and recorded the vocational outcome.

Results

Change in Skills and Self-Efficacy

Before training, 85% of the clients were motivated to work, but less than 5% had enough self-efficacy for the job interview. With regard to nonverbal behavior, 40.7% were observed to have severe problems with eye contact, 74.1% with facial expression, 59.3% with body posture, and 40.7% with movement of arms or legs. With regard to paralinguistic behavior, 40.7% were observed to have severe problems with voice volume, 40.7% with intonation, 51.9% with speed and fluency, and 59.3% with length of responses. With regard to verbal behavior, 81.5% were observed to have severe problems with the amount of information, 55.6% with relevancy, 77.8% with self-disclosure, and 59.3% with propriety. The subjects participated in an average of 5.2 sessions. After the training, 55.6% were effective, 37.0% moderately effective, and 7.4% questionable in overall evaluation. Most of the nonverbal behavior except for facial expression improved (88.9% for posture, 66.7% for movement, 55.5% for eye contact, and 14.8% for facial expression). As for paralinguistic behavior, voice volume improved in 55.5% of the clients (37.5% for length of response, 33.3% for intonation). As for verbal responses, propriety (74%), self-disclosure (63.0%), and information (63%) were improved in more than 60% of the clients, but relevancy was improved in only 3.7%. Self-efficacy for the job interview was fairly improved in 51.9%, moderately improved in 44.4%, and worsened in 3.7%.

Generalization and Outcome

Staff members who accompanied the clients in real job interviews reported that 63.0% performed mostly as they had learned, 25.9% partially. As for vocational outcome of the subjects, 81.5% were employed in competitive settings with disclosure of disability and maintained employment for three months. One was hospitalized because of a psychotic relapse.

Case Vignette: a Woman with Schizophrenia

After she graduated from high school, the patient experienced verbal hallucinations and delusions of persecution, which were the onset of her psychosis. She had no experience with job interviews. She received antipsychotic medication at the psychiatric outpatient clinic of Tokyo University Hospital. Her positive symptoms subsided with the pharmacotherapy, but she was markedly withdrawn. She hoped to work but had low self-esteem.

She was referred to the Day Hospital program for two hours a day at first, and it took two months for her to participate in the full program, with much individual care by a staff member in charge. She looked tense and had poor social skills. Gradually she was accepted by the other Day Hospital clients, and she tried successfully to take easier roles, like preparing for a ball game. She made a few intimate friends in the Day

Hospital, and her self-esteem improved gradually. In the following year, she became one of the leaders of the members.

When she was 22, she wished to work at a clerical job with little self-efficacy. A meeting with her family, the psychiatrist, the staff member in charge, and herself was held, and she agreed to try job finding with disclosure of disability. She started attending a job-finding training group as well as the ordinary Day Hospital program. Before training, she showed poor facial expression and eye contact, tending to lean forward, with low voice volume, and giving humble and disorganized responses with high anxiety. The staff member in charge visited the nearest public employment security office and asked an officer for assistance. The target behaviors in training were good body posture, answering with mouth wide open, and appropriate verbal responses in job interview. Special attention was paid by the trainer to frequent modeling, step-by-step shaping, videofeedback, and positive feedback.

After four training sessions, she visited the office with a Day Hospital staff member and was interviewed for registration. She performed mostly as she had learned. It took two months to find a workplace that was appropriate for her and agreed to interview her. In the course of the stressful transition, she regularly attended the Day Hospital. Individual support by staff and peer support by other Day Hospital members helped to decrease her stress.

After several trials, she learned more interviewing skills and accepted an easier and more realistic job to seek. She was interviewed at a company with referral by the officer, and they decided to employ her. Before the first day of work, she learned initial adjustment skills, including following instructions and making positive requests to the manager. In the first month, she worked less than four hours a day, which was supported by a daily telephone call from the staff. The superior in the company also received technical support from Day Hospital staff and the officer. She gradually worked longer: four months later she worked for seven hours a day, 4.5 days a week. She maintained the position for two years.

Discussion

Effectiveness of the Integrated Approach

The results show that job-finding-related skills were learned by clients and were generalized. The procedure of vocational rehabilitation was relatively safe, because of the low relapse rate during training. In the course of the Day Hospital group activities and the job-finding training group, the clients improved in self-esteem, which helped them to accept realistic choices. This occurred as they acquired skills necessary for the realistic goals and achieved them step by step. They maintained motivation for work, with peer support from the Day Hospital group and individual care by the staff. Antipsychotic medication was maintained by the well-formed relationships among clients, staff, and psychiatrists.

Limitations of This Study

This study had several limitations. It was an open trial with no control. It was based on naturalistic observation by the staff in charge. The subjects were younger and had less severe schizophrenia. The use of the Day Hospital was rather long. Different kinds of skills might be necessary for maintaining work, although the group taught skills related to job-finding.

Conclusions

In conclusion, there is an absolute shortage of vocational rehabilitation resources in Japan, and the Normalization Plan is the minimal and emergent goal for 2003. Cognitive-behavioral therapy, combined and integrated with group activity, individual care, and maintenance pharmacotherapy is useful in connecting clients' needs with rehabilitation resources and enhancing quality of life. Finally, knowledge of the neurobehavioral basis of schizophrenia is expected to promote psychosocial techniques and increase useful resources in vocational rehabilitation in Japan.

Acknowledgments. I thank staff of the Psychiatric Day Treatment Unit of Tokyo University Hospital and the late Dr. Masaru Miyauchi for assistance in my clinical practice.

References

1. Okagami K (ed) (1993) Current state of vocational rehabilitation of "Persons with Mental Disablement," Zenkaren, Tokyo, Japan (in Japanese)
2. Miyauchi M (1997) Psychiatric day care manual, 2nd edn. Kongo-shuppan, Tokyo, Japan (in Japanese)
3. Liberman RP (ed) (1988) Psychiatric rehabilitation of chronic mental patients. American Psychiatric Press, Washington D.C., USA

Innovative Practice in Psychiatric Community Care in Sawa Hospital and Japan

Yutaka Sawa

Summary. Four components are required to maintain community life for handicapped persons: residential facilities, activity programs in the daytime, supporting staff and their involvement as a team, and being understood and accepted by the community. Following other developed countries, community care and treatment programs that include these four conditions have been developed in Sawa Hospital since 1986. Since 1995, new places and activity programs called "From 'to be Supported' to 'to support'" have been developed: food delivery services for the elderly at home; volunteers in day care for the demented; training and education for home helpers; and observers in the home of the demented, which enhances the self-esteem of patients. As well as the rehabilitation programs, psychiatric emergency services have been developed in Sawa Hospital to compensate for community care. Expanding community care or rehabilitation services and intensifying psychiatric emergency services have changed Sawa Hospital. In 17 years, the total number of beds has decreased gradually from 603 to 505. The annual number of admissions has increased from about 300 to 1400. The average length of stay per year has decreased from 700 to 120 days. Nonetheless, 3400 outpatients (170% of the number in 1990) are accepted.

Key words. Psychiatric community care, Hospitalization, Self-esteem, Team therapy, Psychiatric emergency services

Introduction

The Mental Hygiene Act was passed in 1950 in Japan. It was much revised in 1965, and it was changed to the Mental Health Act in 1988. It was revised again in 1994. It was then much revised again into the Mental Health and Welfare Act in 1995. It was revised again in April 2000.

The Mental Hygiene Act induced the admission of psychiatric patients, and the Mental Health Act respects human right and promotes rehabilitation. The Revised

Sawa Hospital, 1-9-1 Shiroyama, Toyonaka, Osaka 561-8691, Japan

Mental Health and Welfare Act provides a social support system and a system for transporting psychiatric patients to the hospital. This history shows the philosophy regarding people with mental illness in Japan, which has lagged 30 years behind that in western countries.

Delayed Progress of Psychiatry in Japan [1]

In Japan there are 309 public psychiatric hospitals, which have 40 419 beds, and 1360 private hospitals with 320 013 beds. The numbers of schizophrenics in a one-day survey were 216 600 inpatients and 47 700 outpatients, according to the report from the Ministry of Health and Welfare in 1996.

The Organization for Economic Cooperation and Development (OECD) in 1999 reported that the average length of hospital stay of mental patients in Japan was 330 days in 1995, which is as 3.8 to 37.1 times high as that in other developed countries (Fig. 1). The first reason for the long length of stay in Japan is the poor rehabilitation facilities and poor support system. The second reason is the different method of calculation. The third reason is that the figures for the length of stay in Japan include senile demented patients.

According to numbers for the psychiatric beds per 10 000 population in six developed countries given by OECD in 1999, the number of beds in Japan increased by 1990, unlike the tendency in other countries (Fig. 2). In nonpsychiatric hospitals, the average number of acute care staff members per bed in Japan is between 23.7% and 61.9% of that in other countries (Fig. 3). The average number of acute-care nurses per bed in Japan is between 23.6% and 71.9% of that in other countries (Fig. 4).

Table 1 shows the progress of the number of residential facilities according to the budget. The Mental Health and Welfare Act provides for four kinds of residential facility. Twenty people can live in a support house, 10 in a welfare home, 30 in a sheltered workshop, and between 5 and 6 in a group home. Table 2 shows the years when the goals are to be reached. According to the annual goal of each facility, the total number of people who can live in all facilities in each year can be calculated. The annual increase then gives the year for each goal of the number of discharges to be reached.

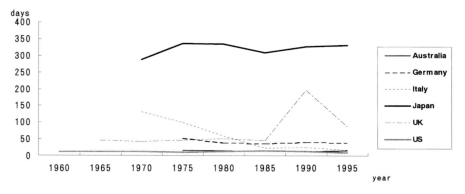

FIG. 1. Average length of hospital stay of patients with mental disorders [1]

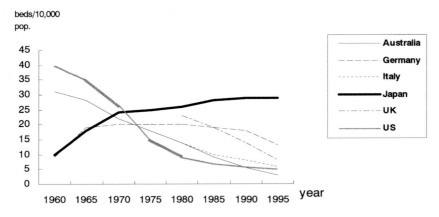

FIG. 2. Numbers of psychiatric beds in six developed countries [1]

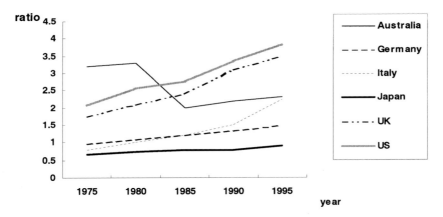

FIG. 3. Acute care hospital staff ratio (average no. of staff members/bed) [1]

For instance, according to the 2000 budget, 100 000 people will be able to live in residential facilities in 2022. But according to the budget of 1999, it can be in 2184, which means this plan is not for patients who are now alive. From these data, the reason for the long length of stay in Japan can be understood.

Rehabilitation Programs in Sawa Hospital

The author insists on four indispensable components of psychiatric community care. The first is residential facilities, which include rehabilitation houses, group homes, and apartments. The second is places and programs for activity in the daytime, which include day care, night care, day and night care, group work, sheltered workshops, welfare factory, and ordinary job. The third is the support staff, specialists consisting

ratio

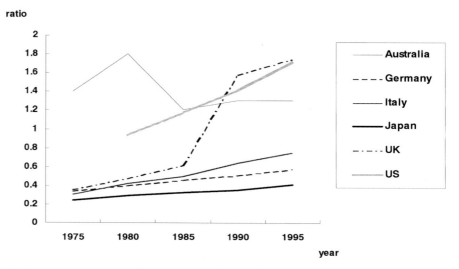

FIG. 4. Acute care nurses ratio (average no. of nurses/bed) [1]

TABLE 1. Progress in number of residential facilities (from the Budget)

Facility	1988	1989	1990	1991	1992	1993	1994	1995	1996 (1)	1996 (2)	1997	1998	1999	2000
Supporting house	0	10	32	41	46	49	62	83	99	99	119	142 (155)	176	232
Welfare home	31	62	51	59	64	68	74	80	88	88	102	121 (102)	109	205
Sheltered workshop	0	0	0	0	5	2	4	7	14	14	24	36 (26)	26	67
Group home	0	0	0	0	50	100	150	220	290	430	540	620	662	795

TABLE 2. Years to reach goals of discharging patients

No. of discharges	1993	1994	1995	1996 (1)	1996 (2)	1997	1998	1999	2000
100 000	2336	2169	2086	2092	2049	2061	2061	2184	2022
80 000	2176	2133	2067	2072	2038	2047	2047	2144	2017
50 000	2161	2079	2039	2041	2021	2027	2027	2082	2009
30 000	2090	2043	2020	2021	2010	2013	2013	2042	2004

of doctors, nurses, psychiatric social workers, clinical psychologists, etc., constituting a team, and volunteers. The fourth component is being understood and accepted by community people, including the movement against stigma and for psychoeducation for the inhabitants. Small incidents bring better outcomes, but big accidents make worse results, in order to enhance understanding and acceptance by community people.

New Places and Activity Programs

New places and activity programs are called "from 'to be supported' to 'to support,'" which is the example of the second of the four indispensable components shown above. This program enhances the self-esteem of patients. For instance, food delivery services for the elderly at home are called "Freudessen," which means "joyful meal" in German. This program also includes volunteers in day care for the demented, training and education for home helpers, and observers in the homes of the demented. Food delivery services can not only enhance self-esteem but also decrease stigma. Part-time workers ride on their bicycles for delivery (schizophrenics are not permitted to drive a car in Japan).

Old people cannot live alone without the help of people with mental illness in the community near the hospital. Volunteers in day care for the demented are also effective. For example, a person with mental retardation showed self-mutilation and bulimia. After playing the role of volunteer, he has never shown self-mutilation. Thus, the integration of the support for several handicapped was shown to be important and effective.

Psychiatric Emergency Services in Sawa Hospital [2]

The more community care expands, the more medical services, especially psychiatric emergency services, should be expanded. Without psychiatric emergency services, people in the community cannot rely on the hospital or accept the philosophy of community care of people with mental illness.

The author also proposes three indispensable components of medical services: rapid response to emergency cases, responsibility for emergencies and rehabilitation or community care, and continuity of treatment and rehabilitation.

The mental health services need not only the three components of the medical services but also the medical model before the legal model, especially in psychiatric emergency services. The Hippocratic oath says, "Whenever I go into a house, I will go for the benefit of the sick . . .". This means that the outreach services are the origin of the emergency services and the emergency services are the origin of the medical services.

The psychiatric emergency service system in Sawa Hospital since 1995 consists of at least an accredited psychiatrist and a visiting nurse on duty for 24 hours, 365 days a year. The number of admissions to the psychiatric emergency services in Sawa Hospital at night and on holidays in 1999 was 438, which is about one-third of the number of admissions per year. In addition to admissions at night and on holidays, there were more patients for the outpatient clinic and much more phone counselings. Much more than half of the patients were not transported by ambulance or police to the outpatient clinic. On the other hand, a little more than half of the patients were transported by ambulance or police in admission cases (Fig. 5).

Outreach services are important to provide rapid intervention for the mentally ill. Because the mentally ill sometimes do not have insight into mental illness, psychiatric services should be given to them where they are. The present state of outreach services in Sawa Hospital for 28 months between September in 1997 and December in 1999 shows that less than half of the patients were hospitalized (Fig. 6). This tendency

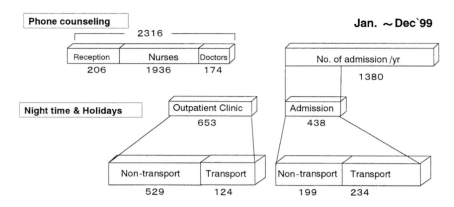

* **Transport:transported by ambulance or police**

FIG. 5. Present state of psychiatric emergency services in Sawa Hospital

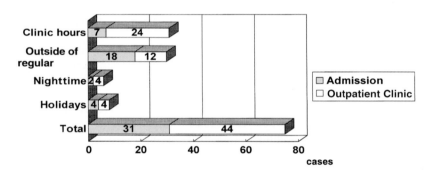

FIG. 6. Present state of outreach services in Sawa Hospital (Sept 1997–Dec 1999). (Regular clinic hours, 9:00–11:30; outside of regular hour, 11:30–17:00; night time, 17:00–9:00)

is found at any time except outside of regular clinic hours. These outreach services are thought to be much more important than the transport system for admission determined by the new Mental Health and Welfare Act.

As examples of the third of the four indispensable components of psychiatric community care, nurse visits and day care are important. The effects of nurse visits or day care on readmission are shown in Fig. 7. The mirror image method was used to calculate the index of total days of hospitalization, times of hospitalization, and days of each hospitalization. The index is calculated by dividing the value after by the value before. Table 3 shows that every index is less than 1, which means that nurse visit or day care prohibits readmission and decreases the days of hospitalization. Compared with the effects of day care, that of the nurse visit is much more effective in prohibiting readmission and decreasing the duration of hospitalization [3].

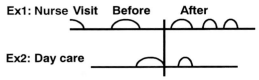

After/Before is calculated in each item

	No. of patients	Total days of hospitalization	Time of hospitalization	Days per hospitalization
Day care	1 2 8	0. 6 7±0. 1 9	0. 5 5±0. 0 8	0. 4 8±0. 1 3
Nurse visit	1 1 3	0. 1 7±0. 0 6	0. 3 2±0. 0 6	0. 1 4±0. 0 4

Mean±SEM

FIG. 7. Effects of nurse visit or day care on readmission [3]

Changes in Sawa Hospital

Expanding the community care or rehabilitation services and intensifying the psychiatric emergency services have changed Sawa Hospital. For 17 years, the total number of beds has decreased gradually from 603 to 505. The annual number of admissions has increased from about 300 to 1400. The average length of stay per year has decreased from 700 to 120 days. Nonetheless, 3400 outpatients (170% of those in 1990) are accepted. The more the residential facilities have increased, the more the supporting services, especially day care and nurse visit, have increased. (Fig. 8).

Conclusions

The cost of admission to a psychiatric ward in Japan is between 1/3 and 1/5 of that in other developed countries. Therefore, the Japanese government has not had an incentive to decrease the number of psychiatric beds, and the hospitals have not decreased the number of beds, because about 90% of the psychiatric hospitals in Japan are managed by private organizations. Many families of patients expect to have the patients admitted in the hospital for life because of the stigma of psychosis and psychotics.

The characteristics and history of psychiatric care in Japan, the history and progress of SAWA Hospital, which has developed these four indispensable components and the new rehabilitation working programs, and the effects of these programs, especially the decrease in the length of stay in the hospital and enhancement of self-esteem brought by the new program, have been shown above. Furthermore, the effect of the psychiatric emergency services and the effect of nurse visits or day care have been shown.

These programs have been prepared in other developed countries since the 1960s, except for the new activity programs shown above. Ironically, this was accomplished

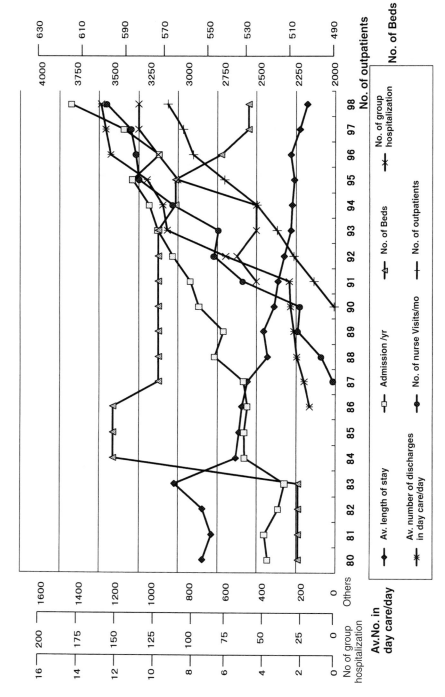

Fig. 8. Changes at Sawa Hospital

in Sawa Hospital because the cost of hospitalization is almost the same as the cost of supporting services in the community in Japan.

References

1. OECD health data 99—a comparative analysis of 29 countries. OECD, 1999
2. Sawa Y (1999) The actual situations and the point at issue of psychiatric emergency services in Osaka and Sawa hospital. In: De Clercq M, Andreoli A, Lamarre S et al (eds) Emergency psychiatry in a changing world (Proceedings of the 5th World Congress of the International Association for Emergency Psychiatry). Elsevier, Amsterdam, pp 443–447
3. Sawa Y (1991) Statistical analysis of the effects of using various means of rehabilitation on the length of stay in the psychiatric hospital (in Japanese) Psychiatry Neurol Jap 93: pp 1042–1052

Optimal Utilization of Resources

Radha Shankar

Summary. The research literature suggests that the key elements in the comprehensive management of schizophrenia should include early detection of illness, relapse prevention, reduction of chronicity and disability, and social reintegration of patients. Delivery of such an optimal treatment would require both a wide range of mental health facilities and trained professionals with the appropriate competencies. India is a populous developing country with a limited mental health infrastructure and a marked paucity of mental health professionals. The existing facilities are geared towards providing assistance during the acute phases of the illness, and organized aftercare and psychosocial services are minimal. In addition, there is a compelling diversity in the demography, attitudes, beliefs, and needs of service seekers. This chapter highlights the challenges involved in the delivery of optimal and culturally appropriate services to people with major mental illness in India. The structural limitations of the formal mental health system suggest that a wide spectrum of community resources needs to be utilized to deliver psychosocial services to people with major mental illness. The discussion will focus on the identification and utilization of those resources that will work in synergy with the mental health system and help offset the limitations imposed by the existing infrastructure and scarcity of trained professionals.

Key words. Limited infrastructure, Scarcity of trained manpower, Community resources

Optimal Utilization of Resources

There are no universal models for mental health care, and the development of mental health care delivery systems is influenced by national, regional, and local factors [1]. In determining mental health policy and identifying both appropriate and optimal mental health intervention programmes for a country, several factors need to be taken into account. These include not only the scientific advancements in the field of psychiatry and allied specialties, but also the prevailing economic conditions of that par-

---

Swaram Hospitals, No 70, First Avenue, Indira Nagar Chennai, India

ticular society, the availability of skilled manpower, public awareness related to mental health issues, and the opinion of the people [2]. Most low-income countries are characterized by a limited mental health infrastructure, a paucity of trained manpower, and economic constraints. Therefore, translating gains in knowledge derived from neurobiology, pharmacology, and psychology into effective treatment practices remain a constant challenge for mental health professionals. This challenge is experienced in the management of all mental health problems, but is perhaps best exemplified in the current efforts to deliver optimal treatment for schizophrenia. In the last two decades, research has produced a better understanding of the several biological and psychosocial factors that impact the course and outcome of schizophrenia. Simultaneously, a range of pharmacological and non-pharmacological interventions has been identified that could possibly contribute to a better course and outcome of this disorder. These include both early treatment [3] and continuation of medication, especially with the newer drugs [4], personal therapy, and skills training [5], Cognitive-behavioral therapy [6] and family psychoeducation and support [7–9]. In a country with a population of one billion people, it is important not only to identify priorities among this array of treatment approaches, but also to develop appropriate models of care using innovative strategies and available community resources This chapter will discuss some of these strategies that will help reduce the distorted fit between the needs for care and the distribution of services. An appropriate prelude to this discussion is an understanding of the organization of psychiatric care and the epidemiology of the disorder.

Organization of Psychiatric Care in India

Treatment Facilities

Over the last 50 years, the mental health sector in India has grown in size and in the variety of settings where services are provided. The bulk of mental health treatment facilities are managed by the state, and the services are either free or heavily subsidized. These include the large mental hospitals and the psychiatric units attached to general hospitals. In cities and towns, psychiatric treatment is available from private practitioners on a fee-for-service basis. However, in the absence of health insurance, the utilization of these services, especially for the management of serious and long-term mental illness, is likely to be limited only to those who can afford to pay.

The earliest state-run mental hospitals in India were built by the British and functioned primarily as custodial institutions. The country currently has 42 mental hospitals with 20200 beds. Psychiatry units in general hospitals and teaching hospitals contribute an additional 3000 beds. There is one bed for each 40000 people. This figure is in stark contrast to that in developed countries, which have more favorable ratios. Although most facilities provide both inpatient and ambulatory services, the dominant medical model emphasizes stabilization of patients during the acute phase of illness. Consequently, there is no effort to link up post-discharge management with ambulatory services, and only a few institutions offer basic rehabilitation programs in the form of prevocational training and sheltered workshops [10].

Community-Based Specialized Facilities for Aftercare and Rehabilitation

Reports in the Western literature emphasize that patients suffering from schizophrenia and other psychoses need a broad spectrum of services and supports to facilitate a smooth transition from the hospital to the community [11,12]. These services are also required to promote recovery from psychoses for patients who have never been hospitalized. In India these reports have not been translated into the creation of appropriate facilities, and it is estimated that only about a dozen community-based day centers and short-stay residences that offer rehabilitation programs and prevocational training are available in the entire country [10].

It is also important to note that mental health services are located primarily in urban areas, and the 70% of India's population that is rural does not have access to even basic mental health services on a regular basis

Health utilization statistics suggest that despite the growth in mental health services over the last two decades, only an estimated 10% of patients with severe mental illness receive treatment, and the big gap between the needs for care and the availability and distribution of services continues to widen [13].

Mental Health Manpower

The country has about 3500 psychiatrists, and 150 medical graduates are trained to become psychiatrists each year. The total number of allied mental health professionals, which includes clinical psychologists, social workers, and nurses, does not exceed 3000. The literature has drawn attention to the role of specialized personnel, such as case managers, vocational counselors, and cognitive psychologists, who are needed to optimize the community functioning of patients with schizophrenia. In India these specialized groups of professionals are present in negligible numbers. The extreme limitations in trained mental health manpower and the nearly total absence of specialized manpower suggest that many of the patient-focused interventions in schizophrenia, which are resource intensive and require specialized knowledge or training, need to be applied in a judicious manner. In identifying and developing appropriate treatment strategies for schizophrenia, it is also important to understand both the course and the outcome of the disorder as well as existing patterns of care available in the current Indian context.

Epidemiological Studies of Schizophrenia in India

Several epidemiological studies have been carried out in different parts of India and have examined both rural and urban populations [14–16]. The authors have reported an average prevalence rate of 2 to 3 per 1000, which is in keeping with international trends. Importantly, no significant rural-urban differences in prevalence have been noted. The Indian Council of Medical research, which conducted an incidence and prevalence study in an urban metropolis, reported an incidence of 3 per 100 000, and a higher prevalence rate in urban slums [17]. Although these reports support the universality of the presence of schizophrenia and the similarity in symptom patterns in both rural and urban centers, there appear to be some differences in both the course and the outcome and in the provision of care between urban and rural settings.

Course and Outcome of Schizophrenia in India

The International Pilot Study of Schizophrenia and the Determinants of Outcome of Severe Mental Disorder were among the earliest studies that pointed to a better course and outcome in India and other developing countries, and suggested the importance of psychosocial factors in influencing the course and outcome [18,19]. The latter study also reported that the vast majority of patients continued to live with their natural caregivers during the follow-up period, a finding that has been replicated in other long-term follow-up studies as well as cross-sectional reports.

Two recent cross-cultural comparisons between urban patient populations living in India with those drawn from study sites in the United Kingdom and the United States have also highlighted differences in community care for patients with schizophrenia [20,21]. Almost the entire group of patients from India (pooled $n = 107$) were living with their families, who were the primary caregivers. By contrast, only 40% of patients from the two Western countries lived with their families. Both studies highlighted the fact that more patients from India were married and were also integrated into the work force. One-quarter of the patients in the United States and 16% of the patients in the United Kingdom lived in supervised residences as part of a community care program. In sharp contrast, not a single patient from the two study sites in India was a resident of a professionally managed community-care facility. This could be interpreted to mean either that there was no felt need for supervised residential care in the community or that such facilities were simply not available.

The Indian Council of Medical Research initiated a comprehensive five-year follow-up study in several rural and urban areas to identify sociocultural and clinical variables that could mediate the course and influence the outcome of the disorder [22]. The study enrolled 386 patients satisfying modified Fighter's criteria, and five-year follow up data were available for 75% of the original cohort. The authors reported a good outcome in 24% of patients and an intermediate outcome in 74% of patients on various clinical, social, and global outcome parameters. Only 5% of the original cohort made very poor recovery at the end of the follow-up period. Using a discriminant function analysis, the study identified 14 variables that could significantly discriminate a good outcome in schizophrenia. These included a shorter duration of untreated illness, compliance with medication, rural domicile, and a rise in the socioeconomic status of the patient and the family. More patients in rural areas were employed than in urban areas, and patients in rural areas exhibited lesser degrees of impairment in overall job performance.

The Madras Longitudinal Study, which followed up 76 urban patients for 10 years, also reported a favorable outcome on most clinical and social dimensions [23]. The study supported the hypothesis proposed by Bleuler that patients with schizophrenia reach a plateau of psychopathology and disability early in their illness. Positive and negative symptoms tended to stabilize at between two and five years and remained moderately independent in both cross-sectional and longitudinal assessments. It is important to note that this cohort was part of a research study conducted in a teaching hospital in which patients were followed up vigorously. This facilitated early detection of relapse and ensured both medication compliance and continuity of care. However, the prevalence study conducted by the Indian Council of Medical Research in the same metropolis yielded somewhat different results. Twenty-eight percent of patients with schizophrenia who were identified in this study were severely disabled and were also untreated, although they were residing within a 4-km radius of three large mental health treatment facilities [17].

Wig and co-authors studied the impact of Expressed Emotion (EE) on the course of schizophrenia in rural and urban patients in North India [24]. This was part of a larger study that aimed at elucidating a better outcome for schizophrenia patients in India, as suggested by the International Pilot Study of Schizophrenia. In comparison with families of first-episode patients in London, relatives from the study sites in India showed a significantly lower proportion of high-EE ratings. However, rural–urban differences in the magnitude of the EE index were significant, both at intake and at the end of the two-year follow up. At intake, 30% of urban families were rated as high EE, compared with 8% of rural families. At the end of the two-year follow up period, not a single rural family was rated as high EE. This was in contrast to the 12.5% of the urban families who were assessed to be high EE.

The literature has also reported on the different components of disability as an outcome variable [25]. Global disability tends to be mild or moderate. Higher levels of disability are related to noncompliance with medication, and men are more disabled than women. The importance of disability in the areas of occupation and wage-earning has also been highlighted [26–28]. Studies on the needs of patients with schizophrenia living in urban areas have documented the felt need for employment and vocational rehabilitation, and being gainfully occupied has been related to a better-perceived quality of life [29]. Reports on the burden experienced by caregivers have suggested that urban families may experience a higher burden, although the studies were not conclusive [30,31].

The long-term follow-up studies suggest that the prevailing economic and social forces allow most patients to be cared for primarily by their families in the community. This is likely to reduce social isolation, provide work opportunities, and enhance social reintegration. The literature also suggests that good outcome is linked to patients accessing services early in the course of the illness and continuing to receive care and support from both professionals and families. However, assessment of needs and family burden, as well as the data from prevalence studies in the community that identified a substantial number of untreated patients, tends to suggest that families cannot provide unconditional care without effective guidance and support from the mental health delivery system. An understanding of these social and cultural contexts provides the basis for expanding the service delivery system so that all patients with schizophrenia receive optimal care.

Experiments in Community Psychiatry

Most of the formal institutions involved in the delivery of mental health services are located in urban areas, and the vast majority of the Indian population lives in rural areas. In an attempt to redress this unequal distribution of resources, experiments in community health care for rural areas were launched over two decades ago. One of these experiments was conducted under the aegis of the World Health Organization's collaborative study on strategies for extending mental health care to previously unserved areas [32]. A rural catchment area in north India known as the Raipur Rani Block was identified as the demonstration site for this study. The Raipur Rani project examined the feasibility of including mental health services as part of general health services. The authors reported that it was possible to deliver basic mental health treatment utilizing the services of the existing general health infrastructure and non-specialist personnel [33]. The success of this and other pilot projects in different parts of the country served as the impetus for the formulation of the policy document for mental health, which is referred to as the National Mental Health Programme (NMHP) [34].

National Mental Health Programme

In 1975, the World Health Organization drew attention to the need for delineating national priorities in mental health and establishing national mental health programs that would define both the objectives and the modalities for meeting the health needs of the population [35]. In 1982, policy planners in India adopted the National Mental Health Programme with the key objectives (1) to ensure availability and accessibility of minimum mental health care to all sections of society, (2) to ensure application of mental health knowledge in general health care and in social development, and (3) to promote community participation in mental health service development and to stimulate efforts towards self help in the community.

The main approaches suggested in the program to achieve the objectives were (1) diffusion of mental health skills to the periphery of the health service system, (2) appropriate appointments of tasks in mental health care, (3) equitable and balanced territorial distribution of resources, (4) integration of basic mental health care into general health services, and (5) linkage to community development.

Following the formulation of the National Mental Health Programme, a wide range of activities was undertaken to test both the objectives and the different approaches suggested for the delivery of mental health services. Among them was the development of a model community-care program in an administrative unit comprising a population of 1.5 million people. This large-scale community project was taken up to evaluate the efficacy of the integration of mental health programs with the primary care infrastructure. The key elements utilized in this project included (1) decentralized training, (2) provision of mental health care in all health facilities in the administrative unit, (3) involvement of all categories of health and welfare personnel, and (4) built-in systems of monitoring and supervision. The results of this experiment in community mental health have been extensively reported, and the authors suggest that it is possible to provide basic mental health services by integrating them with the primary care infrastructure [13]. One component of this experimental service system pertained to the delivery of psychiatric services in the small town that served as the headquarters of the administrative unit. Three hundred twenty-six patients with schizophrenia were registered over a 10-year period, and details of interventions provided to them were systematically recorded. Most patients were managed with drugs like chloropromazine and the provision of basic information and guidance to families. No special efforts were made to offer rehabilitation and aftercare services to the patients, and it was the responsibility of the family to provide ongoing support and facilitate reintegration. This management strategy had a positive impact on 70% of patients. It was noted that the vast majority of patients lived with their families, and problems in providing care arose when natural caregivers were not available or were unwilling to provide for the patient. In spite of these favorable reports, concern and reservations have been voiced about using nonskilled manpower to deliver mental health care that involves complex issues of diagnosis and pharmacotherapy. Some of these concerns have been addressed by the concerted focus on training and the provision of referral support as an important component of integration, especially in the management of complex situations. While emphasizing the importance of using paraprofessionals in strategies to extend mental health care in India, Murthy [13] has identified the following reasons to illustrate the utility of paraprofessionals: (1) Most villages are unable to access mental health services, and primary health personnel are often the only source of help in any type of mental disorder. (2) Rural populations have many traditional beliefs about mental disorders that may prevent them from using the limited services and resources that exist. Primary health workers who are drawn from local communities could be effective in altering the attitudes and beliefs of the community so as to encourage the use of these services. (3) Involvement of primary care personnel promotes medication acceptance and compliance.

The experiences from the community projects have also suggested that although paraprofessionals do not need to acquire very specialized expertise in order to deliver basic mental health services, the formal mental health system must involve paraprofessionals in the planning process and develop mechanisms for review and supervision [13]. Delivery of mental health services through the primary care network is possible in rural communities, in spite of little or no mental health infrastructure and extreme limitations of trained manpower, because of several intrinsic advantages. These include stability, cohesiveness, greater tolerance of limitations in role functioning, and more opportunities for social reintegration [36].

The success of the model projects conceived under the National Mental Health Programme has stimulated initiatives for mental health care among professionals, nongovernmental organizations, and citizens and resulted in a wide array of community-care initiatives in both urban and rural areas [37,38].

The literature has reported favorable results in the training of general practitioners for the front-line management of mental illness in urban areas, although it was not possible to implement specialist plans of management in the primary care setting of general practice [39]. There is growing recognition of the importance of the family as an essential component of mental health care, and this has translated into efforts to provide them with information, support, training, and opportunities for networking [40–42].

The National Mental Health Programme has emphasized the involvement of the community in the implementation of services and has suggested that community members can be used to create awareness and eradicate misconceptions, act as pressure groups to develop facilities, and provide support by way of organizational and material help. The principle involved in all these efforts is the optimal utilization of the available resources, particularly nonpsychiatric medical professionals, lay volunteers, student volunteers, and nonpsychiatric welfare agencies [43,44].

Conclusions

The primary impetus for the formulation of the National Mental Health Programme as a vehicle for the delivery of noninstitutional services was the lack of institutions as well as the resource and manpower constraints in India. Today, there is growing acceptance of interventions that are not located in institutions, are less restrictive, and facilitate social reintegration within the primary group of the individual. This is particularly applicable to patients suffering from severe mental illness who faced the possibility of treatment only within institutions. Murthy has reviewed community-care programs in India and drawn attention to the difference between community approaches as practiced in the West and in India [45]. In developed countries, community care is often an extension of the larger mental health infrastructure into nontraditional mental health settings, and it utilizes mental health manpower. In developing countries, community care is delivered by nonspecialists whose knowledge of biological and psychosocial treatments and the service systems will have to be infused into the primary care network on a context-specific basis. In addition to political commitment, overall economic development, and public and family involvement, the critical success factors for the successful implementation of community care programs have been identified [45]. These include (1) willingness of mental health professionals to accept professional roles and responsibilities that are wider in scope than direct patient care and include training and supervision of community workers; (2) Willingness of mental health professionals to accept an enhanced role for nonspecialist physicians in handling complex mental health disorders; and (3) willingness of mental health professionals to provide clear role definitions for paraprofessionals, facilitate enhanced role status for this group, and develop mechanisms for providing nonintrusive supervision and logistical support for this group of individuals who are involved in the delivery of mental health services.

References

1. Sartorius N (1990) Mental health care in continental Europe. Medley or mosaic. In: Marks IM, Scott RA (eds) Mental health care delivery. Innovations, impediments, and implementations. Cambridge University Press, New York
2. Narayana Reddy GN (1992) Mental health planning and policy development at national level. In: Srinivasa Murthy R, Burns B (eds) Proceedings of the Indo–US symposium on community mental health. Sponsored by the National Institute of Mental health and Neurosciences India and Alcohol, Drug Abuse and Mental Health Administration, USA
3. Falloon IRH, Coverdale JH, Laidlaw TM, et al (1998) Early intervention for schizophrenic disorders. Implementing optimal treatment strategies in routine clinical services. Br J Psychiatry 172(Suppl 33):33–38
4. Kane JM, Marder SR (1993) Psychopharmacological treatment of schizophrenia. Schizophr Bull 19:287–302

5. Penn DL, Mueser KT (1996) Research update on the psychosocial treatment of schizophrenia. Am J Psychiatry 153:607–617
6. Chadwick P, Birchwood M (1994) The omnipotence of voices. A cognitive approach to auditory hallucinations. Br J Psychiatry 164:190–201
7. Xiong W, Philips MR, Hu X, et al (1994) A family based intervention for schizophrenic patients in China: a randomized clinical trial. Br J Psychiatry 165:239–247
8. Tarrier N, Barrowclough C, Proceddu K, et al (1994) The Salford family intervention project; relapse rates of schizophrenia at five and eight years. Br J Psychiatry 165:829–832
9. Szmukler GI, Hermann H, Colusa S, et al (1996) A controlled trial of counselling intervention for caregivers of relatives with schizophrenia. Soc Psychiatry Psychiatr Epidemiol 21:149–155
10. Murthy RS, Kumar K, Chatterji S (1997) Schizophrenia: epidemiology and community aspects. In: Kulhara P, Avasthi A, Verma SK (eds) Schizophrenia: the Indian scene. Post Graduate Institute of Medical Education and Research, Chandigarh
11. Bachrach LL (1993) Continuity of care and approaches to case management for long term mentally ill patients. Hosp Commun Psychiatry 44:465–468
12. Brekke JS, Test MA (1992) A model for measuring the implementation of community support programs. Results from three sites. Commun Ment Health J 28:227–247
13. Srinivasa Murthy R (1992) Integration of mental health with primary health cares—Indian experience. In: Srinivasa Murthy R, Burns B (eds) Proceedings of the Indo-US Symposium on Community Mental Health. Sponsored by the National Institute of Mental Health and Neurosciences India and Alcohol, Drug Abuse and Mental Health Administration, USA
14. Dube KC (1970) A study of prevalence and biological variables in mental illness in rural and urban communities in Uttar Pradesh, India. Acta Psychiatr Scand 46:327
15. Padmavathi R, Rajkumar S, Manoharan A, et al (1987) Prevalence of schizophrenia in an urban community in Madras. Indian J Psychiatry 31:233–239
16. Isaac MK, Kapur RI (1980) A cost-effective analysis of three different methods of psychiatric case finding in the general population. Br J Psychiatry 137:540–546
17. Indian Council of Medical Research (1990) Final report on the longitudinal study of functional psychosis in an urban community. ICMR, New Delhi
18. Dube K, Kumar N, Dube S (1984) Long term course and outcome of the Agra cases in the International Pilot study of Schizophrenia. Acta Psychiatr Scand 170:170–179
19. Jablensky J, Sartorius N, Emberg G, et al (1992) Schizophrenia. Manifestations, incidence, course in different cultures. A World Health Organization ten country study. Psychol Med Monogr Suppl 20:1–97
20. Dani MM, Thienhaus OJ (1996) Characteristics of patients with schizophrenia in two cities in the U.S. and India. Psychiatr Serv 47:300–301
21. Sharma V, Murthy S, Kumar K, et al (1998) Comparison of people with schizophrenia from Liverpool, England and Sakalwara Bangalore, India. Int J Soc Psychiatry 44:225–230
22. Indian Council of Medical Research (1988) Report on the multicentre study of factors associated with course and outcome of Schizophrenia. ICMR, New Delhi
23. Eaton W, Thara R, Ferdman B (1995) Structure and course of positive and negative symptoms in schizophrenia. Arch Gen Psychiatry 52:127–134
24. Wig NN, Menon DK, Bedi H, et al (1987) Expressed emotion and schizophrenia in North India. 2. Distribution of expressed emotion components among relatives of schizophrenic patients in Aarhus and Chandigarh. Br J Psychiatry 151:160–165
25. Thara R, Rajkumar S (1993) Nature and course of disability in schizophrenia. Indian J Psychiatry 35:33–35
26. Shankar R, Kamath S, Joseph A (1995) Gender differences in disability. A comparison of married patients with schizophrenia. Schizophr Res 16:17–23

27. Gopinath PS, Chaturvedi SK, Murali T, et al (1985) Work programme of schizophrenic day boarders in an outpatient therapy unit. Indian J Psychiatry 27:201–212
28. Srinivasan TN, Thara R (1997) How do men with schizophrenia fare at work? A follow up study from India. Schizophr Res 25:149–154
29. Nagaswami V, Valecha V, Thara R, et al (1985) Rehabilitation needs of schizophrenic patients. A preliminary report. Indian J Psychiatry 27:213–220
30. Mubarak Ali R, Bhatti RS (1988) Social support system and family burden due to chronic schizophrenia in rural and urban background. Indian J Psychiatry 38:349–353
31. Chakraborty S, Raj L, Kulhara P, et al (1995) A comparison of the extent and pattern of family burden in affective disorders and schizophrenia. Indian J Psychiatry 23:174–180
32. Sartorius N, Harding T (1983) The WHO collaborative study on strategies for extending health care. 1. The genesis of the study. Am J Psychiatry 140:1470–1479
33. Wig NN, Srinivasa Murthy R, Harding TW (1981) A model for rural psychiatric services—Raipur Rani Experience. Indian J Psychiatry 23:275–290
34. National Mental Health program for India (1982) Directorate General of Health Services. Ministry of Health and Family Welfare, New Delhi
35. Organization of Mental Health Services in Developing Countries (1975) Technical Report Series 564. World Health Organization, Geneva
36. Srinivasa Murthy R (1998) Rural psychiatry in developing countries. Psychiatr Serv 49:967–969
37. Thara R, Islam A, Padmavathy R (1996) Management of psychosocial problems in an urban community. In: Hunt L (ed) Proceedings of the Third Asia Pacific Conference on the Social Sciences and Medicine. Edith Cowan University, Perth, Australia
38. Sharma S, Palit M (1991) National Mental Health Programme. A progress report (1982–1990). Directorate General of Health Services. New Delhi
39. Shyam Sundar C, Kapur RL, Isaac MK, et al (1983) Orientation courses for GP's. Indian J Psychiatry 22:295–297
40. Pai S, Kapur RI (1983) Evaluation of home care treatment for schizophrenic patients. Acta Psychiatr Scand 67:80–88
41. Shankar R, Menon MS (1991) Interventions with families in the management of schizophrenia. The issues facing a community based rehabilitation center in India. Psychosoc Rehabil J 15(1):85–89
42. Shankar R, Menon MS (1993) Development of a framework of interventions with families in the management of schizophrenia. Psychosoc Rehabil J 16(3):76–91
43. Ranganathan M (1989) A study on college student volunteers participation in the services and rehabilitation programs at the National Institute of Mental Health and neuro sciences. Ph.D. Thesis, Bangalore University
44. Issac MK (1992) Role of paraprofessionals and non professionals in mental health care in India. In: Srinivasa Murthy R, Burns B (eds) Proceedings of the Indo–US Symposium on Community Mental Health. Sponsored by the National Institute of Mental Health and Neurosciences India and Alcohol, Drug Abuse and Mental Health Administration, USA
45. Murthy RS (1992) Mental health. In: Mukhopadyaya A (ed) State of India's Health. Voluntary Health Association of India

Applying Effective Treatment Strategies in Day Hospitals: A Nursing Perspective

Franca Berti, Fabrizia Pizzale, Angela Gallerani,
Cristina Mantoan, Monia Simani, Claudia Mantovani,
Monica Zanforlin, Monica Cavallini, Alessandra Spettoli,
Gino Targa, and Ian R.H. Falloon

Summary. The closure of psychiatric hospitals in Italy, as in other countries, has led to many chronically disabled patients living relatively impoverished lives in residential homes. There has been an increasing demand to provide day centers for them to enrich their lives in the community. In general, these centers have provided recreation, care, and support. Some have become a focus for developing cooperatives where the less impaired patients have been engaged in constructive work activities. Few centers have attempted to introduce effective treatment strategies and to develop a day-treatment program. Il Ponte in Ferrara is one center where a team of mainly professionally trained nurses, supported by psychiatrists, has implemented a rehabilitation program for patients with chronic schizophrenia disorders. The program is based on the application of effective pharmacotherapy, mental health education, goal-oriented problem-solving, interpersonal communication and social skills training, and cognitive-behavioral family treatment approaches. The development of this program, its benefits, and its limitations will be discussed from a nursing perspective. The importance of engaging nurses throughout the development of innovative practice is often overlooked but is always crucial.

Key words. Day treatment, Nursing, Innovation

Background

Despite limited evidence for its benefits, the day hospital remains a core component of many models of community mental health services. A major limitation appears to be the continued lack of a clear definition of the goals of psychiatric day treatment [1]. Day care, partial hospitalization, resocialization, vocational rehabilitation, and mere recreation have been considered legitimate goals of such programs [2]. All of these goals may be reasonable for specific cases of serious mental disorders. However, the limited research evidence suggests that most day-treatment programs are not effective in meeting the needs of the most seriously mentally disordered people that they are designed to assist and dropouts are unaccepably high [3,4]. Those day-

---

USA Ferrara, Centro Diurmo "IL PONJE", via Fulvio Testi, 17, 44100 Ferrara, Italy

232

treatment programs that have shown the greatest benefits have usually included specific living skills training and cognitive-behavioral strategies combined with optimal drug therapy [1,5-7]. These strategies have traditionally been provided by trained psychiatrists and clinical psychologists. However, there is growing evidence that nurses, social workers, and rehabilitation therapists can achieve similar benefits when they are adequately trained and supervised in psychosocial strategies [8-10].

This paper describes a day-treatment program in Ferrara, Italy, where the application of evidence-based strategies is provided to former residents of long-term mental hospitals by a multidisciplinary team of nurses and rehabilitation therapists who are trained and supervised in these methods. Their impressions of the utility of the strategies used and their satisfaction with their work will be discussed.

The Program

The day-treatment program, Il Ponte, is located in the center of Ferrara, a medieval city with 200 000 inhabitants on the river Po near Bologna in northeast Italy. The program is located in a community mental health center, that provides a full range of mental health services to half the city. It is staffed by seven professionally trained nurses and one rehabilitation therapist. Psychiatric, psychological, and social work services are provided in consultation within the community mental health team. However, the day-treatment center is managed almost exclusively by the nonmedical team, with weekly group and individual case supervision provided by a psychiatrist who has a special interest in cognitive-behavioral therapy.

Twenty patients regularly attend the service from 8:30 to 13:30. In the afternoon, specific treatment sessions are arranged, in particular, family interventions and in vivo assignments with patients attending the day center as well as others from the community mental health program. All patients have a diagnosis of a functional psychosis, usually a bipolar or schizophrenic disorder, and are usually aged between 30 and 50 years. Most are single, live with their families, are not employed, and have poor social skills.

The treatment is based on the integrated mental health care approach. One or two personal goals are set for each patient after a detailed semi-structured assessment of his or her functional status, key problems, and medical and psychosocial needs. These goals are usually associated with developing friendships and enduring close relationships, and treatment plans usually focus on enhancement of interpersonal social and leisure skills. The needs and goals of families and other key caregivers are routinely assessed.

The treatment program includes a full range of cognitive-behavioral strategies: patient and family education about mental disorders and their treatment; problem-solving groups for patients that incorporate social skills training for independent living, leisure activity, and work; communication skills training in groups for patients that target the development of friendships and intimate relationships; medication management, including strategies for adherence and early warning signs; cognitive-behavioral family therapy in single-family as well as multiple-family groups; in vivo practice of social skills in the community; psychomotor therapy to assist in the recognition of stress responses, relaxation, and to promote physical health; and specific cognitive-behavioral therapy strategies for anxiety management, mood management, anger management, sleep and appetite problems, persisting psychosis, low self-esteem, underactivity, and overactivity.

Training

Staff members have received intensive training courses in evidence-based integrated mental health care since 1990. These courses have been conducted in several centers throughout Italy by national and international experts. Each course has been between two and five days long. They have focused on teaching the practical skills of the methods described above in a series of lectures, demonstrations, and role-played practice sessions. Specific topics have included cognitive–behavioral assessments of patients and families, medication management, compliance and early warning signs, psychoeducation of major mental disorders, behavioral family and marital therapy, structured problem-solving training, social and work skills training, assertive case management and intensive treatment in the community, and specific strategies for mood disorders, anxiety, sleep and eating problems, and suicide risk management.

After the courses on site, peer supervision has been provided on a weekly basis, with case discussion, role-played practice, and problem-solving to resolve difficult therapy issues. Patient handouts for assessments, education, and homework have been prepared for everyday use in the service. Most are based on the book *Intervento Psicoeducativo in Psichiatria* by Falloon and colleagues [11].

Case Management

Each patient has one key worker who conducts regular assessments of progress towards his or her personal goals. The duration of treatment for each person depends on his or her goal achievement and usually lasts for six to eight months. However a few patients continue in treatment for several years as they progress towards more and more ambitious goals.

Survey of Staff Satisfaction

A frequent criticism of evidence-based practice in Italy is that it is tedious and therapists become bored with it. By contrast, psychodynamic approaches are considered exciting, stimulating, and sexy. As a result, the penetration of highly effective cognitive-behavioral strategies has been limited by this lack of staff satisfaction. In order to test this impression, we devised a small investigation of the attitudes of our team to those mental health strategies commonly used in day-treatment services. In addition, we asked them about their stress and satisfaction with the service and invited them to make comments on how the service might be improved.

The eight nonmedical staff at the center (seven nurses and one rehabilitation therapist) completed a self-reported questionnaire survey of their impressions of the service and their job satisfaction. Table 1 summarizes the demographic characteristics of the sample. Each person's impressions of her application of 25 treatment strate-

TABLE 1. Staff background

Professional training
  Professional nurse = 7
  Rehabilitation therapist = 1
Age (yr) mean = 34.5
Sex
  Female = 8 (100%)
  Male = 0
Mouth status
  Single = 3
  Married = 4
  Separated = 1
Years of service: mean = 11.3

gies were surveyed by self-report questionnaire. These included the main evidence-based core strategies that were used most frequently in the day-treatment program, as well as other psychosocial strategies used commonly in other centers in Italy, such as supportive, psychodynamic, and family systemic therapies. Each item was rated from 0 to 3 (0 = not at all; 3 = very much) on how much the nurse enjoyed applying it, and from 0 to 3 on how much she thought it helped the patients.

The five strategies that nurses enjoyed the most were problem-solving, communication training and education with patients, education of families, and psychomotor training. Those they rated least enjoyable were psychodynamic psychotherapy, psychiatric and psychosocial evaluation, pharmacotherapy, and recreational therapy. The strategies considered most valuable to the patients were the education strategies for patients and families, early warning signs, crisis management, social skills training, and specific cognitive-behavioral therapy strategies. Psychotherapy, recreational activities, and psychiatric evaluation were considered the least helpful. Training and administrative aspects of the program were considered highly satisfactory by almost all staff.

Stress and Burnout

Stress levels were very low, with only 25% of the staff rating their work stress as moderate. Few considered that work stress accounted for the time they were ill and away from work. All except one person rated themselves as moderately or very satisfied with their work and were happy to continue in their present jobs.

Discussion

It can be concluded that the evidence-based strategies were well accepted by the nursing staff of the day-treatment program. They showed high levels of enjoyment and considered them highly valuable in the treatment of a very disabled psychiatric population. Stress levels and burnout seemed minimal, despite the high level of disability of most of the patients attending the center. It was clear that with relatively brief training and weekly case supervision by a psychiatrist, evidence-based cognitive-behavioral strategies, including family interventions, social skills training, and specific strategies for mood, anxiety, anger, substance use, and eating and sleeping disorders, could be applied by a team of nurses, social workers, and educational therapists. These findings replicate those of other services that have employed teams of well-trained nurses to apply evidence-based treatment strategies [12–15].

Comments on how the program could be improved focused upon a wider use of psychoeducational and family strategies, particularly with major affective disorders. These included the use of early detection and intervention with major episodes of a non-psychotic type. At present there has been little clinical research on innovative treatment strategies for the affective psychoses. The interest of our group in this area was triggered by a training course one year ago directed by Professor David Miklowitz from the University of Colorado. He showed us that small adaptations in the psychoeducational and cognitive-behavioral family approaches could lead to similar reductions in major affective episodes as those observed in research with schizophrenic disorders.

In recent times, most day-treatment programs have been poorly defined, with vague objectives. The structural aspects of the programs have received the same criticisms. It is evident that the most important aspects of these centers is the treatment strategies that they deliver. Day treatment provides an opportunity to deliver intensive biomedical and psychosocial treatment in a setting more pleasant and more acceptable than an acute care hospital unit. Users are able to return to the sanctuary of their own homes and carers at the end of each session. When social and work skills are core parts of their personal goals, the ability to carry out real-life practice of these skills is facilitated. Families feel more at home in these settings and are more readily included in the treatment programs.

The assertive community treatment programs that enable intensive crisis and rehabilitation work to be conducted in the home or other community settings may be considered a specialized form of day treatment. Once again they have been criticized as focusing on the location of the treatment, not on the quality of the treatment strategies that are provided [16]. It is clear that evidence-based treatment is the essential component that leads to recovery from all forms of mental disorders and their associated disabilities and handicaps. However, it seems important that these strategies be delivered in a highly flexible way that is clearly aimed to help patients achieve their personal goals [1]. Poor adherence to day treatment seems associated with inflexible group-oriented approaches that lack individualized application of effective strategies and do not develop a teamwork approach among patients, families, and professionals [4] Day-treatment centers that provide a full range of these strategies on an intensive daily basis, especially if this is based on the personal goals of the patients and their key caregivers, and has the possibility of being delivered in the home or other settings in the community, would seem to be an important component of the modern mental health service.

Although there has been a strong push in some areas to convert all day treatment to an employment focus [5], it should be noted that this is only one of the commonly expressed needs of disabled people, and that seeking friendship, developing independent living skills, as well as creative and constructive hobbies and leisure activities are all among the personal goals that a comprehensive skills training program can assist with evidence-based treatment strategies [1,17,18]. An additional consideration might be the provision of evening and weekend sessions, not only for families, but also for those people who may be continuing to work while experiencing mild exacerbations of their disorders or who wish to continue to work on enhancing their social, interpersonal, and recreational skills.

References

1. Falloon IRH, Talbot RE (1982) Achieving the goals of day treatment. J Nerv Men Dis 170:279–285
2. Oka K, Maeda M, Hirano T, et al (1999) Multicenter study on the effects of day care therapy on schizophrenia: a comparison of day care patients with outpatients. Psychiatry Clin Neurosci 53:505–510
3. Oyama H (1999) The effect of psychiatric day care on positive and negative symptoms in schizophrenia. J Clin Psychiatry 41:635–642
4. McGonagle IM, Gentle J (1996) Reasons for non-attendance at a day hospital for people with enduring mental illness: the clients' perspective. J Psychiatr Men Health Nursing 3:61–66
5. Drake RE, Becker DR, Clark RE, et al (1999) Research on the individual placement and support model of supported employment. Psychiatr Q 70:289–301
6. Milne D (1984) A comprehensive evaluation of two psychiatric day hospitals. Br J Psychiatry 145:533–537
7. Wing JK (1982) Long-term community care: experience in a London borough. Psychol Med Monogr Suppl
8. Neal MT (1986) Partial hospitalization. An alternative to inpatient psychiatric hospitalization. Nursing Clin North Am 21:461–471
9. Paykel ES, Mangen SP, Griffith JH, et al (1982) Community psychiatric nursing for neurotic patients: a controlled trial. Br J Psychiatry 140:573–581
10. Sensky T, Turkington D, Kingdon D, et al (2000) Arch Gen Psychiatry 57:165–172
11. Falloon IRH, et al (1992) Intervento psicoeducativo integrato in psichiatria. Erickson, Trento, Italy
12. Corrigan PW, Williams OB, McCracken SG, et al (1998) Staff attitudes that impede the implmentation of behavioral tretament programs. Behav Modif 22:548–562
13. Falloon IRH, Fadden G (1993) Integrated mental health care. Cambridge University Press, Cambridge, England
14. Hafner RJ, Crago A, Christensen D, et al (1996) Training case managers in cognitive-behaviour therapy. Aust N Z J Men Health Nursing 5:163–170
15. Lancashire S, Haddock G, Tarrier N, et al (1997) Effects of training in psychosocial interventions for community psychiatric nurses in England. Psychiatr Serv 48:39–41
16. Holloway F (2000) Mental health policy, fashion and evidence-based practice. Psychiatr Bull 24:161–162
17. Andrews G (1999) Efficacy, effectiveness and efficiency in mental health service delivery. Aust N Z J Psychiatry 33:316–322
18. Torrey WC, Mead S, Ross G (1998) Addressing the social needs of mental health consumers when day treatment programs convert to supported employment: Can consumer-run services play a role? Psychiatr Rehabil J 22:73–75

Interpersonal Caring Techniques: Concepts and Quasi-Experimental Research

SUSIE KIM

Summary. Based on Peplau's interpersonal theory, Kim developed interpersonal caring techniques (ICTs) that may be used to motivate patients in the community to gain vitality in life and help them care for themselves. ICTs are intended to help patients feel better and gain creative energy through the nurses' love and attention. ICTs include eight techniques: noticing, participating, sharing, active listening, companioning, complementing, comforting, and hoping. This study used a quasi-experimental, pretest/posttest design to assess the effects of nursing interventions using ICTs on the mentally ill. There were two experimental groups (ICT and non-ICT) and one control group. Statistical analysis showed that compared with the non-ICT and the control group, the ICT group showed significant improvement in self-care, interpersonal relationships, and social functioning between pretest, 6 months later (post 1), 12 months later (post 2), and 24 months later (post 3). Additional data from family members also support the above results. These results suggest that ICTs are effective in rehabilitating the mentally ill.

Key words. Caring, Interpersonal caring, Interpersonal caring technique, Chronic schizophrenia, Community mental health

Introduction

The number of psychiatric patients, according to official statistics released by the Korean government, was estimated to be approximately 1 000 000 in 1995, accounting for 2.2 percent of the nation's population [1]. Of the officially reported patients, 90 000 (9.0%) need to be hospitalized, but only 35 370 are accommodated in the limited space of mental health institutions. The remaining 960 000 patients, including almost 70 000 who require intermediate treatment, are at home without proper health care. The government's mental health policy had focused on the expansion of large-scale, national or public and private mental hospitals. The capacity of these hospitals is still far short

College of Nursing Science, Ewha Woman's University, 11-1 Daehyun-dong, Seodaemoon-ku, Seoul, Korea 120-750

of the needs. In recent years the government has realized the importance of social rehabilitation programs that link hospitalization and normal social life.

Mental health problems are more serious among the economically underprivileged. The morbidity rate is twice as high among economically poor segments of Korean society on the average [2]. Nevertheless, only 5.3% of hospitalized mental patients are from families supported by state welfare, while the proportion of families supported state welfare is 8.9% of the total population [3]. This suggests that a large number of mental patients from the economically underprivileged segment are at home without proper treatment or care. Therefore, it is imperative to develop easily accessible, cost-effective alternatives that would offer effective mental health care as well as useful social rehabilitation programs for the mentally ill [4]. One solution is to establish community-based mental health nursing programs designed to break the cycle of revolving-door hospitalizations and to increase the psychosocial functioning and community integration of these vulnerable individuals [5–7]. This research was undertaken in such a community program, which includes home care, day care, and psychoeducational programs for patients, families and health professionals, provided by psychiatric nurse practitioners.

Development of Interpersonal Caring Techniques

Peplau [8], a leading psychiatric nursing educator, suggested that the nurse plays an important role in rehabilitating the mentally ill. The nurse is in a unique position to influence the mentally ill to have positive experiences and personal insights. Peplau also emphasized observation, interpretation, and intervention as essential aspects of the nurse–patient interaction, and how nurses need to focus on the process of recovering and enhancing the health and well-being of patients. However, the content of such interactions, i.e., how such interventions should be carried out, has not been explained, leaving a vague definition of specific caring actions [9,10].

On the basis of Peplau's conceptualization, Kim [11–13], using Strauss and Corbin's grounded theory approach, developed eight interpersonal caring techniques (ICTs) to help long-term mentally ill patients rediscover motivation and a zest for life, as well as facilitate their independence and self-care. Interpersonal caring is based on loving concern for and interest in the patient and is posited to encourage patients, to make them feel happy and energized, and to increase creative motivation for action. These techniques are as follows.

Noticing

Noticing is the skill of integrating mental abilities with attitudes through sensory information gained from sight, hearing, smell, taste, and touch, in order to become aware of subtle changes, expressions, and feelings. In this sense, noticing is an active means of taking interest in another person. It is like the insightful inquiry a mother tenderly has for her young children. It is a skill of comprehensively yet profoundly discerning and being attentive to all actions open to observation, such as dressing styles, facial expressions, voice tone, emotional changes, gait, special habits, personality, hobbies, and interpersonal relationships, as well as the patient's strengths, interests, areas of low self-confidence, people they may dislike, and family relationships.

Participating

Participating is the skill of jointly observing the other person's physical, psychological, and existence and being involved in their experience. It includes physical and psychological realities and experiences. Participating is being a partner, being involved in and caring for the other person, through becoming directly involved in his or her actions or life at appropriate periods. For example, taking interest in the problems patients face in life, conversing with them, and being a part of their specific treatment plans. Such participatory action helps patients to recognize how much someone is supportive in the distressful realities they face, and thus helps them to face and overcome their problems.

Sharing

Sharing is the skill of joining in the other person's presence, possessions, feelings, experiences, and what they learn. In other words, it is jointly claiming and experiencing life's knowledge, interests, time, talent, dreams, and hopes and is different from a unidirectional act of offering from one person to another. Examples include talking about problems, sharing empathy in the issues the patient faces, sharing different perspectives on common topics, and crying together. The nature of sharing is found in the old Korean saying "When sorrow is shared it halves, and when joy is shared it doubles." Responses to this technique have been expressed as "not feeling lonely" and "feeling strength."

Active Listening

Active listening means consciously and intently paying attention to what truly needs to be heard. It implies an active process of concentration and persistence. Therefore, active listening not only entails hearing spoken words, but extends to the person's inner thoughts and feelings, and seeks to discover the meaning behind actions and words as well as underlying issues through this process. Examples of active listening include assessing mood, facial expressions, feelings, etc. while listening, keeping eye contact while focusing, listening with a therapeutic and proactive attitude, not interrupting the patient's conversation, and observing verbal and nonverbal responses while listening. Active listening helps patients to realize how they are being treated as valued individuals and increases their self-esteem.

Complimenting

Complimenting means finding and acknowledging the other person's strengths and potential, boosting self-confidence, and building growth and development. Such complimenting extends to encouraging, the act of trusting in, affirming, and supporting the person's strengths. In this way, complimenting supports patients to have courage and "can-do" spirit in their daily life, work, and relationships with other patients, family members, and health care providers. Helping patients to discover their strengths and potential and recognizing them, praising good actions, telling them with confidence that they can do it, encouraging them in areas that they lack confidence, reminding them of good things in the past, and discovering and talking about positive aspects, are all examples of complimenting.

Companioning

Companioning means joining in the solitary path the person is taking alone. This is accomplished through words, actions, spirit (*ma-eum* in Korean, and physically being close, so that the patient may feel emotionally supported and be able to recognize positive aspects. Examples include being together with them as a way of helping them realize they are the focus of attention. This helps patients to realize that they are neither isolated nor forgotten, but feel cared for as important human beings, increasing their quality of life.

Comforting

Comforting is the skill of acknowledging the person's feelings through his or her perspective, of accepting the person, and of pulling together his or her greater strength. For example, accepting without criticism when patients share their problems and emotional difficulties, being on their side, and supporting them to take heart. In this way, comforting is a skill of providing what they need, offering additional strength and shelter. Comforting helps patients to have courage in interacting with other people and fosters hope.

Hoping

Hoping means shedding light on possibilities for the person. Examples include telling patients that today will be a good day, seeking together things that can be done now as preparation for the future, emphasizing that they can do it, expressing the belief that the current situation will improve, and seeking the meaning behind the pain or disease they face. With hope it is possible to overcome even the worst difficulties.

Figure 1 is a schematic diagram showing how caregivers' behavior using ICTs influences patients' rehabilitation. It shows that ICTs give rise to patients' self-esteem, which in turn motivates patients to undertake self-care more seriously, increases the interpersonal relationship between caregivers and patients, and helps them to conduct social functions better.

Quasi-Experimental Research Methodology

This study used a quasi-experimental, pretest/posttest design to assess the effects of nursing intervention using ICTs on long-term psychiatric patients in the community. Subjects included both patients and their family members in two experimental groups—the ICT group and non-ICT group (patients who were in the rehabilitation program but not under the nursing intervention using ICTs)—and a control group. The sample sizes of these three groups are presented in Table 1.

Interpersonal
relationships
⇕

Fɪɢ. 1. A conceptual model

- Interpersonal ⇨ Self-esteem ⇨ Self-care
  caring techniques

Social functioning

TABLE 1. Participants in quasi-experimental design

Group	No. of patients	No. of family members	Total
ICT group	40	154	194
Non-ICT group	303	1707	1910
Control group	20	32	52
Total	363	1893	2156

As presented in Fig. 1, three dependent variables—self-care activities, interpersonal relationship skills, and social functioning—were used in assessing the effect of ICTs. In addition, family satisfaction was measured to see the effect of ICTs from an objective third person's perspective. This variable was measured at the end of the experiment among family members of the ICT and non-ICT group subjects.

Owing to difficulty in finding instruments appropriate for the given population and culture, several Western and Korean instruments were revised to meet the needs of this study. These four variables had 46, 15, 15, and 21 items. An analysis shows that these variables are quite reliable, with high internal consistency scores. Cronbach's alpha was 0.9200 for self-care activities, 0.9214 for interpersonal relationship skills, and 0.8997 for social functioning.

Results

There were no significant differences among groups before the program trials. That is, three groups were identical in all demographic variables, such as sex, age, number of admissions, length of hospitalization, and diagnosis (all schizophrenia according to DSM-IV).

Table 2 shows changes in self-care activity scores among the three groups over 24 months. The ICT group had a far higher increase in self-care activities than the non-ICT and control groups. There is no significant difference between the non-ICT and the control groups. It is interesting to note that the score of self-care activities for the ICT group shows a dramatic increase between the 6th month (post 1) and the 12th month (post 2), but a minor improvement after the 12th month. This might mean that it took about six months for nurse practitioners to establish a rapport. But once a positive relationship was established, the patients showed a significant improvement in self-care activities. After 12 months, the behavior stayed stable. As for the non-ICT group, a slight increase occurred between post 1 and post 2 when the patients were

TABLE 2. Self-care activities: group comparisons

Time (mo)	ICT	Non-ICT	Control
Pre	2.65 (.98)	2.41 (.32)	2.41 (.54)
Post 1 (6)	2.61 (.69)	2.45 (.43)	2.49 (.62)*
Post 2 (12)	2.96 (.61)	2.64 (.49)	2.46 (.68)**
Post 3 (24)	2.98 (.51)	2.46 (.68)	2.47 (1.21)***

*$P < 0.05$, **$P < 0.01$, ***$P < 0.005$

TABLE 3. Interpersonal relationship: group comparisons

Time (mo)	ICT	Non-ICT	Control
Pre	1.56 (.72)	1.62 (.68)	1.58 (.71)
Post 1 (6)	2.12 (.42)	1.98 (.59)	1.56 (.68)
Post 2 (12)	2.96 (.48)	2.14 (.61)	1.52 (.72)*
Post 3 (24)	3.29 (.69)	2.42 (.61)	1.48 (.81)**

*$P < 0.05$, **$P < 0.01$

TABLE 4. Social functions: group comparisons

Time (mo)	ICT	Non-ICT	Control
Pre	1.64 (.26)	1.67 (.31)	1.61 (.29)
Post 1 (6)	1.82 (.29)	1.71 (.28)	1.58 (.78)
Post 2 (12)	2.43 (.73)	1.98 (.42)	1.42 (.67)*
Post 3 (24)	2.85 (1.23)	2.12 (.71)	1.23 (.95)**

*$P < 0.05$, **$P < 0.01$

under a rehabilitation program, but they regressed back to post 1 in the 24th month (post 3). This might mean that ICTs are effective in improving self-care activities of the mentally ill.

Table 3 shows changes in interpersonal relationships among the three groups. The score of the ICT group increased from 1.56 to 2.12 in the first six months (from pre to post 1). A dramatic increase is seen from 2.12 to 2.96 in the following six months (post 1 to post 2). In other words, the growth rate was slow in the beginning, as the nurse and patients developed a personal rapport. After 12 months, the growth rate slowed down, showing the stability of interpersonal behavior.

Table 4 presents changes in the social functions score among the three groups. The score of the ICT group increased steadily over the 24 months, far more than that of the other two groups. The score of the non-ICT group also showed some improvement, particularly between post 1 and post 2. But the score of the control group in fact decreased over the experimental period. The results show that ICTs are effective in increasing social functioning skills of the mentally ill.

Table 5 shows the evaluation of the family's satisfaction with the improvement of the patients on the four variables plus self-esteem variable among the ICT and non-ICT groups. This test was additionally made to confirm the effectiveness of the ICTs from a third person's perspective. Scores for the control group could not be obtained

TABLE 5. Family satisfaction scale: group comparisons

Variable	ICT $n = 14\%$	Non-ICT $n = 18\%$	Control $n = 10\%$
Self-care	84.83	77.08	77.5
Self-esteem	87.45	76.39	70
Interpersonal relationships	91.07	70.83	67.5
Social functioning	83.93	69.44	77.5

TABLE 6. Institutionalization: group comparisons

Variable	Group	Pre	Post 12 mo	Post 24 mo
No. of admissions	ICT	13.10	.40	0.10
	Non-ICT	12.94	.60	.32
	Control	12.80	14.01	12.10
No. of days in institution	ICT	236.81	49.21	6.43
	Non-ICT	227.15	55.05	21.13
	Control	228.72	218.45	187.21

because of difficulty in developing relationships with family members of the patients outside the rehabilitation program. Table 5 shows that the percentage of the families that indicated satisfaction is greater in the ICT group than in the two other groups on all of the four variables.

Table 6 presents differences in institutionalization among the aforementioned three groups. Both the number of admissions and the total number of days in the institution per year are lowest in the ICT group, followed by the non-ICT group and the control group. The number of admissions in the ICT group before the program (13.10) dropped dramatically to 0.40 at post 12 months and 0.10 at post 24 months. That is, ICTs are effective not only in improving self-care, interpersonal relationships, and social functioning, but also in reducing the frequency and duration of institutionalization. One of the critical roles of psychiatric nurse practitioners is to educate and help family members to develop good relations with their patients [14,15].

Conclusions

This chapter presents the concept of ICTs nurses could use in community-based mental health centers and the results of a quasi-experimental research design to assess the effect of such tools. The results of the quasi-experimental study have several implications for mental health rehabilitation programs.

First, ICTs are useful tools for promoting self-care of long-term psychiatric patients. Effective day-care programs are important, but such programs, if supplemented by ICTs, can be far more effective in rehabilitating mental health patients than otherwise.

Second, ICTs are effective not only in improving self-care, interpersonal relationships, and social functioning, but also in reducing the frequency and duration of institutionalization. This is a very significant finding for overall mental health policy. After a pilot program developed by this author was proven to be very effective, both central and local government agencies have replicated a similar program in different locations in Korea. It appears that community-based programs will be a major alternative to large-scale institutionalization for the future of mental health care in Korea.

Third, well-trained psychiatric nurse practitioners can play an important role in rehabilitating the mentally ill.

References

1. Korean Ministry of Health and Welfare (1995) Community Mental Health Policy
2. Kim B (1994) Community mental health: How can we do it. Seminar Proceedings on Policy and Trend of Community Mental Health, Seoul Central Hospital
3. Suh D (1998) Understanding of community mental health in Korean society. In: Textbook for Mental Health Practitioners. Korean National Institute of Health
4. Nam J (1993) A study of community-based mental health practice, Korea Institute of Health and Social Affairs
5. Lee K (1993) A study on roles and utilization of psychiatric nurses. J Psychiatr Nursing 2:1, 13–21
6. Lee S (1996) Effect of rehabilitation nursing program for home-bound psychiatric patients, Doctoral dissertation, Ewha Woman's University, Seoul, Korea
7. Kim S (1999) Helping the mentally ill become active again. Health Care Travel Professionals 6:5, 22–26
8. Peplau H (1952) Interpersonal relations in nursing. Putnam, New York
9. Fitzpatrick J (1997) Interpersonal relationships in nursing: concepts and applications. Proceedings of International Conference on Interpersonal Relationships in Nursing, Korean Association of Psychiatric Mental Health Nurse Practitioners, Seoul, Korea, pp 45–51
10. Sills G (1975) Psychiatric nursing theory and practice, milieu: 1946–1974. In: Psychiatric Nursing 1946–1974—A Report on the State of the Art, N.Y.: American Journal of Nursing Co.
11. Kim S (1997) Care for long-term psychiatric patients: a community-based nursing model. Proceedings of International Conference on Interpersonal Relationships in Nursing, Korean Association of Psychiatric Mental Health Nurse Practitioners, Seoul, Korea
12. Kim S (1997) Application of interpersonal relationship theory to Korean psychiatric patients in community. Proceedings of International Conference on Interpersonal Relationships in Nursing, Korean Association of Psychiatric Mental Health Nurse Practitioners, Seoul, Korea, 61–78
13. Kim S (1998) Out of darkness. Reflection. 3rd Quarter, pp 8–13
14. Beam S (1984) Helping families survive. Am J Nursing 229–232
15. Cobb S (1976) Social support as a moderator of life stress. Psychosom Med 38:5

Implementing Community-Based Psychiatry in an Urban District of Tokyo: Report on Minato Net 21

Masaaki Murakami[1], Masafumi Mizuno[2], and Tomoko Kanata[1]

Summary. There has been a rapid growth of community-based psychiatric treatment in many countries, owing to the worldwide movement of deinstitutionalization. This chapter reports on the activities of Minato Net 21 in Tokyo. Japan had a long history of long-term hospital care in mental health, starting from the Mental Hygiene Law (1950). However, the emphasis was changing from relying on long-term institutional care towards protecting human rights and establishing social rehabilitation facilities in the late 1980s. The Japanese government set up the target figures of rehabilitation facilities for the mentally disordered to be constructed from 1995 to 2002. However, the major characteristics of the Japanese health delivery system, such as the national insurance system, which covers most of the hospital charges, and the private psychiatric hospitals, which own 90% of beds, are not much in favor of community-based treatment. Recently the government has been trying to change this situation gradually by supporting community-based psychiatry. Although the network systems that support community-based treatment are not yet well constructed, partly due to the lack of availability informal social resources, Minato Net 21, a comprehensive community care program for people with mental disorders, has started to work on implementing community-based psychiatry in an urban area of Tokyo, where very few social resources for the mentally disordered exist. A multidisciplinary team consisting of medical doctors, nurses, social workers, and a clinical psychologist was organized. They work with the mentally disordered and the family members in order to improve their problem-solving abilities. They are also trying to develop a network system by integrating information. Minato Net 21 is an innovative clinical model that will promote community-based psychiatry, even in an area where informal social resources are scarce.

Key words. Minato Net 21, Comprehensive approach, Community care, Multidisciplinary team

[1] Faculty of Sociology and Social Work, Meiji Gakuin University, 1-2-37 Shirokanedai, Minato-ku, Tokyo 108-8636, Japan
[2] Department of Neuropsychiatry, School of Medicine, Keio University, 35 Shinanomachi, Shinjuku-ku, Tokyo 160-8582, Japan

Introduction

To implement a comprehensive approach that has already been proven effective in one particular community, several barriers have to be overcome if the same approach is to be implemented in different sociocultural situations, especially taking into account the historical background of the legal and mental health delivery systems, which themselves can contribute to the present state of the study group. The characteristics of the community, the stigma against mental disorders, and the family system in the society also have to be considered.

Sociocultural Background

Legal System

For a long time, the basic law administering mental health was the Mental Hygiene Law (1950) from just after the Second World War until a scandal involving the violation of human rights came to light in a private mental hospital in 1984. The Mental Health Law (1987) was enacted, emphasizing protection of human rights of inpatients and establishing social rehabilitation facilities. At this time the government had no social welfare measures for the mentally disordered. In 1993, the Fundamental Law of People with Disabilities was enacted. The law clearly defined for the first time that the mentally disordered are people not only with diseases but also with disabilities, for example, physically handicapped and mentally retarded people. In order to assure the consistency of the law, the government had to guarantee social welfare measures, because the mentally disordered were defined as people having disabilities. The law was revised to the Mental Health and Welfare Law (1995) in order to position social welfare policy for the mentally disordered in the law system.

After this law, Plans for Disabled People—A 7 Year Action Plan for Normalization was officially manifested by the government, making a recommendation for a barrier-free community under the idea of normalization. Concrete figures were shown (Table 1) for several rehabilitation facilities for the mentally disordered to be

TABLE 1. Types of rehabilitation facilities and numbers to be constructed in 7 years' time shown in the Plan for Disabled Persons (1995)

Name of facility	1995		2002	
	Places	Persons	Places	Persons
Life training facility	83	1 660	300	6 000
Welfare home	80	800	300	3 000
Sheltered work institution	7	210	100	3 000
Welfare workshop	1	30	59	1 770
Day care	372	18 600	1000	50 000
Group home	220	1 210	920	5 060
Foster parent system for vocational training	2356	3 770	3300	5 280
Community life supporting center	0	0	650	13 000

constructed in 7 years' time. However, as soon as these figures were introduced, they were said to be too modest to meet the aim of the plan, even if it was fully realized.

Health Delivery System

The characteristic of the health delivery system in Japan is universal coverage for every citizen at reasonable cost. A fee is paid for every service, and the delivery system is functionally undifferentiated. The financing system is strictly regulated by a nationally uniform schedule, and the expense is covered by national insurance and public expenditure [1]. What is additionally most important is that almost 90% of the psychiatric beds are operated privately. As an example of how reasonable the cost is, the fee for a chronic schizophrenic patient admitted to hospital for a month is about ¥250000–300000, that is, about US$2000–2500 per month, depending on what kind of hospital the patient is admitted to. Hospitals are classified into five ranks according to the ratio of the nursing staff, including fully qualified nurses to assistant nurses, to the number of the mentally disordered. The price schedule differs for each rank. The payment is expensive if the ratio of the nursing staff is high. Information regarding the type of hospital is very seldom disclosed, however, so it is almost impossible for patients to know to what rank of hospital they are being admitted prior to admission. Since almost 100% of the citizens have some kind of health insurance, they actually pay 0–30% of the above-mentioned fee in the example, depending on the kind of insurance they possess. At most, this comes to ¥75000–90000, the equivalent of US$600–750. The amount is quite low compared with the cost in America and European countries. This means that even though the length of stay of the mentally disordered is long, the economic burden is not so heavy for the family. The government thought the financial mechanisms were successful with regard to cost compared with the care they supplied, compared with, for instance, the huge asylums that used to exist in the United Kingdom in the 1950s and the state hospitals in the United States in the 1960s. This was true, although it disregarded the patients' point of view that they would want to be back living in the community. Moreover, the hospital-based services were also against the principle of The Protection of Persons with Mental Illness and the Improvement of Mental Health adopted by the United Nations in 1991, which stated that "Every patient shall have the right to be treated and cared for, as far as possible, in the community in which he or she lives" (Principle 7.1).

When the stigmas associated with mental disorders and these economic factors were combined, some family members, especially those in nuclear families, thought it was convenient to isolate mentally disordered persons in private hospitals, because all they had to do was to pay a relatively cheap fee for long hospitalization. Otherwise they would have to care for the mentally disordered by themselves because there was no systematic legal support from the government or from the weakened community care system.

Transition to Community Psychiatry

Current figures show that the Japanese psychiatric system is still hospital-based psychiatry. It has 29.1 beds per 10000 population, which is quite high compared with other advanced nations (Fig. 1). The mean length of stay is 492.1 days. This is also

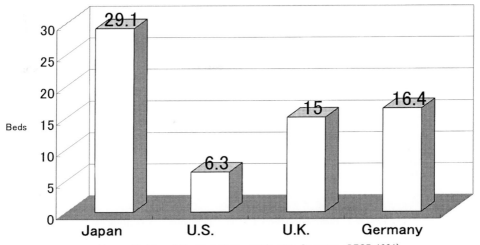

(Japan–Ministry of Health & Welfare; U.S., U.K., Germany– OECD 1991)

FIG. 1. Comparison of psychiatric beds per 10000 in Japan and other advanced countries

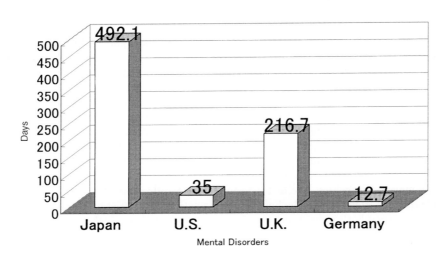

(Japan–Ministry of Health & Welfare; U.S., U.K., Germany– OECD 1991)

FIG. 2. Comparison of mean length of stay in Japan and other advanced countries

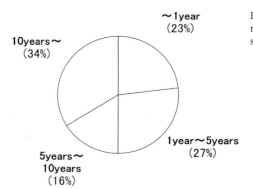

~1year
(23%)

10years~
(34%)

1year~5years
(27%)

5years~
10years
(16%)

FIG. 3. Percentage of inpatients in Japanese mental hospitals with different lengths of stay. [3]

TABLE 2. Basic admission fee paid per patient according to length of stay per day in a hospital that is ranked 5 according to the number of then nursing staff

14 days>: 427 pt
15–30 days: 230 pt
31–90 days: 125 pt
91–180 days: 40 pt
181–365 days: 25 pt
365 days<: 0 pt

One point is worth 10 yen. The hospital is paid at a high rate when the stay is short, but as the patient stays for a longer time, the admission fee per day decreases. 1 pt-10 yen

exceptionally long compared with other advanced countries (Fig. 2). Among the inpatients, 50% stay more than 5 years (Fig. 3). Approximately 20% to 30% of the inpatients are so-called socially hospitalized people who would be able to live in the community if there were appropriate facilities and programs there [2].

The ministry has tried to change this situation gradually, however, through guiding of policy from hospital-based to community-based psychiatry. The ministry is also changing its uniform mandatory fee schedule to gradually benefit community psychiatry. For instance, reimbursement for day-care fees and community nurses' fees is covered by insurance. Additionally, the basic admission fee for mentally disordered persons decreases as the duration of the stay increases (Table 2). This means that there is no longer any economic benefit in keeping the so-called socially hospitalized mentally disordered persons in the hospital. These patients are easier to manage in wards than acute psychotic patients or severely chronic patients, because they are more independent and need less nursing.

Together with this schedule, the government has set up a new scheme called the "recuperation" ward. Under the scheme, once a hospital can build a facility that meets the government guideline, which is more spacious and has much better amenities than the former psychiatric wards, a higher price is paid through a different payment schedule. This means that those mentally disordered people whose condition is deteriorating should be kept in facilities such as the "ospite" in Italy. However, in this "recuperation" ward lies the danger that this system may lead to the abandonment of the efforts of "socially hospitalized" mentally disordered persons to get back to the community, and lead to keeping them in a different facility that may have amenities a little better than a hospital, secluding them from society for a lifetime. Almost simultaneously, a special high price is set for the "acute ward," which must meet strict regulations in order to qualify. More doctors and nurses have to be allocated to these than to the former ordinary wards. It means that the government's aim is to differentiate between the function of the wards to apply more pressure on returning the "socially hospitalized" patients to the community by means of changing the schedule of reimbursement fees.

In the past, before the policy-guided rehabilitation schemes, there were sporadic unsystematic attempts in a different domain to return mentally disordered persons to the community. There were two main streams.

One was in antithesis to the medical model, in which pioneering family members and social workers in the 1970s developed a unique support system in the community. They tried not to depend on the medical domain, instead starting sheltered workshops, group homes, and Life Supporting Centers, which were originally started unofficially through voluntary work but which were all later legally authorized as rehabilitation facilities by the government. However, as they started keeping their distance from the medical domain, all of them are living a life model that is not medically comprehensive enough. Nevertheless, this attempt has played an important role, making breakthroughs in rehabilitation compared with medical doctors, many of whom maintained a pessimistic attitude against attempts to return the mentally disordered to the community.

The other stream consisted of hospitals taking the initiative. They made arduous efforts to return their patients to the community, especially core hospitals that fulfilled the basic function of mental health in those districts led by innovative directors. They had to face many difficult problems at the same time: for example, returning patients to their community meant downsizing the hospital, and the lack of financial support for community-based psychiatry resulted in the loss of income, bringing the hospital into jeopardy. These innovators had to build residential facilities, develop daytime activity programs, and train staff to support the mentally disordered in the community. In addition, extra efforts had to be made to overcome the stigma of mental disorder in the community. Although some patients did return to the community, they seemed to live in a rather confined relationship, somewhat limited to former hospital peers or mental health professionals. These results mean that more remains to be done, not only in coordinating various facilities that are linked to the hospital, but in constructing the network system that is really open to the community itself.

Our attempt was to implement community-based psychiatry in an urban area where no core hospital existed and there was only one sheltered workshop in the area. What we did have was the rehabilitation program based on a comprehensive approach to the mentally disordered, the Optimal Treatment Project (OTP). Developing an effective comprehensive software system that matches the community is also essential in addition to and together with the "hardware," namely, the facilities that have to be constructed, such as those shown in "The Plan for the Disabled People."

Minato Net 21

A multidisciplinary team consisting of three medical doctors, three nurses, two social workers, and one clinical psychologist was organized, using the comprehensive OTP method. It was called "Minato Net 21" after the name of the ward where Meiji Gakuin University is located.

Psychiatric beds are quite unevenly distributed in Tokyo. There are many in the western part of Tokyo, where land prices are low, but they are scarce in the eastern part, including the center of the city where Minato Ward is located. The ward had a population of 154 370 in 1999. There are only 50 beds in the ward, which belong to a university hospital, so they do not play a large role in community care. Thus, there was no core mental hospital to look after the mentally disordered in the community. If someone becomes ill and is forced to be admitted by commitment in Minato Ward, he or she will be admitted to the designated hospital on duty that day, which is likely to be in the western part of Tokyo, without regard to where the mentally disordered person lives. Social resources are also unevenly distributed, since there is only one sheltered workshop in the ward.

It is difficult for the mentally disordered to live in an urban area because of the following characteristics. These people are the result of the disintegration of the extended family and a weakened local community. In addition to this general situation, Minato Ward has few social resources, as previously mentioned. Inevitably, a severe burden is imposed on members of the family living with the mentally disordered, typically members of nuclear families. One of the main strategies of OTP is stress management for carers together with the mentally disordered. It is thus effective when there is little support from outside and the burden tends to focus on the carer. Building a network system so that the mentally disordered and their carers can get access to all the resources they need is also helpful for efficient management. By integrating information, we are trying to be a "one-stop agency" for psychiatric care and social service in the community.

Challenges and Keys for the Future

Challenges and keys for the future are that all the staff cannot concentrate exclusively on this Minato Net 21 activity. They have other full-time work to do and are working for Minato Net 21 on an entirely voluntary basis. There is no reimbursement schedule for the multidisciplinary team for community-based psychiatry to insure financial support. The net is run by research funds. We have become a social resource ourselves in this ward, constructing the network and exploiting social resources for consumers.

This activity gropes towards an efficient model to realize a comprehensive approach in the urban district of Tokyo, where there are local barriers to overcome. Activities include training of mental health volunteers, organizing a festival for community exchanges, in order to achieve efficient networking and enlighten the community. We have been promoting our Net by distributing pamphlets and internet home pages (http://www.minatonet.min.gr.jp/). We are in pursuit of the possibility of developing this Net into a nonprofit organization in the near future to be an active model for the accumulation of knowhow for urban areas or other areas where mental health social resources are scarce or nonexistent.

References

1. Naoki I, Campbell CJ (eds) (1996) Containing health care costs in Japan. University of Michigan
2. Oshima I, Inomata K, Toita A, et al. (1991) Psychiatr Neurol Jpn 93:582–602
3. Takahashi K (1993) Journal of Japanese Association of Psychiatric Hospitals 12:5–49

Keynote Lecture: Cognitive Remediation in Schizophrenia

Robert Paul Liberman

Summary. The symptomatic, neurocognitive and functional phenomena of schizophrenia are in constant interaction and flux as determined by the activity of the brain, psychotropic drugs, environmental antecedents and consequences, and behavioral repertoires. Neurocognitive functioning has been hypothesized to be "rate limiting" in the learning capacity of individuals with schizophrenia for acquiring and utilizing knowledge and skills for success in everyday life. Interventions to favorably affect neurocognition can be staged from several levels or sources, including medication and direct training, or through more general therapies that may have indirect salutary benefits on brain function. Atypical antipsychotic drugs, such as risperidone and olanzapine, have been documented to enhance neurocognition in schizophrenia; however, whether or not such enhancements result in improved psychosocial functioning may depend upon the concomitant impact and demands of the therapeutic milieu. Direct training of the brain can normalize neurocognition in schizophrenia, but these effects have not been shown to have broad clinical value. Newer methods of cognitive remediation, such as errorless learning, may have more durable and generalizable effects on psychosocial functioning, but their focus will have to be on compensating cognitive deficits that are directly linked to instrumental role activities. Social skills training and a systematic therapeutic environment that reinforces adaptive behavior may also yield both improved neurocognition and higher levels of instrumental role functioning.

Key words. Cognitive remediations, Schizophrenia, Rehabilitation, Train the brain, Skills training

The clinical priorities for psychiatrists and other mental health professionals must be the social and role functioning of persons with disabling mental disorders, as well as on their material and subjective quality of life. Symptoms and cognitive impairments and abnormalities in brain function or structure are only important to the extent that they intrude upon a person's functional capacity and satisfaction in daily living. Con-

School of Medicine, UCLA, Los Angeles, CA 90095, USA

sequently, interventions that are efficacious in ameliorating or removing symptoms and cognitive impairments must be ultimately evaluated in terms of their success in improving independent living skills, social competence, and everyday pleasures. Before homing in on cognitive remediation, the focal point of this presentation, I will provide an introductory context for this approach to clinical intervention.

Despite advances in neuroscientific understanding of schizophrenia during the past "decade of the brain," we are not much further along in our knowledge of the biological underpinnings of this most disabling of the mental disorders. Although hypotheses have been paraded with much fanfare regarding genetic and neurodevelopmental abnormalities that supposedly underlie schizophrenia, the mechanisms that translate these putative predispositions into the onset or relapse of the symptoms and disabilities of the disorder are not known. Examination of the distributions of neurocognitive functioning and structural and functional abnormalities of the brain in persons with the categorical diagnosis of schizophrenia immediately reveals the great overlap with distributions of the same variables among normal samples. Statistical significance in differences between persons with schizophrenia and various normal or psychopathological contrast groups has not yielded the qualitative differences that would be desirable when trying to identify etiological mechanisms. Whether one reviews the research on ventricle-to-brain ratios or the size of the hippocampus, thalamus, prefrontal cortex blood flow visualized by functional magnetic resonance imaging (fMRI), hypofrontality assessed by positron emission tomography (PET), or other neurocircuits, the biological basis of schizophrenia has proven as elusive as the "schizophrenogenic mother."

Moreover, if neurocognitive abnormalities, as genetic markers, are as enduring as they have been posited to be [1,2], how can we explain the recovery from schizophrenia that has been well documented [3–6]? If neurocognitive abnormalities are supposed to be "rate limiting" for psychosocial functioning and endure throughout periods of symptom exacerbation or remission, how are we to explain the gifted intellectual contributions of Dr. William Minor, the "madman" who was as responsible as anyone for the first edition of the Oxford Dictionary of the English Language [7], even as he languished in a British asylum for lunatics?

Determinants of Social and Role Functioning

As shown in Fig. 1, factors within the individual and the environment interact in two directions to determine the social and role functioning and quality of life of persons with schizophrenia. Whereas genetic endowment, premorbid social adjustment, negative symptoms, medication side effects, and cognitive impairments—as attributes of the individual—combine with favorable or adverse environmental variables, such as a supportive and rewarding family climate or stressful life events, to influence social and role functioning, so does functioning in a reciprocal fashion affect these individual and environmental factors.

For example, research conducted at our UCLA Center for Research on Treatment and Rehabilitation of Psychosis has shown that the negative symptoms and subclinical psychopathology of an individual with schizophrenia can provoke emotionally intrusive and critical responses in family members, which, in turn, have an

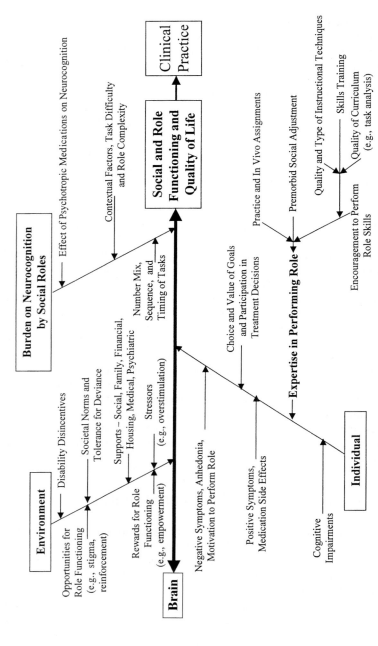

FIG. 1. Factors that influence social and role functioning and quality of life in schizophrenia. The variables or factors that operate from the individual, environmental, and central nervous system levels interact among one another. Thus, environmental factors affect the individual and the brain; the factors within the individual affect the environment and are affected by the functioning of the brain; and the brain is affected by the environment and behaviors of the individual

escalating effect on the individual's symptomatology. If the family interaction continues under these stressful conditions, relapse or exacerbation of psychosis may ensue and the emotional burden on the family may increase [8]. Similarly, imperceptiveness of an individual with schizophrenia to the emotional states of peers may lead the person to awkward or provocative conversational initiatives that may result in rejection or even hostility from peers. As a consequence, the individual may suffer overarousal that even further imperils the accuracy of social perception and decision-making.

As can be seen from Fig. 1, cognitive deficits are but one domain that influences social and role functioning—a multivariate, pluralistic, reciprocal, and probabilistic framework is needed to understand the determinants of an individual's functioning and quality of life. In fact, cognitive dysfunction may not be the most important determinant of social functioning at any one given time and place for an individual with schizophrenia. For instance, among young persons with recent onset of schizophrenia who were treated with risperidone and case management services in an outpatient clinic, high expressed emotion within the family predicted educational and vocational functioning after one year somewhat better than cognitive deficits; furthermore, high expressed emotion also predicted symptomatic relapse, which was not the case with cognitive deficits [9].

Given our genetic endowments and learning histories, we and our patients with schizophrenia share the attributes of dynamic, living organisms in an ever-changing world. We move freely and experience a multitude of antecedents and consequences in our environments that shape our behavior. Our behavior—including cognitions, affects, work, friendships, family relations, recreational activities, and imagery—is always having an impact on our environments, and, reciprocally, our environments are constantly influencing our behavior. The corollary of this science of human behavior [10,11] is that treatment and rehabilitation of persons with schizophrenia, if they aim to achieve durable and substantial improvement, remission of symptoms, and recovery of social functioning, must be multimodal, comprehensive, linked to the phase of the disorder, continuous, coordinated, collaborative, and consumer-oriented [12].

Strategies to Improve Social and Role Functioning

As highlighted in the Practice Guideline for Treatment of Schizophrenia by the American Psychiatric Association [13], treatment and rehabilitation must be keyed to the phase of the individual's disorder. As shown in Fig. 2, during the acute phase of the illness, when symptoms are at their peak, pharmacotherapy is given priority, because it has the greatest efficacy on symptoms. However, interventions that reduce socioenvironmental stressors—such as hospitalization with predictable, low-demand, secure, and stable scheduling of activities and interactions—are also indicated for the acute phase. When symptoms begin to subside in the stable phase of the disorder, treaters give priority to titration of antipsychotic medication to optimal therapeutic effects while minimizing side effects. During both of these phases, it is essential for the psychiatrist and treatment team to engage the family or other natural caregivers in psychoeducational and supportive sessions and to begin educating the patient

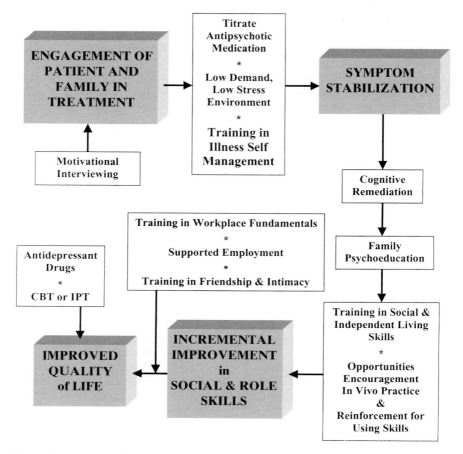

FIG. 2. Phasic progress for clinical improvement in schizophrenia. Treatment and rehabilitation of schizophrenia should be linked to the phase of the disorder. Treatments that are appropriate for the acute phase of the disorder are customarily changed to be suitable for the stabilizing and stable phases of the disorder. *CBT*, cognitive behavioral therapy; *IPT*, interpersonal therapy

regarding the purposes, benefits, side effects, and self-administration of medication. With stabilization of psychotic symptoms, the next goals are to help the patient and family develop an "emergency plan" to thwart relapses and promote the capacity for the patient to connect with and sustain long-term aftercare services in the community.

Regaining social and vocational functioning usually lags behind symptomatic improvement; thus, it is usually advisable to delay active efforts in these domains until the individual has been in the stable phase of the disorder for at least six months. With symptoms in abeyance and the person's social network providing encouragement and positive reinforcement for incremental improvements in daily self-care and instrumental role skills, social functioning gradually improves. However, it is only after considerable time has passed with a successful resumption of involvement in social, educational, and vocational activities that one can expect any improvements in quality of life. The latter is also sensitive to the mood states of the individual; hence, a supportive therapeutic relationship balanced by attainment of realistic yet personally selected goals is an efficient means of bolstering morale and protecting the individual from post-psychotic depression. It is during the stable phase of the disorder that interventions to overcome cognitive deficits can be strategically made.

What are the various strategies for cognitive remediation? There are two direct strategies and one indirect approach. The direct strategies are neurocognitive pharmacotherapy and precision teaching or training of cognitive functions. The indirect strategy aims to compensate for the cognitive deficits that are present, either through use of social skills training or social support that can provide substitutes for deficits in memory, learning, problem-solving, or perception.

Neurocognitive Pharmacotherapy

There is increasing evidence that atypical antipsychotic drugs, especially risperidone and olanzapine, have greater salutary effects on a range of neurocognitive functions than conventional or typical antipsychotic agents. This overall conclusion must be tempered, however, by the fact that most of the extant studies have been sponsored by pharmaceutical companies and, thus, must be replicated by independent investigators supported by governmental or foundation grants. A recently published meta-analysis [14] and a thorough review of the literature [15] have documented the spectrum of benefits of the atypical antipsychotics on specific cognitive mechanisms.

It appears that clozapine improves attention and verbal fluency; that risperidone improves working memory, executive functioning, attention, reaction time, and motor and verbal learning; and that olanzapine improves verbal learning and memory, verbal fluency, and executive function. The significantly greater effects of these atypical drugs remain even after the reduced use of anticholinergic agents (e.g., benztropine) has been partialed out statistically. Although the improvements found with these psychoactive agents have been statistically significant when compared with baseline functioning or with the effects of typical agents such as haloperidol, residual cognitive impairments in patients, even after optimal doses of pharmacotherapy, point to the need for better drugs or supplementary behavioral interventions for further remediation.

It is encouraging, however, that the direct effects on cognitive remediation produced by clozapine, olanzapine and risperidone have been found even with patients who were previously treatment refractory and who had been institutionalized for many years [16]. A number of caveats regarding methodology for research on neurocognitive pharmacotherapy are apt when interpreting the significance of findings that are reported in the scientific literature. These include the needs to register the baseline medication and symptomatic status of the patients, conduct studies with random assignment and double-blind conditions, evaluate the changes in neurocognition after varying periods of treatment, use appropriate dosing strategies and levels with adequate sample size, use appropriately selected and standardized neurocognitive test batteries, and prevent confounding from concurrent changes in symptoms, adjunctive medications, medication side effects, and psychosocial or behavioral treatments

Little is known about the neuropharmacology of cognitive functions in human beings; hence, the use of medications to remediate deficits in neurocognition will remain an empirical enterprise, devoid of theory-driven and hypothesis-testing efforts, for the foreseeable future. As we open the opaque curtain on the functioning of the brain, it is very likely that "designer drugs" will be forthcoming from the laboratories of academia and the pharmaceutical industry that will revolutionize the cognitive remediation of schizophrenia. Until then, there are many new atypical antipsychotic drugs in the pipeline and other drugs that are reasonable candidates to study for their effects on cognition: selegiline, donepezil, modafinil, methylphenidate, dextro-amphetamine, pemoline, and combinations of psychoactive medications. Moreover, little research has been done on the long-term cognitive benefits that may accrue from electroconvulsive therapy or from transcranial magnetic stimulation, even though some evidence exists for better outcomes for persons with schizophrenia who do not respond to any of the available drugs but who do respond to initial and maintenance electroconvulsive therapy [17,18].

Direct Training of Cognitive Functions

One might view effective direct modes of cognitive remediation, using either drugs or behavioral training, as building a higher platform for individuals with schizophrenia to mount as a point of departure for broader and more comprehensive psychosocial and vocational rehabilitation [19]. One of the first efforts to directly train a cognitive function was undertaken about 100 years ago by Carl Jung, who gave frequent assignments to a schizophrenic patient to read and memorize passages from the Bible. Jung tested her recall of the passages and reported that this "treatment kept alert the patient's attention, appeared to improve her functioning and reduce her hallucinations." [19a] Research on cognitive remediation can be divided into two main training strategies: improvements aimed at focused neurocognitive functions, with training taking place under highly controlled laboratory conditions; and more clinically ambitious training of a hierarchy of cognitive and sociobehavioral deficits. The latter strategy has been pursued mainly by Brenner and his associates, with only ambiguous and indecisive effects on both the neurocognitive and clinical outcomes targeted for intervention [20–22]. The laboratory studies of direct training of sustained attention, executive function, and other neurocognitive domains, while in some cases showing changes that approximated normalization of the functions, have not been associated with demonstrable improvements in psychosocial functioning, and it is possible that the training effects reflect nonspecific enhancement of motivation to perform the tasks rather than specific improvements in the cognitive functions per se [23].

Computer-assisted training of performance on cognitive tasks has yielded improvements in the tasks, and on more general problem-solving exercises, with patients reporting satisfaction with the exercises [23a,23b]. Educational techniques such as contingent reinforcement for task engagement were used to facilitate learning. An example of computer-aided cognitive remediation is shown in Fig. 3.

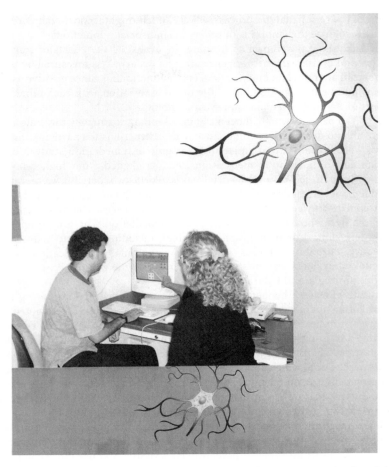

FIG. 3. Recent advances in cognitive remediation include computer-assisted training of neurocognitive functions and abilities

Cognitive Remediation of Social Perception

A study conducted by our group attempted to bridge the gap between the laboratory and the clinic [24] by targeting for remediation an interrelated set of cognitive functions related to social perception that were considered broad enough to have clinical significance. For example, one of the targeted cognitions was accuracy in perceiving the emotions of others, which required learning how to filter relevant from irrelevant stimuli. A second function targeted for remediation was learning how to recall memories of past events that might aid the individual in understanding the cues, context, norms, and rules for appropriate behavior in social situations. Another function included in the training was accuracy in understanding the meaning of facial expressions through a serial analytic process, which we felt might improve patients' ability to rapidly recognize the emotions of others during social interactions.

In our analysis of the impact of training, we evaluated the effects of training on perception and examined whether generalization occurred, as measured by pre-post assessments of attention, memory, and executive functioning. Since positive psychotic symptoms and neurocognition have little or no association with each other, we did not expect to find improvements in psychopathology.

Hospitalized patients who had been stabilized for approximately three months and who were able to demonstrate compliance with instructions for participating in role play tests were invited to participate in the cognitive remediation study. Most were taking atypical antipsychotic medications, had graduated from high school, and showed deficits in self-care and social skills. Forty-two patients were randomly assigned to either 22 sessions of cognitive remediation (20 minutes each, twice weekly for approximately three months) or similar amounts of leisure activities supervised by the same staff who conducted the cognitive remediation. The two groups did not differ on any clinical or demographic variables, including baseline neurocognitive performance, duration of illness, severity of symptoms, or medication dosage in haloperidol equivalents. Patients were maintained on their initial type and dose of medication throughout the duration of the study.

The results showed a beneficial effect of training on measures of perception, but not on attention, memory, or executive functioning. The improvements noted in perception were substantial (increases of 2.5–3.5 standard deviations), with the patients who received training approximating the performance of normal samples at the time of post-testing. The training effects that we discerned may be explained by several possible mechanisms, which at this point must remain speculative: similarity between the training materials and the pre-post materials used to test for emotion perception; use of inductive reasoning and compensatory procedures in the training; or use of homework between sessions and role play exercises in the training.

At this point in the early development of direct training of cognitive functions in schizophrenia, it will be important to identify those neurocognitions which are most closely linked to various types of psychosocial activities and use those cognitions as targets for intervention; [24a] to design and test environmental supports that will enable individuals with schizophrenia to compensate for deficits that are not malleable; to determine if training social and independent living skills at the molar level (e.g., as in the UCLA modules for skills training) will translate into improvements in neurocognition at the molecular level; and to develop new and more powerful methods of precision teaching that will have greater efficacy and generalized impact on neurocognition as well as on broader social functioning. Two examples of the last-named strategy are exemplified by the use of two innovative approaches to teaching now being studied at our UCLA Center for Research on Treatment and Rehabilitation of Psychosis: errorless learning methods, and shaping of sustained attention for rehabilitation readiness.

Errorless Learning of Neurocognitive Functions and Work Skills

Building on previous work that documented the relatively normal capacity of individuals with schizophrenia in procedural learning and memory, errorless learning procedures were adapted for teaching patients to perform the Wisconsin Card-Sorting

Task, a test of dorsolateral prefrontal lobe functioning. The procedure required a task analysis of the card-sorting test, followed by hierarchical arrangement of its constituent components according to level of complexity. The training procedure enabled individuals to succeed at low levels of task complexity and to use these successful learning experiences as building blocks for sequential and incremental completion of more complex tasks. Training consisted of guided instruction, modeling (which incorporates procedural learning principles), and reinforcement to minimize the commission of errors. Once the trainee demonstrated initial mastery of a given level of task complexity, the degree of trainer involvement was gradually faded out. The results showed effective and durable performance of the card-sorting task with improvements bringing the trainees to the level of normal controls [25].

The errorless learning paradigm has been applied to teaching individuals with schizophrenia to perform well on entry-level job tasks in a simulated work environment, with the aim of facilitating employability and sustained employment in the competitive job market. Patients were randomly assigned to either errorless learning or standard, trial-and-error learning conditions. Training was conducted in small groups during the course of a single session lasting approximately 45 minutes for each of two tasks—sorting index cards using various rules and assembling a toilet tank flush mechanism. These tasks had previously been validated by employers and vocational rehabilitation counselors as representative of entry-level jobs available in the community [26]. The results from the first 30 subjects (out of a total of 100) support the effectiveness of errorless learning for these job tasks. Performance was very high for the subjects trained using errorless learning, with accuracy of more than 98% for each task. Three month follow-ups revealed no appreciable drop in performance by the subjects who were exposed to errorless learning. Errorless learning appeared to have compensated for the subjects' neurocognitive deficits, since measures of neurocognition showed a stronger relationship to performance for subjects given standard training than for those involved in errorless learning.

Shaping Sustained Attention for Conversation Skills

Because individuals who are relatively unresponsive to even the new atypical antipsychotic drugs are often thought-disordered, highly distractible, and less able to benefit from verbally mediated treatments, we have initiated a multisite demonstration study at our UCLA Research Center to use behavioral shaping procedures to extend the sustained attention of such individuals as they participate in a conversation skills training module. Investigators at sites in New York, Missouri, Nebraska, and California are utilizing a common protocol aimed at increasing the attentional capacity of thought-disordered and disorganized schizophrenic patients by using "shaping tokens." As each patient meets or exceeds a previously determined threshold of eye contact and appropriate responsiveness to the instructions of the conversation skills trainer, he or she receives both a shaping token and positive social reinforcement (e.g., praise). A cotherapist is responsible for monitoring the attention span of each participant in the group and for dispensing the shaping tokens on a contingent basis, initially every few minutes. Later, after sustained attention has been demonstrated by the patient for increasingly longer periods, the shaping tokens and associated praise are given more sparsely. At the end of the sessions, the patients can trade in their accumulated tokens for special treats and privileges.

The findings thus far have been very encouraging, with the vast majority of these very regressed and institutionalized patients making significant progress in their attention spans—from less than a minute at baseline to an average of 45 minutes after three months [27]. These individuals were then able to participate constructively in a Basic Conversation Skills module [28], without intensive supervision. Similar favorable results from modeling and shaping procedures have been seen in studies of thought disorder, on-task behavior, completion of academic assignments in a remedial education classroom, and appropriate verbal behavior [29–31]. Thus, it appears that shaping procedures, combined with modeling and social reinforcement, can enhance the participation level of patients who had previously been written off as treatment failures unable to benefit from psychosocial rehabilitation. Whether the improvements are specifically a result of improvements in the target neurocognitive and linguistic behaviors or whether the therapeutic effects are mediated through more general enhancement of the motivation and alertness of patients, the point remains that previously refractory patients can now be brought into the mainstream of comprehensive and standard treatment and rehabilitation services.

Compensatory Strategies for Overcoming Cognitive Impairments

In compensatory strategies that seek to overcome cognitive deficits, more indirect interventions are employed to enable individuals with schizophrenia to cope with their cognitive impairments or to function despite being hampered by neurocognitive deficits. These include social skills training, cognitive adaptive training, social learning programs (token economy), and supported employment.

Social Skills Training

In social skills training, the basic learning principles that are helpful for human beings to acquire knowledge and skills are organized and structured so that even patients with cognitive deficits can have their deficits overridden or compensated for, with the result that learning can occur [32]. For example, if a patient has severe memory problems and has difficulty sustaining attention to questions or videotaped models, the trainer can repeat the sequence once or twice or more, or have other group members with more efficient memories to serve as models until the individual responds correctly. Then, drills can be offered that give an individual with problems in memory retention an opportunity to practice what has been presented so that it is overlearned. There is evidence that social skills training can compensate for patients' learning disabilities, enabling individuals with a wide variety of psychiatric symptoms to acquire social and independent living skills [33]. Although evidence has accumulated that there are significant predictive relationships between verbal learning, verbal memory, and executive functions with laboratory analogues of skills training, these analogues are simple questions and answers and do not realistically mirror the actual clinical use of skills training procedures [23].

One of the reasons that social skills training is effective with schizophrenic persons comes from the fact that learning social skills, in large measure, depends upon procedural or implicit learning. This type of learning and memory is unimpaired in schizophrenia and is not significantly different than that in normal persons [34]. Procedural learning does not require conscious awareness or the processing of complex verbal or abstract information; rather, it takes place automatically or effortlessly outside the person's awareness, much like when people learn a new dance step or how to ride a bicycle [35]. Implicit learning is similar to imitative learning which utilizes neural circuitry in the pre-motor cortex and Broca's area. These brain regions have not been shown to be reduced in size or activity in schizophrenia, accounting for the efficacy of social skills training in schizophrenia. Thus, the cognitive skills practiced and utilized in social skills training are based on neural circuits that have been "spared" from impairment in schizophrenia.

The modules in the UCLA Social and Independent Living Skills Program capitalize on the intact neural systems underlying implicit and procedural learning. These modules include Medication Management, Symptom Management, Basic Conversation Skills, Friendship and Intimacy, Recreation for Leisure, Community Re-Entry, and Substance Abuse Management [28]. Each module comprises seven recurring learning activities which are used to teach the skills in each topical area and which are designed to overcome or compensate for cognitive impairments. The learning activities that enable the modules to exert prepotency over all but the most severe cognitive and symptomatic impairments include motivational interviewing and induction of therapeutic but realistic expectations; video models with Socratic questions and answers; role play exercises with coaching and video feedback of "self-as-model"; problem-solving exercises related to gathering resources for using the skills and overcoming unexpectedly encountered obstacles en route to using the skills; and in vivo and homework exercises to promote generalization. The ability of the modules and other modes of skills training to compensate for cognitive impairments is reflected by the international dissemination of the modules [36], their translation into 16 different languages [37], and their demonstrated effectiveness in a range of naturalistic settings. Although further systematic study is required, preliminary data from a controlled study of social skills training at our Research Center at UCLA, Keio University, and Fukushima Medical College [see chapter by Mizuno and Kashima, this volume; S. Niwa, unpublished paper] revealed that improvements occurred in selected neurocognitive functions as a result of the skills training. This suggests that "top-down" cognitive remediation may be a possibility which is congruent with basic neuroscience studies of the plasticity of the brain.

Cognitive Adaptive Training

Cognitive Adaptive Training (CAT) consists of a battery of neurocognitive and behavioral assessments paired with manual-driven interventions that are designed to compensate for the specific deficits in executive functions, attention, and memory that were detected during the assessment phase. CAT interventions include such environmental supports as posted signs, checklists, signaling devices (e.g., beepers), specially labeled containers for organizing belongings, and palm-held computers or other scheduling tools. These compensatory methods are established in the patients' homes and maintained and updated during weekly home visits by a therapist. Empirical evaluations of CAT found that the interventions improved adaptive functioning and quality of life, as well as reducing relapse rates by approximately 45% in comparison to control conditions [38].

A case vignette illustrates how CAT can be helpful to patients who are pursuing vocational goals. A 41-year-old university graduate, who had formerly worked in jobs that required business acumen, had been unemployed since the onset of his schizophrenia 12 years previously. His neurocognitive testing revealed unimpaired intelligence but significant impairments in organization, planning, sustained attention, and working memory. His assets included normal or above-normal verbal fluency, language abilities, psychomotor speed, visual-motor sequencing, concept formation, and cognitive flexibility (e.g., normal performance on the Wisconsin Card Sorting Test). With the help of a palm-held computer, which he was taught to use, and daily to weekly telephone reminders, prompts, and reinforcement, he was able to obtain and sustain a job as a clerk in an upscale bookstore, which he enjoyed because it brought him into contact with fellow college graduates and enabled him to use his language and vocabulary skills. In Fig. 4 is shown a spectrum of electronic communication devices that can promote continuity and coordination of mental health services, adherence to treatment, and application of social and independent living skills into everyday life.

Other Compensatory Programs

Two other compensatory programs that can enable patients with schizophrenia to overcome or accommodate to their cognitive deficits and symptoms while achieving their personal goals with higher levels of psychosocial functioning are supported employment and social learning programs (token economy). Supported employment is characterized by a "place, then train" ideology of rehabilitation, which has been documented to enable individuals with severe and persisting mental illness to obtain ordinary jobs in the competitive marketplace much more frequently than the old-fashioned, transitional, or sheltered employment programs that featured a "train, then place" philosophy [39].

Jobs are found for patients, or patients find their own, with the help of the vocational specialist, who continues to provide follow-along emotional and professional support to the individual indefinitely while the individual continues to work. If a job is lost, the debacle is viewed as a learning experience, and the vocational specialist and patient persevere in finding another job. Other attributes of supported employment include integrating the activities of the vocational specialist or job coach within the services of a comprehensive psychiatric treatment team; frequent consultation between the employment specialist and the other members of the treatment team, especially with the psychiatrist, who must often make judgments regarding adjustments in the patient's type and dose of medication and provide crisis intervention; a positive and informed expression of desire to work by the patient prior to beginning a job search; and matching the person with the job, using the person's preferences, interests, assets, and deficits to optimize compatibility.

When a structured, manual-driven approach to supported employment is used with high fidelity by staff members, evidence to date suggests that upwards of 40% of persons with schizophrenia can obtain competitive employment. Because of fears of

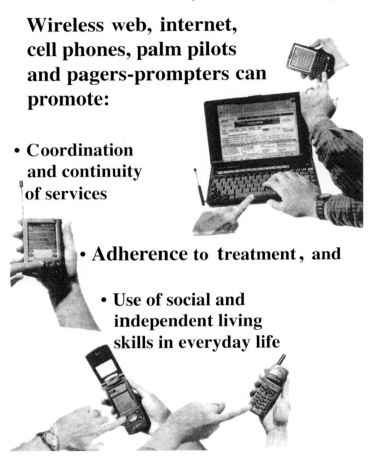

Wireless web, internet, cell phones, palm pilots and pagers-prompters can promote:

- **Coordination and continuity of services**

- **Adherence to treatment, and**

- **Use of social and independent living skills in everyday life**

FIG. 4. Electronic communication devices useful in mental health services

jeopardizing their Social Security benefits, most of these individuals choose part-time jobs not exceeding 10–20 hours per week [40]. It is likely that the supportive role of the employment specialist and the "wrap-around" and well-coordinated services of the psychiatric team permit the schizophrenic patient to compensate for cognitive deficits in obtaining and maintaining work. Unfortunately, follow-up studies have found that fewer than 50% of those participating in supported employment who do get to work are still working at that job six months later. Inadequate job tenure may derive from deficits in work or social skills, neurocognitive impairments, loss of interest or motivation, or exacerbations of psychosis.

The Workplace Fundamentals Module was designed to improve the job tenure and satisfaction of persons with mental disabilities. As shown in Table 1, this module consists of four major skill areas, the first of which aims to establish motivation for working and the subsequent ones to improve job performance. An evaluation of this

TABLE 1. Skill areas of the Workplace Fundamentals Module

Why work? Identifying the benefits and demands of working
Getting comfortable on the job: What is this job and this
    workplace?
Anticipating stressors on the job: What problems may occur?
Coping with stressors on the job: How am I going to solve this
    problem?

The Workplace Fundamentals Module has four major skill areas
which focus on establishing motivation for the individual's decision
to work, followed by preparing participants to anticipate and cope
with stressors at the workplace. The primary coping technique
taught in the Workplace Fundamentals Module is social problem-
solving

module documented a doubling of the knowledge and skills among patients participating in a group, accompanied by almost 20% more hours in competitive work
during the 3 months of training [40a].

Round-the-clock social learning or token economy programs have been among the
best-replicated and validated psychosocial interventions for schizophrenia [41]. These
programs create an ongoing "learning environment" for patients with schizophrenia
where the involvement of participants in educational programs aimed at improving
self-care, personal hygiene, social relations, academic skills, and adaptive behavior is
supported by a motivational climate wherein tangible, material, and social reinforcers
are delivered contingent upon appropriate behavior by the patients [42–44].

One study carried out at the longest-lived token economy, the Camarillo-UCLA
Clinical Research Unit of the UCLA Center for Research on Treatment and Rehabilitation of Psychosis, showed the prepotent effectiveness of the social learning procedures in overcoming neurocognitive deficits in patients with treatment-refractory
forms of schizophrenia. Patients were randomly assigned to receive risperidone or
haloperidol in a double-blind evaluation of the effects of these two antipsychotic
drugs on a spectrum of neurocognitive functions. Whereas risperidone had significantly greater effects on a wide range of neurocognitions (including verbal fluency,
verbal learning, working memory, and emotion perception), these advantages were
not translated into better ward functioning for the risperidone-treated patients compared to those who received haloperidol. Presumably because the token economy was
such a powerful motivational force, patients under both drug conditions showed
similar improvement in activities of daily living and aggressive and destructive behavior. Similar prepotency of psychosocial intervention was reported for supported
employment programs that observed the differential effects of atypical antipsychotics
on cognition.

Conclusions

We should not heed the skeptical, cynical, and disbelieving views of colleagues who
would turn away from the challenge of developing techniques for directly modifying
neurocognition in schizophrenia. Challenges abound in science and medicine that
deter the faint of heart. Advances cannot and should not be blocked by dissenters and

Philistines who publish their nay-saying in the guise of sound, critical expertise. Practical applications in science and medicine have always had to await the development of scientific breakthroughs and new technology to bring about further advances in practice.

Our knowledge of the brain, its structure and functions, is in its infancy. One only need to ponder the extraordinary complexity inherent in the brain to appreciate the discoveries that are still beyond the horizon; the brain has 100 billion neurons, each of which has 200,000 synapses. Each synapse probably has a minimum of 200 different neurotransmitters affecting its excitation and inhibition, but we only know something about 25 of these chemical messengers at present. Each neurotransmitter very likely articulates with 50 different receptors, and each connection of neurotransmitter with receptor opens a flood of secondary and tertiary changes in the cell membrane, transporter systems, protein and enzymatic synthesis or inhibition and further chemical changes that we may not fully appreciate at present. With the plasticity of the brain reflected by well over 200 billion neural circuits, why can't we be optimistic of gaining greater mastery over cognitive impairments in schizophrenia in the future?

Without the scientific discoveries of Michael Faraday, Alessandro Volta, and Humphrey Davy, the development of the electric light bulb and the movie camera by Thomas Edison would not have been possible. Without the basic anatomical work of Thomas Harvey and the discovery of ether and nitrous oxide as anesthetics, modern surgery would not have been possible. Without the basic theoretical and experimental work of von Neumann, Aiken, Mauchly, and Eckart, the omnipresent computer would not be available to us. Without the pioneering research of Pavlov and Skinner, behavior therapy would not be in widespread use; and without the serendipitous discovery of chlorpromazine by the French physicians Henri Laborit, Jean Delay, and Pierre Deniker 50 years ago, we would still be treating persons with schizophrenia by anachronistic custodial and constraining methods in locked wards of large asylums.

Plasticity of the Brain: Procedural or Implicit Learning and Memory

In addition to the infusion of new training techniques that can be drawn from the field of applied behavior analysis (e.g., errorless learning, antecedent control) and precision teaching (e.g., academic learning time, automatic learning, flexible learning environments), we can look forward to new opportunities for cognitive remediation from the basic knowledge that is emerging from the view of the brain as possessing plasticity and redundancy in its own capacities for managing information and for compensating for damaged neural circuits, cells, and regions.

There is increasing evidence that persons with schizophrenia have well-preserved procedural (implicit) capacities for learning and memory that lie outside of conscious awareness and are most likely dependent upon the functioning of the sensory (parietal) neocortex [45], but not the medial temporal structures that may be impaired in schizophrenia. Acquisition of new information via procedural mechanisms appears to activate the parietal, motor, and prefrontal areas, whereas consolidation and memory appear to be mediated by the cerebellar, parietal, and premotor areas, which are not viewed as impaired in schizophrenia [46]. This would suggest that training techniques that utilize implicit procedures—such as errorless learning and probabilistic classification learning—may permit individuals with schizophrenia to improve their neurocognition, through training of compensatory systems that can replace or substitute for impairments in attention, working memory, emotion perception, or executive functions. Developments in educational technology and cognitive neuroscience may soon magnify the therapeutic impact of clinical neurocognition.

New developments in brain plasticity underscore an optimistic view of the future for cognitive remediation of schizophrenia. Reprogramming the brain has been achieved with constraint-induced movement therapy for stroke survivors with hemiplegia or hemiparesis. By involving patients full time in a regimen of planned immobilization of their nonaffected limb, patients were required to feed themselves and carry out a spectrum of exercises and self-care functions with their disabled limb. After a month, not only did the post-stroke patients regain approximately 65% of the use of their disabled limbs, but neuroimaging found that the area of the brain impaired by the stroke had doubled in size. If this type of reprogramming is feasible in the brains of individuals with cerebrovascular accidents, there is good reason to design similar treatment strategies for persons with schizophrenia; for example, in developing constraint-induced therapy for working memory and verbal learning.

Two other studies of the surprising capacity of the brain for functional abilities suggests that procedural or implicit learning and memory may be mobilized for more utilitarian purposes than heretofore in the treatment of schizophrenia. In one of these studies, post-stroke individuals who were unable to articulate or give rationales for observed interpersonal interaction showed an uncanny ability to discern dissimulation when observing videotapes of notorious public figures (e.g., President Nixon lying about his involvement in the Watergate fiasco or President Clinton lying about his involvement with Monica Lewinsky). That implicit learning and memory may also be utilized in remediating emotion perception is suggested by studies that have shown how quickly and unconsciously people can make accurate and reliable "snap" judgments of applicants who are going through job interviews or teachers who are instructing their students in class. Rapid judgments based on viewing 15 seconds of videotape excerpts, where the raters were not able to articulate the reasons for their judgments, were astoundingly sound and consistent with ratings made from entire job interviews or experiences of students at the end of an entire semester with their teachers. The advent of virtual reality methods, based on computer technology, has already led to therapeutic applications for anxiety disorders and behavioral medicine in pain and circulatory management. Given the key role of emotion perception in mediating social and vocational functioning in schizophrenia, virtual reality techniques may have therapeutic potential in improving schizophrenics' perception of emotion through brain mechanisms of implicit learning and memory [47].

Brain Plasticity: Well-Preserved Brain Regions and Neuronal Growth

As noted above, an area of the brain that is well preserved in schizophrenia and that may account for the efficacy of social skills training is the premotor cortex, which is activated during fMRI experiments when subjects are asked to imitate hand gestures demonstrated by a model. In other words, the same regions of the brain that send commands to our muscles when we act also seem able to recognize the same action when performed by others. Providing a bridge from thought and action to the crucial role of imitation in our social behavior, both the premotor cortex and Broca's language area may reveal the neuroanatomy that mediates communication and social skills.

The plasticity of the brain invokes the prospects for new and more effective methods of cognitive remediation. Several recent findings utilizing neuroimaging provide more detailed insights into the scope of neuroplasticity. In a landmark study that demonstrated the normalization of abnormalities in the brain of patients with severe psychopathology, both pharmacotherapy and behavior therapy brought about normal glucose metabolism in the right caudate nucleus among patients with obsessive-compulsive disorder. The normalization of metabolism, viewed by PET scans, was seen only in those patients who responded therapeutically to the two types of intervention [48]. As psychiatric treatment and rehabilitation increases the number of individuals with schizophrenia who recover symptomatically and functionally from their disorders, pre- vs. postneuroimaging studies of temporo-frontal-thalamic regions of the brain (which have been found to be abnormal in size and function in schizophrenia) will become research priorities. Such studies will push back the frontier of the clinical significance of neuroplasticity in schizophrenia.

A plethora of experimental findings have documented the influence of experience, environment, and behavior on brain structure. Just as stimulus deprivation leads to anatomic as well as functional loss, enriched stimulation from the environment produces increased density of neurons and processes in the brain. Engaging subjects in learning tasks leads to synaptogenesis. Remapping of the brain has been found with as little as 15 min of practice on a given task [49], and educational interventions have been shown to increase cognitive capacity [50].

Several processes affecting brain structure, such as myelination, arborization of dendrites and axons, synaptogenesis, formation of new neurotransmitter receptor sites, and neuronal cell structure persist throughout the life span, especially during childhood and adolescence [51]. The corpus collosum increases in size from age 3 to 9 years. Because this structure integrates the activity of the left and right cerebral hemispheres, the increased size may reflect increased ability to perform higher-level cognitive abilities. Longitudinal studies of children and adolescents have charted the growth spurts in the brain between the ages of 3 and 15 years that coincide with important leaps in learning ability. During this age interval, rapid growth is seen in the frontal circuits responsible for focusing attention, maintaining alertness, planning actions, organizing new skills, and learning new behaviors. During adolescence, higher growth rates are seen in the parietal lobe and premotor cortex, areas associated with language skills, mathematical thinking, and understanding of spatial relationships.

Other investigators have found brain growth through age 21, primarily related to additional neuronal columns and progenitor neural cells in the ventricles of older adults. The concept of "reserve brain capacity" suggests that intellectual experience throughout life can have a salutary effect on neural structure and function, even engendering resilience of the brain and protecting the person from the ravages of brain injury or disease. For example, at the older end of the age spectrum, nuns whose language was grammatically and conceptually more complex earlier in life were significantly less likely to develop Alzheimer's disease than nuns with more mundane language capacities. As neuropharmacologists make further progress in the isolation and development of nerve growth factors, we may look forward to a day when the so-called rate-limiting psychosocial adaptations linked to impairments in neurocognition of persons with schizophrenia will only remain as a bad memory.

Even adequate amounts of sleep can have salubrious effects on the brain, and sleep is certainly a modifiable element in the everyday life of a person with schizophrenia. Researchers have shown that when people learn a new skill, their performance does not improve until after they have had more than six and preferably eight hours of sleep. Even new factual information may be encoded more reliably when sufficient sleep has been had. During both deep, slow-wave sleep and dreaming or rapid eye movement (REM) sleep cycles, physical and chemical reactions occur that apparently strengthens memory traces.

The evidence from experimental psychology and neuroscience is that the human brain is not fully formed at birth; rather, the growth of synapses, neurotransmitter receptors, and even neurons is strongly influenced by experience. The frontal lobes, where planning, initiative, learning, emotion, and reasoning are integrated, do not fully develop until adolescence and young adulthood. Every behavioral action, emotional response, personality trait, and neurocognitive function involves both nature and nurture. The timeless and tiresome questions "Is it nature or nurture?" or "Is cognitive remediation possible?" should be replaced by "What forms of pharmacological and behavioral interventions facilitate the most desirable and functional qualities in human nature, schizophrenia, and neurocognition?" As the interrelationships of social and neurochemical influences become more widely recognized and studied, the identification, design, and empirical validation of new interventions for cognitive remediation will mature into an organized scientific effort that will push back the frontier of our ignorance of interactions among brain, behavior, and environment.

Future Directions

Cognitive remediation, like charity, begins at home. This means that our own cognitions and attitudes must change in many ways if we are to effectively offer cognitive remediation to our patients with schizophrenia. What are the attitudes that mental health professionals must adopt for themselves?

- A realistic optimism, based on recent outcome studies, that symptomatic remission and functional recovery is possible in upwards of 50% of persons with schizophrenia. We must surrender outdated stereotypes and beliefs about the deteriorating course of schizophrenia.
- Willingness to provide comprehensive (including cognitive remediation), continuous, coordinated, and consumer-oriented treatment and rehabilitation that involves the patient and family in the treatment enterprise. We must discard former styles of treatment that were patronizing and paternalistic.
- Providing treatment and rehabilitation in the natural environment, using mobile outreach and personal telecommunication technology that has the potential for stretching our limited time and personnel to prompt, reinforce, and monitor progress in our clientele. This approach, grounded in the lives of our patients and

their own personal goals, will also enhance the generalization of skills and cognitive remediation to patients' everyday life.

- Encouraging our patients to manage their own illnesses, by taking more responsibility for learning how to reliably use their medications, identify their warning signs of relapse, and implement relapse prevention plans. The corollary of patients' becoming partners with us in treatment, rather than passive receptacles for our services, is our responsibility to design and validate evidence-based methods for teaching illness- or disease-management skills to patients.
- Helping to erase stigma by discussing openly with patients, relatives, and the general public the names, nature, and treatment of the disorders which we treat. We must avoid euphemisms and stop closeting our own mental disorders. If we cannot speak openly about our own recovery from mood, anxiety, and other disorders, how can we expect the public and media to speak openly about schizophrenia? If we do not become part of the solution to stigma by taking every opportunity to speak directly and candidly about serious mental disorders, then we are part of the problem.

The future is bright with hope for consumers, carers, and clinicians. The twenty-first century will see the control of schizophrenia as a scourge of mankind around the world, just as infectious diseases were controlled or eliminated in the twentieth century.

References

1. Nuechterlein KH, Dawson ME (1984) Information processing and attentional functioning in the developmental course of schizophrenia disorders. Schizophr Bull 10:160–203
2. Green MF, Nuechterlein KH (1999) Should schizophrenia be treated as a neurocognitive disorder? Schizophr Bull 25:309–320
3. Harding CM, Zahniser FH (1994) Empirical correction of seven myths about schizophrenia with implications for treatment. Acta Psychiatr Scand 90 (Suppl 384):140–146
4. Lovejoy M (1983) Expectations and the recovery process. Schizophr Bull 8:605–609
5. Edwards J, Maude D, McGorry PD, et al (1998) Prolonged recovery in first episode psychosis. Br J Psychiatry 172:107–116
6. Nasar S (1998) The beautiful mind. Simon & Schuster, New York
7. Winchester S (1998) The professor and the madman: A tale of murder, insanity, and the making of the Oxford English Dictionary. Harper Collins, New York
8. Rosenfarb I, Goldstein M, Mintz J, et al (1995) Expressed emotion and subclinical psychopathology observable within the transactions between schizophrenic patients and their family members. J Abnorm Psychol 104:259–267
9. Nuechterlein KH, Green MF, Subotnik K, et al (2001) Cognitive factors are highly predictive of work outcome in the early course of schizophrenia. Schizophr Res (in press)
10. Liberman RP (1972) A guide to behavioral analysis and therapy. Pergamon, New York
11. Liberman RP, Bedell J (1989) Behavior therapy. In: Kaplan H, Sadock BJ (eds) Comprehensive textbook of psychiatry, 5th edn. Williams & Wilkins, Baltimore, pp 1462–1481
12. Liberman RP, Kopelowicz A, Gutkind D, et al (2001) Recovery from schizophrenia: operational criteria for defining recovery and factors related to recovery. Psychiatr Serv (in press)

13. American Psychiatric Association (1997) Practice guideline for the treatment of patients with schizophrenia. American Psychiatric Association, Washington, DC

14. Keefe RSE, Silva SG, Perkins DO, et al (1999) The effects of atypical antipsychotic drugs on neurocognitive impairment in schizophrenia: a review and meta-analysis. Schizophr Bull 25:201–222

15. Meltzer HY, McGurk SR (1999) The effects of clozapine, risperidone and olanzapine on cognitive function in schizophrenia. Schizophr Bull 25:233–256

16. Green MF, Marshall BD, Wirshing WC, et al (1997) Does risperidone improve verbal working memory in treatment-resistant schizophrenia? Am J Psychiatry 154:799–804

17. Kramer BA (1999) ECT in treatment-refractory schizophrenia. J Pract Psychiatry Behav Health 5:242–244

18. Cohen D (2000) Absence of cognitive impairment at long-term follow-up in adolescent treated with ECT. Am J Psychiatry 157:460–462

19. Fralish KB, Guercia A (1998) Integrative approaches to cognitive rehabilitation. Brain Source 2:18–40

19a. Jung CG (1989) Memories, dreams, reflections. Vintage Books, New York

20. Brenner HD, Roder V, Hodel B, et al (1994) Integrated psychological therapy for schizophrenic patients. Hogrefe & Huber, Toronto

21. Hermanutz M, Gestrich J (1987) Cognitive training of schizophrenic patients. Nervenarzt 58:91–96

22. Spaulding WD, Fleming SK, Reed D, et al (1999) Cognitive functioning in schizophrenia: implications for psychiatric rehabilitation. Schizophr Bull 25:275–290

23. Bellack AS, Gold JM, Buchanan RW (1999) Cognitive rehabilitation for schizophrenia: problems, prospects and strategies. Schizophr Bull 25:257–274

23a. Medalia A, Aluma M, Tyron M, Merriam AE (1998) Effectiveness of attention training in schizophrenia. Schizophr Bull 24:147–152

23b. Medalia A, Revheim N (1999) Computer-assisted learning in psychiatric rehabilitation. Psychiatr Rehabil Skills 3:77–98

24. Van den Gaag M, Kern R, Liberman RP, et al (2001) A controlled trial of cognitive remediation in schizophrenia. Schizophr Bull (in press)

24a. Hogarty GE, Flesher S (1999) Practice principles of cognitive enhancement therapy of schizophrenia. Schizophr Bull 25:693–708

25. Kern RS, Wallace CJ, Hellman SG, et al (1996) A training procedure for remediating WCST deficits in chronic psychotic patients: an adaptation of errorless learning principles. J Psychiatr Res 30:283–294

26. Zarate R, Liberman RP, Mintz J, et al (1998) Validation of a work capacity evaluation in individuals with psychiatric disorders. J Rehabil 64:28–34

27. Silverstein S, Menditto A, Stuve P (1999) Shaping procedures as cognitive retraining techniques in individuals with severe and persistent mental illness. Psychiatr Rehabil Skills 3:59–76

28. Psychiatric Rehabilitation Consultants (1999) Modules for training social and independent living skills. Available from Psychiatric Rehabilitation Consultants, PO Box 2867, Camarillo CA 93011, USA

29. Massel HK, Corrigan PW, Liberman RP, et al (1991) Conversation skills training of thought disordered schizophrenic patients through attention focusing. Psychiatry Res 38:51–61

30. Menditto AA, Baldwin LJ, O'Neal LG, et al (1991) Social learning procedures for increasing attention and improving basic skills in severely regressed institutionalized patients. J Behav Ther Exp Psychiatry 22:265–269

31. Patterson RL, Teigen JR, Liberman RP, et al (1975) Increasing speech intensity of chronic patients ('mumblers') by shaping techniques. J Nerv Ment Dis 160:182–187

32. Liberman RP, Nuechterlein KH, Wallace CJ (1982) Social skills training and the nature of schizophrenia. In: Curran JP, Monti PM (eds) Social skills training: a practical handbook for assessment and treatment. Guilford, New York, pp 5–56

33. Eckman TA, Wirshing WC, Marder SR, et al (1992) Technique for training schizophrenic patients in illness self-management: a controlled trial. Am J Psychiatry 149:1549–1555

34. Keri S, Kelemen O, Szekerew G, Bagoczky N, Erdelyi R, Antal A, Benedek G, Janka Z (2000) Schizophrenics know more than they can tell: probabilistic classification learning in schizophrenia. Psychol Med 30:149–155

35. Kern RS, Green MF, Wallace CJ (1997) Declarative and procedural learning in schizophrenia: a test of the integrity of divergent memory systems. Cogn Neuropsychiatry 2:39–50

36. Liberman RP (1998) International perspectives on skills training for the mentally disabled. Int Rev Psychia 10:5–9

37. Xu Z, Weng Y, Hou Y (1999) Efficacy and follow-up of research on medication management module training for schizophrenic patients in Beijing. Chin J Psychiatry 32:96–99

38. Velligan DI, Bow-Thomas CC, Huntzinger C, Ritch J, Ledbetter N, Prihoda TJ, Miller AL (2000) Cognitive adaptive training as compensation for neurocognitive impairments in schizophrenia. Am J Psychiatry 157:1313–1323

39. Cook JA, Razzano L (2000) Vocational rehabilitation for persons with schizophrenia: recent research and implications for practice. Schizophr Bull 26:87–103

40. Bond GR, Drake RE, Mueser K, et al (1997) An update on supported employment for persons with severe mental illness. Psychiatr Serv 48:335–346

40a. Wallace CJ, Tauber R, Wilde J (1999) Teaching fundamental workplace skills to persons with serious mental illness. Psychiatr Serv 50:1147–1153

41. Liberman RP (2000) The token economy. Am J Psychiatry 157:1398

42. Glynn SM, Liberman RP, Bowen L, et al (1994) The Clinical Research Unit at Camarillo State Hospital. In: Corrigan PW, Liberman RP (eds) Behavior therapy in psychiatric hospitals. Springer, New York

43. Lecomte T, Liberman RP, Wallace CJ (2000) Identifying and employing reinforcers in motivating the participation and progress in treatment of the seriously mentally ill. Psychiatr Serv 51:1312–1314

44. Paul GR, Menditto AA (1992) Effectiveness of inpatient treatment programs for mentally ill adults in public psychiatric facilities. Appl Prevent Psychol 1:45–63

45. Keri S, Kelemen O, Szekeres G, et al (2000) Schizophrenics know more than they can tell: probabilistic classification learning in schizophrenia. Psychol Med 30:149–155

46. Shadmehr R, Holcomb HH (2000) Procedural memory. Am J Psychiatry 157:162

47. Kee KS, Kern RS, Green MF (1998) Perception of emotion and psychosocial functioning in schizophrenia. Psychiatry Res 81:57–65

48. Baxter LR, Schwartz MJ, Bergman KS, Szuba MP, Guze BH, Mazziotta JC, Alazraki A, Selin CE, Ferng HK, Munford P, Phelps ME (1992) Caudate glucose metabolism rate changes with both drug and behavior therapy for obsessive-compulsive disorder. Arch Gen Psychiatry 49:681–689

49. Eisenberg L (1995) The social construction of the human brain. Am J Psychiatry 152:1563–1575

50. Schaie KW (1994) The course of adult intellectual development. Am Psychol 49:304–313

51. Giedd J (1999) Human brain growth: images in neuroscience. Am J Psychiatry 156:4

Part 8
Innovations in Practice

Cognitive, Social, and Psychopathological Factors in the Comprehensive Treatment of Schizophrenia

TILO HELD

Summary. Recent research findings suggest that the early course of schizophrenia, perhaps even before the outburst of positive symptoms, may be decisive for the outcome of the disorder. In psychosocial treatment programs, besides psychopathological symptoms, cognitive impairments and the nonfulfillment of social roles should be addressed directly. Work with families plays a central role in early rehabilitation. We present research data on the issues of family burden, families' satisfaction, and the efficacy of the Optimal Treatment Program (OTP) program in early psychosis cases.

Key words. Schizophrenia, Psychosocial therapy, Drug therapy, Cognitive factors, Social factors

The Early Course of Schizophrenia

Early detection of and early intervention in schizophrenic disorders are currently the focus of considerable interest in the scientific community. Multiple reasons converge to attract researchers and clinical teams to this field of investigation: First, stigma is a prominent factor of the life quality (or the lack of it) in schizophrenic patients. Because stigma is predominantly related to the chronic stages of schizophrenia, we might hope to help our patients better with early interventions in a nonstigmatizing therapeutic environment. Second, cognitive and social impairment seems often to precede the first outburst of positive symptoms. Third, investigations into the early course of schizophrenia seem to indicate that cognitive deterioration is most important in the first months or years of the disorder and that further decline, if it happens at all, is much slower. Finally, the duration of untreated psychosis has been associated with poor outcome in some studies, but this finding has not yet been consistently replicated. Thus, early and effective treatment has been considered very promising for the amelioration of the overall outcome of schizophrenic disorders.

Rheinische Kliniken Bonn, Kaiser-Karl-Ring 20, D 53111 Bonn, Germany

Neurocognitive Impairment

In a recent review paper, which is the update of a first review in 1996 on the functional consequences of neurocognitive deficits in schizophrenia, Michael Green et al. [1] report a significant association between secondary verbal memory, immediate verbal memory card sorting, vigilance, and measures of functional outcome such as community and daily activity, social problem solving, instrumental skills, and psychosocial skill acquisition. They theorize that an intermediate construct, such as learning ability, might better account for the links between basic neurocognition and functional outcome (Fig. 1). On the other hand, no consistent association between psychopathological symptoms and functional outcome has been found. Because these symptoms are the main target of neuroleptic medication, there seems to be an obvious rationale for other forms of treatment, complementary to neuroleptics, if an optimal functional outcome of schizophrenia is to be achieved.

Of course, the interaction between neuroleptic medication on the one hand, and cognitive and social factors on the other side, has to be examined. Whereas medication influences the social situation of the patient rather indirectly, via symptom reduction and better social acceptance, one can observe a very direct influence of neuroleptics on cognition. Until atypical neuroleptics became available, in clinical practice it was impossible to distinguish between the beneficial effects of neuroleptics on cognitive factors via reduction of the manifestations of the disorder and the detrimental cognitive effects of medication, so often complained of by our patients. By now, there is increasing evidence that typical neuroleptics quite often induce functional impairment of cognitive performance, as compared with their atypical counterparts. At the same time, atypical neuroleptics, on the whole, have a better correcting action on the disorder-specific cognitive disturbances.

From the viewpoint of cognition, a strong case is to be made for the use of atypical neuroleptics. But this overall positive statement has to be tempered by two caveats: First, the anticholinergic effects of some of the atypical neuroleptics (e.g., clozapine, olanzapin) may impair the learning of nonverbal information. Second, D_1 antagonism (e.g., clozapine, risperidon, olanzapine) may impair the speed of concept formation and working memory performance.

An important step forward in the cognitive rehabilitation of our patients has been the introduction of computer-aided neuropsychological training with the software package Cogpack [2], which offers specific and attractive video-play-like lessons in the following psychological domains: Concentration, Reaction, Information, Strategy, Memory, Calculation, Logic, and Language. In our experience, there are specific

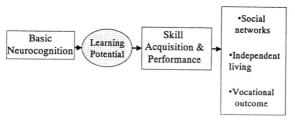

Fig. 1. Learning potential as a mediator for functional outcome [1]

advantages to this form of training: continuous feedback to the patient on his progress and his current limitations, flexibility of the tasks, effects of video-plays, enhanced motivation, and patient–computer interaction (help by the computer, interactive comments by the computer). One lesson (45 minutes) has to be performed every day for at least three weeks. According to the individual's training progress, the lessons become increasingly difficult. Two of the above-mentioned domains are covered every day. Whereas the evaluation of training effects is still under way in a multi-centered German study with our participation, a consistent correlation between some of the training tasks and the outcome of vocational rehabilitation has already been found.

Social Roles of the Patient

The influential ABC study from Mannheim [3] has attracted our attention to the importance of social role fulfillment for the further development of the patient (Fig. 2). If the fulfillment of social roles is so crucially important for the overall outcome, treatment should make a particular effort from the onset to counteract social stagnation and social decline. In women the first psychotic episode occurs about four years later on average than in men and the number of social roles fulfilled by women at that age tends to be much greater, which might contribute to explain the better fate of women in psychosocial rehabilitation.

If social stagnation and social decline are to be counteracted, so is the shrinking of the social network. Typically, the unfavorable evolution is as follows. In the premorbid phase, the social network of future schizophrenics is normal to slightly diminished. In the early stages of the disorder, the proportion of relatives is high. In the chronic stage, the social network is composed mainly of other patients and professional carers. As we have repeatedly said, therapeutic efforts are particularly necessary and promising in the early stages of the illness. This is when highly motivated relatives are at hand, asking for advice and training how to best help the patient. In the past, it has been a major error not to value this natural resource to its full extent. Research on social networks shows that this natural resource is not there forever. In

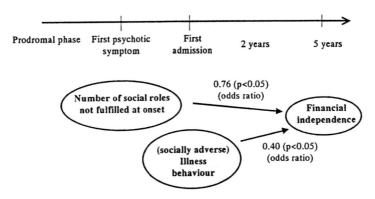

FIG. 2. Predicting the course of schizophrenia [3]

TABLE 1. Burden on the relating: compaison between Bonn and Naples

Bonn	Naples
Lowest values of the five centers	Highest values of the five centers
Global objective burden	Problems at work
Global subjective burden	Neglect of other relatives
Financial problems	Feelings of guilt
Constraints on social activities	Feeling not to be able to stand the situation any longer
Negative effects on family life	
Worries about the future	

TABLE 2. Coping strategies of the families: Comparison between Bonn and Naples

Bonn	Naples
Highest values	Highest values
Maintenance of social interests	Coercion
Practical and emotional support	Social involvement of the patient
Lowest values	Talking with friends
Resignation	Resignation
Seeking spiritual help	Seeking spiritual help

the later stages, very often resignation leads the relatives to be replaced by professional carers and other chronic patients as principal members of the network.

The Burden on the Relatives

This raises, of course, the question of the burden imposed on relatives when they live together with the patient. In a multicentered Biomed study by the European Union, we have examined how cultural factors and differences in service provision might affect the overall level of family burden and the choice of specific coping strategies in five European cities (Naples, Athens, Lisbon, Aylesbury, and Bonn) [4,5]. The results of this study suggest that as far as the overall burden is concerned, there is a continuum, with Bonn at the lowest and Naples at the highest end (Table 1). The coping strategies preferred by families in Bonn and Naples are shown in Table 2.

A conclusion of this study might be that the overall burden and coping strategies are highly dependent on cultural and political factors relating to the stigma imposed on schizophrenia and the availability of financial and professional support. In this respect, the Bonn families seem to be in a better situation. From the patient's perspective, the lower degree of burden in the Bonn families is partly due to the relatives' lesser degree of involvement with the patient and their higher degree of confidence that the professionals will be able to provide services to the patient.

Feedback to the Relatives

The OTP for schizophrenic disorders, which is designed to include any new evidence-based therapeutic strategy, aims at optimizing the overall quality of service provision and including all of the new families and patients. This has not yet been achieved in Bonn. We still have the (hopefully good) usual treatment and OTP treatment for a smaller proportion of families.

We used the questionnaires of the Biomed study to look at the differences in the opinions of families in different contexts on their own situation and on the quality of service delivery. Thirteen families came from a relatives' association, 25 families were attending an expert-directed relatives' group, and 22 families were taking part in the OTP. Three factors emerged from the answers: satisfaction with family life, feeling that the course of the disorder can be influenced, and feeling of being personally supported. Of the three factors, the OTP group had significantly better scores than the three other groups, taken independently or together ($P = 0.05$, $P = 0.001$, $P = 0.04$).

As the data collection and data analysis of all OTP centers progress, more will be known on the crucial question: Is it possible, by the early administration over a five-year period of a package of evidence-based treatment strategies, to alter the course of the disease instead of achieving short-lived ameliorations? Today we are not in a position to answer that question. But we are able to show (Falloon et al., unpublished data) that the benefits of the OTP methods are by no means restricted to chronic patients. On the contrary, the early involvement of highly motivated family members gives promise of better results.

References

1. Green M, Kern RS, Braff DL, et al (2000) Neurocognitive deficits and functional outcome in schizophrenia: are we measuring the "right stuff"? Schizophr Bull 26:119–136
2. Marker K. Marker software: Cognition-1 Im Steg 9, D-68526 Ladenburg
3. Häfner H, Löffler W, Maurer K, et al (1999) Depression, negative symptoms, social stagnation and social decline in the early course of schizophrenia Acta Psychiatr Scand 100:105–118
4. Magliano L, Fadden G, Madianos M, et al (1998) Burden on the families of patients with schizophrenia: results of the BIOMED I study. Soc Psychiatry Psychiatr Epidemiol 33:405–412
5. Magliano L, Fadden G, Economou M, et al (1998) Social and clinical factors influencing the choice of coping strategies in relatives of patients with schizophrenia: results of the BIOMED I study Soc Psychiatry Psychiatr Epidemiol 33:413–419

Family Interventions in Schizophrenia in Italian Mental Health Services

Rita Roncone[1], PierLuigi Morosini[2], Ian R.H. Falloon[3], and Massimo Casacchia[1]

Summary. This chapter, after discussing some of the issues that slow down the implementation of psychosocial family strategies in schizophrenic disorders in Italian mental health services, also reports the preliminary results of the Italian research project "Involvement and Support of Relatives of Persons Affected by Mental Illness." The design was a randomized controlled-trial comparison of two methods of family-based treatments in schizophrenia. Thirty-nine subjects with a diagnosis of schizophrenic disorder were randomly assigned to single-family (SF) and 35 were assigned to multi-family (MF) psychoeducational intervention. Clinical variables, quality of life, social functioning, and satisfaction with the mental health services were assessed in the patients, and burden of care, quality of life, and satisfaction with the mental health services, were assessed in the relatives. All the evaluations were carried out at the beginning and after six months of treatment by trained independent raters. The 12-month follow-up data are not yet available. The preliminary data from only a third of the sample (25 subjects) show a good reduction in symptoms and a good improvement in social functioning at the six-month follow-up. For social functioning alone, a greater improvement was observed in women and in the multifamily intervention. This ongoing study demonstrates that psychosocial family interventions may be easily introduced in the routine activities of Italian mental health services. The six-month partial results seem to confirm the clinical and social benefits of both the individual and the group approach.

Key words. Schizophrenia, Family interventions, Burden of care, Mental health services, Randomized controlled trial

[1] Psychiatric Department, University of L'Aquila, Coppito, Nuovo Ospedale S. Salvatore, 67100 L'Aquila, Italy
[2] National Health Institute, Laboratory of Epidemiology and Biostatistcs, Viale Regina Elena 299, 00161 Roma, Italy
[3] Optimal Treatment Project (OTP), Department of Psychiatry and Behavioural Science, University of Auckland, New Zealand

Introduction

Evidence-based family psychosocial interventions to help people suffering from schizophrenia and their relatives are not often considered an essential element of good practice in mental health services, even if they are only comparable to the introduction of psychotrophic drugs.

The Italian psychiatric reform, called "Low 180," dated 1978, established four principal components: a gradual phasing out of mental hospitals, with the cessation of all new admissions; the establishment of General Hospital Psychiatric Wards (GHPW) for acute admission, each having a maximum of 15 beds; the restriction of compulsory admissions; and the setting up of Community Mental Health Centers (CMHC) proving psychiatric care to geographically defined areas. Nowadays in most cases the Mental Health Departments, which include the psychiatric wards in general hospitals, emphasize community and network interventions. In Italy families, even if they have become smaller and smaller, keep close ties, and children do not leave the parental home till relatively late. The Italian scenario could be considered very favorable for the routine inclusion of such treatments. However, psychosocial treatments are still available in only a few centers and they are not generalized [1].

What are the main factors that may have hindered the acceptance and dissemination of this approach in the Italian mental health departments? First and foremost, there is a problem of cultural models that can be so grossly synthesized: a distaste for too structured and too technical and not sufficiently political approaches; a kind of ambivalent dislike for the behavioral and cognitive-behavioral approaches, which have always been regarded as too simple and limited by the psychodynamically or systemically oriented mental health professionals. They are still the majority among Italian psychotherapists and may have an understandable reluctance to accept a new and competitive approach [1].

The main aim of the Italian project "Involvement and Support of Relatives of Persons Affected by Mental Illness" is the controlled comparison of the efficacy of two methods of family-based treatment for patients affected by schizophrenia and their relatives, who are considered as 24-h "informal" caregivers and as persons who may experience a severe burden. The second objective, relevant to the above discussion, was to investigate the difficulty in the implementation of the approach in routine practice. The project has been deliberately carried out in public mental health departments, and the intervention was delivered by the mental health professionals of the departments, who would also continue to do their normal work. No extra staff or other resources were provided, except for the research assessments.

Materials and Methods

The criteria for the inclusion of the patients in the study were a diagnosis of schizophrenia or schizoaffective disorder according to the DSM-IV criteria; having lived in a family with relatives or with a spouse for at least the three months preceding inclusion in the study; age 18–49 years; receiving continuous care from public mental health out-patient services; and consent to participate from both patients and relatives.

The assessment tools for the patients were the Community Health Record (CHR) for psychiatric history and treatment [2]; the 24-item Brief Psychiatric Rating Scale (BPRS) 4.0 expanded version (Italian edition by Morosini and Casacchia [3]) and Current Psychiatric Status 50, CPS 50 [2], for symptoms; the MOS 36-Item Short Form Health Survey, SF-36 (Italian version, Apolone et al. [4]) on quality of life; a simple questionnaire on satisfaction with the mental health services [5]; one of the Italian versions of the Disability Assessment Scale II [6] for social functioning. This tools includes a Global Rating of Overall Community Functioning, or GROCF, on a scale from 80 (good functioning in each area) to 1 (inability to maintain basic functioning and severe health risk, e.g., very dirty, dressed in an inappropriate way, at risk of dehydration). The relatives' assessment included the subjective and objective burden of care (Questionnaire for Family Problems [7]), and again the quality of life (SF-36), and satisfaction with the psychiatric services [5]. The assessments were performed by university-independent raters, who were not involved in and were blinded to the treatments and who were visiting the services periodically.

The patients and their families were randomized by an externally developed and managed randomization protocol to a single-family intervention group or a multi-family psychoeducational intervention group. The multi-family had to include at least three families. In both treatments, the patients and relatives were seen together. The family psychoeducational integrated intervention included a number of strategies: education about the disease, improvement of communication skills, problem-solving, and social skills. No attempt was made to modify the usual patterns of drug prescription. All the professionals were trained to deliver both treatments according to a manual for individual treatment [8], to which a special section on multifamily treatment had been added.

Results

The study is still ongoing; 74 patients (52 men and 22 women) and their relatives (140 subjects) were included in the multicenter study. Thirty-nine patients were allocated to the single-family and 35 to the multifamily intervention. Some preliminary results at six months will be reported here, which concern only one-third of the patient' sample (25 subjects; 18 men and 7 women). The main sociodemographic features of the subjects are shown in Table 1. Only symptomatology and social functioning outcomes will be described here. No statistically significant differences in symptoms or social functioning between the two treatment groups were present at time 0 (Table 2).

Symptoms

In our subsample at six months, the BPRS total score showed a remarkable reduction (Table 2). No statistically significant difference was observed between the two treatment groups.

Social Functioning

In the subsample here considered, the GROCF showed a remarkable improvement in the whole sample (Table 2). The women seemed to obtain greater benefits, improving

TABLE 1. Demographic and clinical characteristics of the 25 patients with schizophrenic disorders of our subsample

Characteristic	Single-family intervention ($n = 13$)	Multifamily intervention ($n = 12$)
Age (yr) (SD)	30.5 (6.3)	34.6 (6.9)
Sex		
Male (%)	8 (61.5)	10 (83.3)
Female (%)	5 (38.5)	8 (16.7)
Marital status		
Single (%)	9 (69.2)	9 (75.0)
Married (%)	2 (15.4)	2 (16.7)
Divorced or separated (%)	2 (15.4)	1 (8.3)
Education		
Years of education (SD)	12.0 (3.3)	10.1 (2.4)
Working condition		
Unemployed (%)	6 (46.1)	7 (58.3)
Employed (%)	2 (14.4)	2 (16.7)
Sheltered work (%)	2 (14.4)	—
Housewife (%)	2 (14.4)	2 (16.7)
Student (%)	1 (7.7)	1 (8.3)
Diagnosis (DSM-IV)		
Schizophrenia Paranoid Type	7 (53.8)	6 (50.0)
Schizophrenia Disorganized Type	1 (7.7)	2 (16.7)
Schizophrenia Undifferentiated Type	2 (14.4)	2 (16.7)
Schizophrenia Residual Type	1 (7.7)	1 (8.3)
Schizophrenia Disornder	2 (14.4)	1 (8.3)
Length of illness (mo)	101.6 (80.7)	130.0 (116.7)

TABLE 2. Clinical and social functioning results after six months of treatment in our sub-sample of 25 patients

Result	Single-family intervention ($n = 13$)	P^a	Multifamily intervention ($n = 12$)	P^a	Total sample ($n = 25$)	P^b
Symptoms (Brief Psychiatric Rating Scale, BPRS, total score), mean (SD)						
T0 BPRS total score	41.6 (9.9)	—	42.2 (11.3)	—	41.9 (10.4)	0.03
T6 BPRS total score	38.1 (6.5)		37.5 (7.5)		37.8 (8.1)	
Social functioning (Global Rating of Overall Community Functioning, GROCF score), mean (SD)						
T0 GROCF score	39.5 (17.0)	—	37.0 (10.1)	0.02	38.2 (13.6)	0.006
T6 GROCF score	46.3 (15.4)		47.9 (17.3)		47.1 (16.1)	

[a] Paired t-test

[b] t-test for independent samples

in their social disability much more than the men (the GROCF for women at T_0 was 37.4 and the SD was 11.2; at T_6 it was 54.1 and the SD was 7.9; $P = 0.003$, t-test).

In this small sample at six months a moderately greater improvement was observed in the patients included in the multifamily groups than in the patients receiving single-family intervention.

Discussion and Conclusions

The very preliminary data at six-month follow-up show a good clinical and social improvement for patients, the latter being markedly greater for women and slightly better for patients included in the multifamily treatments.

In an unpublished work by Veltro et al. [9], a controlled, randomized family behavioral trial in Benevento, a town in south Italy, performance of the family intervention according to Falloon caused a significant and marked reduction in relapses and readmissions. Apart from this work, no other research has been carried out in Italy on the efficacy and effectiveness of the approach. Good results were obtained in the training of professionals [10,11]. However, trained and motivated staff found it difficult to implement what they had learned. The main obstacles were the indifference or hostility of their colleagues and the rigid organization of the mental health services. This would make it difficult to provide family intervention at home outside normal working hours, especially by nurses.

In our study, the treatment was carried out mainly in the outpatient setting, except for the first two or three encounters, and this may have contributed to the success of the implementation. The mental health departments participating in our study are situated in different Italian regions, and despite the differences in organization and staff provision, none had particular difficulties in performing the intervention. However, it must be stressed that the department managers were very supportive and that the participation in research may have increased the staff motivation.

These preliminary results seem to confirm the feasibility and the clinical and social benefits of psychosocial family treatment. The complete 12-month results will clarify the advantages of this kind of implementation and may or not confirm that the multifamily treatment is at least of equal efficacy.

Acknowledgments. Support for the research described in this chapter was provided by a grant from the National Mental Health Project, National Institute of Health, Grant No. 96/Q/T/30, Rome, Italy. We also wish to thank the mental health professionals of the following Italian mental health services involved in the project for their cooperation and support: Mental Health Department of Ferrara, Mental Health Center Codigoro, Region Emilia-Romagna (Ferrara); Mental Health Department AUSL 5-Region Marche, Jesi (Ancona); Mental Health Unit District 96 Region Campania Salerno; Mental Health Center Sora (Frosinone), Region Lazio; Mental Health Service AUSL 6-Region Marche, Fabriano (Ancona); Mental Health Services of Perugia and Marsciano (Perugia), Region Umbria; and Mental Health Department of Arezzo, Region Toscane.

References

1. Casacchia M, Roncone R (1999) I trattamenti psicoeducativi familiari nella schizofrenia: esterofilia o applicazione di trattamenti basati sull'evidenza? Epidemiologia e Psichiatria Sociale 8(3):183–189
2. Falloon IRH (1999) Optimal treatment for psychosis in an international multisite demonstration project. Optimal Treatment Project Collaborators. Psychiatr Serv 50: 615–618
3. Morosini PL, Casacchia M (1995) Traduzione italiana della Brief Psychiatric Rating Scale, versione 4.0 ampliata (BPRS 4.0). Rivista di Riabilitazione Psichiatrica e Psicosociale III:199–228
4. Apolone G, Mosconi P, Ware JE (1997) Questionario sullo stato di salute SF-36. Manuale d'uso e guida all'interpretazione dei risultati. Guerini e Associati Editore, Milano
5. Morosini PL, Gigantesco A, Bianchetti F, et al (1998) Studio di riproducibilità di uno strumento per la valutazione dell'opinione degli utenti dei servizi di salute mentale. Giornale Italiano di Psicopatologia 1:61–68
6. Morosini PL, Veltro F, Cerreta A, et al (1988) Disabilità sociale. Adattamento dello strumento in lingua italiana. Rivista Sperimentale di Freniatria 3:541–563
7. Morosini P, Roncone R, Veltro F, et al (1991) Routine assessment tool in psychiatry: a case of questionnaire of family attitude and burden. Ital J Psychiatry Behav Sci 1(1): 95–102
8. Falloon IHR (1993) Intervento psicoeducativo integrato in psichiatria. Erikson, Trento
9. Veltro F, Magliano L, Morosini PL, et al (1996) Behavioural Family Therapy (BFT) for patients with schizophrenia: a randomised controlled trial (RCT). Proceedings V Congress World Association for Psychosocial Rehabilitation, Rotterdam, p 173
10. Magliano L (1995) L'intervento psicoeducativo familiare: l'esperienza italiana. Epidemiologia e Psichiatria Sociale 4(2):103–105
11. Magliano L, Veltro F, Morosini P (1993) L'approccio psicoeducativo territoriale. Un'esperienza di formazione integrata per gli operatori di un servizio di salute mentale. Rivista Sperimentale di Freniatria 4:562–579

Early Intervention for Schizophrenic Disorders: Implementing Optimal Treatment Strategies in Clinical Services

Rolf W. Gråwe[1], Jan H. Widen[2], and Ian R.H. Falloon[3]

Summary. Integrated pharmacological and psychosocial interventions with adults who show early signs and symptoms of schizophrenic disorders may lower the incidence and prevalence of major episodes of acute disturbance. These programs combine early detection of psychotic symptoms by general practitioners with close collaboration with mental health professionals who are trained to conduct comprehensive psychiatric assessments and to apply without delay those medication and psychosocial strategies that have proven effective in reducing the prevalence of psychotic symptoms and associated disability in randomized, controlled studies. Long-term monitoring of early signs of recurrence of these subthreshold psychotic episodes, with further intervention aimed at reducing biological vulnerability and managing the detrimental effects of excessive stress, appears essential to maintain these benefits. A large-scale international study, the Optimal Treatment Project (OTP), aims to apply these effective treatment strategies to all incident cases of psychosis throughout a 5-year period, with repeated assessments of clinical, social, and economic benefits. Preliminary 2-year results from a Norwegian center reveal, in spite of the small number of patients and low statistical power, that this kind of optimalized treatment approach has an effect on rehospitalization rates, and that 40 percent of the recent-onset cases have a very good outcome.

Key words. Schizophrenia, Recent-onset, Treatment outcome

Introduction

In recent years, evidence has been accumulating that suggests that primary prevention of functional psychotic disorders may already be occurring. The falling incidence of these disorders in several countries with well-developed public health services may be associated in part with improvements in obstetric care, control of epidemics of

---

[1] Norwegian University of Technology and Science, Department of Psychiatry and Behavioural Medicine, PO Box 3008, Lade, 7441 Trondheim, Norway
[2] Telemark sentralsykehus, Clinic for Early Intervention of Psychosis, 3700 Skien, Norway
[3] Villa Ariete, Mikliano 10, 06050 Marsciano (PG), Italy

neuro-viruses, and better management of high fevers that sometimes lead to convulsions [1–4]. Another factor that could be hypothesized as leading to the reduced incidence of disabling episodes of psychosis may be improved early detection and effective clinical management of emerging psychotic symptoms by general practitioners.

Early intervention with initial presentations of psychosis would appear to make good sense. Full and lasting recovery from most medical disorders is associated with early detection and intervention with effective treatment strategies before irreparable organ damage occurs. However, despite the current wave of enthusiasm for such services in mental health, it should be emphasized that at present there is no clear evidence that early detection and intervention improves the long-term outcome of schizophrenia or other psychotic disorders [5,6].

Epidemiological studies show that the most consistent predictors of clinical and social recovery include many that would tend to expedite the initiation of effective treatment early in the course of the disorder. These include acute onset, onset triggered by major life stress, associated symptoms of major mood disorder, later onset in women at a time when they are often married and caring for children, onset in people with good premorbid psychosocial adjustment, and onset of mainly psychotic rather than negative symptoms [7,8]. One common feature is that these factors are all likely to lead to earlier detection of abnormality and effective seeking of help by patients or their caregivers.

Detection is likely to be delayed in cases in which the onset is gradual, occurring in a person with poor premorbid psychosocial adjustment, without any obvious triggering events, with deficit symptoms leading to social withdrawal, and with little overt unusual behavior. The delay in recognizing that this presentation is associated with a serious mental disorder may last months or even years. Effective treatment may not be sought until profound handicaps in social and work functioning have occurred.

Early recognition of cases of functional psychoses that result in rapid and unexpected declines in social functioning is not difficult. Patients, friends, families, work mates, teachers, and general practitioners are all likely to promote immediate assessment and treatment. The more gradual onset, with slower functional decline, presents a considerable challenge for early detection and intervention strategies.

A second concern that has been raised about early intervention is that early treatment is likely to be helpful only if that treatment is highly effective and readily available. Improvement in the effectiveness of treatment of the functional psychoses in controlling florid psychotic symptoms and reducing the risks of recurrent episodes and their associated social disabilities and handicaps ranks among the greatest medical achievements of the past century [9]. This has occurred in three stages. In the first stage, the provision of psychosocial rehabilitation resources enabled even those persons most impaired by these disorders to lead a constructive life in the community. Second, the discovery of the antipsychotic effects of the neuroleptic drugs enabled most (75%–80%) acute psychotic episodes to be controlled, and the rate of recurrent episodes to be halved. Finally, the development of stress management, involving persons caring for the patient, reduced the risk of recurrent episodes even further, to at least half that achieved with optimal neuroleptic drug treatment alone (Falloon et al., chapter in this volume).

In summary, it can be concluded that a three- to fourfold decrease in major impairments from psychotic symptoms can be achieved by integrated pharmacotherapy and effective psychosocial strategies. One study of continued treatment has shown that full clinical and social recovery from schizophrenic psychoses may be achieved in a high proportion of cases when treatment is continued for at least 2 years [10].

It should be noted that most of the research upon which this optimism is based has been conducted over relatively brief periods, with seldom more than one year of active treatment, few field trials, and relatively unsophisticated assessments of benefits. However, the consistency of the results and indications that benefits can be sustained, especially when provided within a continued care model [11], provides strong support for the widespread application of such methods [12,13]. Despite consistent demonstration of the cost-effectiveness of integrated drug and psychosocial strategies, few clinical services deliver this approach in a competent manner. This poses a serious international problem [9,12,14,15]. It is evident that lasting improvements in the outcome of functional psychoses will not occur until all services provide the most effective and efficient treatment strategies to all their consumers at all stages of these disorders. At present, few mental health teams are trained and equipped to undertake such treatment, even for well-established cases of psychotic disorders [9].

It may be hypothesized that the early detection of functional psychoses, followed by rapid application of the integrated treatment strategies, would enhance the rates of recovery from these disorders. However, continued long-term treatment with the same strategies may be essential to achieve lasting stable benefits, including full recovery of social functioning. In one small epidemiological pilot study of early detection and intervention with integrated effective biomedical and psychosocial strategies, the observed incidence of schizophrenia (DSM-III-R) was reduced from 7.4 cases per 100 000 per annum to 0.75 per 100 000 [16]. A much lower than expected incidence of major depressive disorders was also observed [17]. A substantial number of cases with early features suggestive of a psychosis or subsyndromal major affective symptoms were detected. It was concluded that early detection and intervention had prevented the full-blown development of an impending episode, resulting in a milder form of the disorder that responded remarkably well to optimal treatment. Continued monitoring of the early intervention cases revealed very few recurrences, all of which responded to the combined biomedical and psychosocial regimen. Those first episode cases that were detected at the syndromal level were almost all successfully treated, with very few showing residual symptoms at 12-month follow-up [18].

There is an urgent need to study this approach under rigorous controlled trial conditions. Unfortunately, our own attempts to secure funding for such a trial have proved unrewarding. The Melbourne group led by Alison Yung and Patrick McGorry are in the process of performing such a study, with encouraging results.

The present study aimed to provide optimal treatment for patients referred by general practitioners from the city of Trondheim and the surrounding mountainous countryside. Early detection and referral was encouraged through community education programmes. However, almost all patients were clearly suffering from their first major psychotic episodes when they entered the study. They were provided with combined medication and psychosocial interventions for a period of 5 years, during which time their clinical, social, and family outcomes were repeatedly assessed to monitor the benefits of the program.

Methods

Subjects

Recent-onset patients were selected for the study if they were diagnosed as having recent onset DSM-IV schizophrenia, schizoaffective, or schizophreniform disorders; were between 18 and 35 years of age; were prescribed antipsychotic drugs; did not have any substance use disorders; and were not mentally retarded. Recent onset was defined as having psychotic symptoms for less than 2 years. After written informed consent had been obtained, 50 patients were randomly assigned to the outpatient treatment program. Most of the patients were referred to the project from hospital wards (57%), other outpatient clinics (23%), and primary health care practititioners (21%). Of 168 consecutive referrals, 72 were excluded because of age or diagnosis, and another 46 were excluded for other reasons (most were not of recent onset). Of the 50 patients who fulfilled the inclusion criteria, 30 were randomly assigned to an Assertive Community Mental Health Treatment group (ACT) (experimental group) and 20 to a Treatment-as-Usual condition (TAU) (comparison group). The patients were included after hospital discharge and after they had recovered from the psychotic episode.

Of the included patients, 81 percent had schizophrenic disorders, 62 percent were men, and their mean age was 25 years. The mean Global Assessment of Functioning (GAF) and Brief Psychiatric Rating Scale (BPRS) scores at baseline were 50 and 40, respectively. Forty-three percent of the patients lived in high-Expressed Emotion (EE) environments. The two groups did not differ at baseline with respect to sex, age, total score on the BPRS, time previously hospitalized, or time living in high-EE families. However, the patients in the ACT group had higher global functioning on the GAF at baseline ($t = 2.3$, df $= 48$, $p < 0.05$).

Treatment Program

Assertive Community Mental Health Treatment

The patients were treated by a multidisciplinary mental health team with a low case load (patient-staff ratio about 1:10). Each patient had a case manager to assist with the provision of basic social support needs, and in addition received structured psychoeducation, family communication skills and problem-solving skills training, neuroleptic drug management, mobile intensive crisis management provided at home, and individual cognitive-behavioral strategies for residual symptoms and disability. This approach is described in several published manuals [18]. In contrast to the most comprehensive ACT programs, the team did not provide 24-hour service and did not have a vocational specialist.

Treatment-as-Usual

This group received standardized treatment provided by the traditional outpatient mental health care system and the community mental health care services. The patients received regular clinical case management with provision of drug management, supportive housing and day care, crisis management provided by the psychiatric hospitals, rehabilitative programs focusing on promoting independent living and work activity, and simple and brief psychoeducation and supportive psychotherapy. Four patients in this group received less intensive follow-up and treatment, and none received the problem-solving training components of structured behavioral family treatment, comprehensive psychoeducation, or assertive outreach follow-up, as provided to the ACT group. The groups did not differ significantly with respect to antipsychotic drug treatment or drug adherence during the 2-year treatment period.

Assessments

A battery of measures was applied at baseline, 12 months, and 24 months. Assessment of individualized target psychotic symptoms (1–7 score) and medication side effects was performed monthly. Drug compliance was registered continuously. Psychopathology was assessed bimonthly by the BPRS (24-item version) [19]. The BPRS ratings were made from videotaped interviews by raters who were independent and blinded to treatment conditions. In addition to the biweekly ratings, the BPRS was applied every time an increase in symptoms was suspected.

A composite clinical index to define good or poor outcome was computed, based mainly on the continuous BPRS ratings. A good outcome was scored when a patient had no major episodes of any form of psychopathology (including suicide attempts), remained free of any persistent psychotic symptoms, and showed continuous optimal adherence to all aspects of the treatment program during the entire 24-month follow-up period.

Recurrent Psychotic Episode Criteria

A major psychotic episode was defined as an exacerbation of psychotic symptoms occuring after a period of remission (i.e., having no psychotic symptoms). This was confirmed by at least a two-point increase and a score of 6 or 7 on the Target Symptom ratings scale and a score of 6 or 7 on one of the key psychotic symptom items on the BPRS. Finally, a major episode had to be confirmed by an independent person (researcher, family member, clinician, case manager, etc.) as a significant worsening of psychotic symptomatology. A minor episode was defined in a similar way. However, the scores on target symptoms should be in the 4–5 range and follow a period of remission.

Results

With respect to rehospitalization data, 33 percent of the patients in the experimental group and 50 percent of those in the comparison group were not readmitted to a hospital during the 2-year follow-up period. Although 65 percent (n = 13) of those in the comparison group had a minor or a major episode during the period, 43 percent (n = 13) of those receiving assertive community mental health treatment (ACT group) relapsed. However, because of the low statistical power of the study, none of the differences were statistically significant. The same applied for the GAF scores. However, there were very large group differences with respect to rehospitalization times.

The mean number of days of rehospitalization was 32 in the ACT group and 78 in the TAU group. The TAU group also received twice as much involuntary treatment as the ACT group (means of 56 and 24 days, respectively). Therefore, even if the differences with respect to psychotic episodes are not very large, there are significant differences with respect to rehospitalization data.

On a clinical composite index reflecting good outcome with respect to absence of suicide attempts, rehospitalizations, persistent psychotic symptoms, or relapses, 40 percent in the ACT group and 30 percent in the TAU group had a good outcome, with remission of psychotic symptoms without relapse, suicide attempts, or rehospitalization. However, this difference was not statistically significant.

Conclusion

The main result of this study is that assertive community mental health treatment using the integrated biomedical and psychosocial approach reduces hospital use. Hospital admission is a complex outcome variable and should be interpreted with care. It is probably influenced by the treatment, the amount of stress experienced by the individual and his or her key caregivers, their coping skills and psychosocial support, individual decisions made by their therapists about the need for rehospitalization, and so on. For most patients, rehospitalization was involuntary. This may confirm that rehospitalizations reflected exacerbations of psychotic or life-threatening symptoms.

The advantages for the integrated assertive treatment approach according to other clinical outcome variables were notable but did not achieve statistical significance. Schizophrenia is a disorder of low incidence and high prevalence. Thus, it is difficult to conduct comparative treatment studies of early intervention that have enough cases to obtain adequate statistical power. In addition, a substantial number of first episode patients will recover fully and remain well without any specific interventions at all. Thus, the finding that 40% of patients had excellent and stable recovery from all psychiatric symptoms at 2 years could be considered a substantial clinical achievement. In contrast, 30% of the generally well-treated control group had similarly good outcomes.

However, a substantial proportion of patients in the assertive community mental health treatment program continued to experience persistent psychotic and negative symptoms throughout the 2-year period reported here. Specific pharmacological strategies were targeted to these patients, with limited success. However, the newer psychological approaches for persistent psychotic symptoms had not yet been introduced in this phase of the project (see Fowler et al. and Tarrier et al., in this volume).

It may be concluded that 2 years of continued optimal treatment with the latest biomedical and psychosocial treatment strategies produces some worthwhile clinical benefits. However, these benefits were limited, and it would seem necessary to continue comprehensive treatment for more than half the first-episode cases for more than 2 years. Even more effort may be necessary to restore social functioning. This is only obtained through multimodal intensive and continued long-term, goal-oriented treatment by teams of well-trained and committed mental health professionals.

There is a clear need for more randomized, controlled treatment studies of early intervention for this group of patients in order to reveal which patients will profit most from assertive treatment programs and to refine the treatment strategies. Our present understanding does not permit us to recommend any specific approach to early intervention. However, we believe that it is important to adopt an evidence-based approach and to utilize those treatment methods that have been proven effective in the treatment of established cases of schizophrenic disorders. These include assertive case management, neuroleptic medications, psychoeducation, carer-based stress management, goal-oriented living skills training, and cognitive-behavioral strategies for residual symptoms (see Falloon et al., this volume). These strategies have demonstrated their efficacy and should form the basis for all early intervention services.

References

1. Deer G, Gupta G, Murray RM (1990) Is schizophrenia disappearing? Lancet 335:513–516
2. Eagles JM, Whalley LJ (1985) Decline in the diagnosis of schizophrenia among first admissions to Scottish mental hospitals from 1969–1978. Br J Psychiat 146:151–154
3. Joyce PR (1987) Changing trends in first admissions and readmissions for mania and schizophrenia in New Zealand. Aust NZ J Psychiat 21:82–86
4. Munk-Jorgensen P (1986) Decreasing first admission rates of schizophrenia among males in Denmark
5. Crow TJ, MacMillan JF, Johnson AL, Johnstone EC (1986) A randomised controlled trial of prophylactic neuroleptic treatment. Br J Psychiat 120–127
6. McGorry PD, Edwards J, Mihalopoulos C, Harrigan S, Jackson HJ (1996) EPPIC: an evolving system of early detection and optimal management. Schizophr Bull 22:305–326
7. Johnstone EC, MacMillan JF, Frith CD, Benn DK, Crow TJ (1990) Further investigations of predictors of outcome following first schizophrenic episodes. Br J Psychiat 157:182–189
8. Kraus M, Muller-Thomsen T (1993) Schizophrenia with onset in adolescence: an 11-year followup. Schizophr Bull 19:831–841
9. Lehman AF, Carpenter WT, Goldman HH, Steinwachs DM (1995) Treatment outcomes in schizophrenia: implications for practice, policy and research. Schizophr Bull 21:669–675
10. Falloon IRH (1985) Family management of schizophrenia. Johns Hopkins University Press, Baltimore
11. Falloon IRH, Coverdale JH, Brooker C (1996) Psychosocial interventions in schizophrenia: a review. Int J Mental Health 25:3–23
12. Lehman AF, Steinwachs DM (1998) Patterns of usual care for schizophrenia. Initial results from the Schizophrenia Patient Outcomes Research Team (PORT) client survey. Schizophr Bull 24:11–20
13. Kane JM, Marder SR (1993) Psychopharmacologic treatment of schizophrenia. Schizophr Bull 19:287–302
14. Falloon IRH, Held T, Roncone R, Coverdale JH, Laidlaw TM (1998) Optimal treatment strategies to enhance recovery from schizophrenia. Aust NZ J Psychiat 32:43–49
15. Lehman AF, Steinwachs DM (1998) Translating research into practice. The Schizophrenia Patient Outcomes Research Team (PORT) treatment recommendations. Schizophr Bull 24:1–10
16. Falloon IRH (1992) Early intervention for first episodes of schizophrenia: a preliminary exploration. Psychiatry 55:4–15

17. Falloon IRH, Shanahan WJ (1990) Community management of schizophrenia. Br J Hosp Med 43:62–66
18. Falloon IRH, Fadden G (1993) Integrated mental health care. Cambridge University Press, Cambridge
19. Lukoff D, Nuechterlein KH, Ventura J (1986) Symptom monitoring in the rehabilitation of schizophrenic patients. Schizophr Bull 12:594–602

From Randomized Controlled Trials to Evidence-Based Clinical Care for Severe Mental Illness

Ulf Malm, Nils Gustaf Lindgren, and the OTP Research Team at Göteborg University

Summary. From systematic Cochrane reviews of primary scientific research, we know that the most effective setting for the management of severe mental illness is the Assertive Community Treatment (ACT) model. The aim of this study was to evaluate the efficacy of treatment by the ACT program "Integrated Care" in comparison with the best established clinical care. The study was a randomized, controlled trial with two years of follow-up. The trial was carried out during 1994–2000 and included 84 patients with schizophrenic disorders (DSM-IV). Analysis was by both intention-to-treat and attention-to-content-of-care. Between-group comparisons indicated significantly improved consumer satisfaction and social function in favor of "Integrated Care" at follow-up. A technology achievement was a computer-aided tool kit for instantly delivered outcome reports for the monitoring and planning of mental health services. We conclude that good clinical care for patients with schizophrenic disorders can be improved by introducing the community-based program "Integrated Care." To promote putting effective services into practice, and achieving further improvements in outcome, structural changes in the delivery systems of services in harmony with the provider program have to be introduced.

Key words. Schizophrenia, Integrated care, Evidence-based management, Outcome research, Computer-aided outcome reporting

Introduction

Effective settings for schizophrenic patients usually require far more than a doctor or a particular treatment; they require a system of care, the foundation of which includes both pharmacological and psychosocial treatment approaches [1]. The support for patients with severe mental illness should be comprehensive, continuous, and person-intensive. From systematic Cochrane reviews of primary scientific research, we know that the most effective setting for the correct management [2] of severe mental illness is the Assertive Community Treatment (ACT) model [3,4].

Sahlgrenska University Hospital, Bla Straket 15, SE-41345 Göteborg, Sweden

Our Research I: A Two-Year Controlled Study on Outcomes of Integrated Care in Schizophrenia

Introduction

As one site in the international collaborative Optimal Treatment Project [5] we began the OTP-project in western Sweden in September 1994. The project includes several studies on the implementation of Integrated Care (IC) in various treatment contexts and services, and local delivery systems. The aims were to study the long-term efficacy of intervention by a new program, Integrated Care (IC) in comparison with Rational Rehabilitation (RR), a program well established as the best clinical practice.

Patients and Methods

Study Participants. Our randomized study took place in the central Gothenburg area from 1994 to 2000. The sector has a total population of about 97,000. The patients fulfilled the following criteria: DSM-IV diagnostic classification for schizophrenic, schizophreniform, schizoaffective, or delusional disorders. We included all patients aged 18 to 55 years. Patients had to give consent to participate in the study and state that they had been fully informed of all the expected benefits and risks. No other selection procedures were employed. In particular, no patient was excluded on the basis of sex, race, or severity of disorder.

A total of 100 patients participated in one urban efficacy study and two rural effectiveness studies. This paper reports on the 84 patients who have completed the two-year randomized outcome study. Patients were randomized to one of two community-based treatment modalities: IC or RR.

The Integrated Care Program (IC). The main ingredients in the Swedish IC study program for patients with schizophrenic disorders have been assertive team case management by multidisciplinary teams trained in the program, optimal pharmacotherapy, and psychoeducation of patients and informal carers about the disorder and its treatments. Further ingredients are stress management, structured communication training and structured problem-solving, living skills training, specific cognitive behavior strategies for selected problems such as persisting symptoms, and anxiety management (Table 1) (See the chapter by Falloon et al., this volume).

The Rational Strategy for Rehabilitation Program (RR). The RR program was carried out according to guidelines and protocol. This program contains dynamic and group psychotherapies added to a combination of medication and other psychosocial interventions (Table 1) [6]. The RR program was provided by a long-established multidisciplinary team specializing in psychoses' and with well-established case-management services.

Study Design. The urban patient groups were allocated by a randomized parallel design with a comparison of outcome between groups. The patient group whose duration of illness was less than 10 years ($N = 31$) was randomised. The IC:RR ratio was 4:1. In the group of patients whose duration of illness was more than 10 years ($N = 53$), the randomization ratio was 1:1.

TABLE 1. Main features of the two Assertive Community Treatment (ACT)[a] programs studied

Integrated Care	Rational Rehabilitation
Assertive case management	Assertive case management
Reach-out services	Reach-out services
Social network resource groups	Social network meetings
Collaboration with psychiatrist	Collaboration with psychiatrist
	Individual supportive psychotherapy
Structured problem-solving	Early detection and crisis intervention in
Development and maintenance of	community settings
effective social network support	
Early detection and crisis intervention	
in community settings	
Structured communication training	
Minimally effective antipsychotic drug	Minimally effective antipsychotic drug
strategies	strategies
Education	Education
Adherence	Adherence
Prevention of side effects	Prevention of side effects
Early warning signs written down	
Education of informal carers	Education of informal carers
Living skills training	Living skills training
Specific strategies	Specific strategies
Cognitive-behavorioral thereby for selected	Communication-oriented group
patients with persistent psychotic symtoms	therapy
	Individual dynamic psychotherapy
	(for seleceted cases)
	Body awareness training
	Vocational rehabilitation

[a] Due to premises and budgetary reasons, a 24-hour reach-out service could not be established. Neither program was in control of admissions and discharges

Assessments and Outcomes. Methods of evaluation by case managers were an integral part of clinical treatment. Seven assessors (two nurses, three psychologists, and three psychiatrists) conducted independent assessments primarily based on semi-structured interviews with patients and informal carers every 3 months during the first 24 months of the project, then every 6 months. The battery of measures applied contains 10 domains and 21 measures, rated respectively and self-reported (Table 2).

Statistics. For the data based on the ordinal ratings scales, the statistical estimates were carried out by nonparametric tests of significance. The two-sample Wilcoxon matched-pairs signed-ranks test was used to test differences before and after two years. The Mann-Whitney rank sum test for two independent samples was used to test differences between the experimental and control groups. For the statistical testing of effectiveness, an end-point analysis was applied. According to the nature of the data, *t*-tests, mean SD and alternative mean, confidence interval, and the quartiles

TABLE 2. Primary and secondary outcome domains and measures

Outcomes	Domains	Measures[a]
Primary	Global assessments	CGI [7]
		GAF DSM-IV [8]
	Symptoms and signs	BPRS-24 [9]
		GAF-Symptoms subscale [8]
	Side effects	UKU-SERS (Side Effect Rating Scale) [10]
	Social function	Disability Index [5]
		WHO-DAS [11]
		GAF-Disability subscale [8]
	Consumer satisfaction	UKU-ConSat Scale [12]
	Course of illness	Remission by GAF-Disability [8]
		Hospital admission
		Psychotic episodes [13]
		Days-in-hospital
		Unnatural deaths/suicides
Secondary	Distress	Global Distress Scale [5]
		Self-reported perceived distress (SERS-Pat) (manuscript in preparation)
	Quality of life	QLS-100 [14]
		SF-36 [15]
	Impact on informal carers	Global Household Stress [5]
		GHQ-28 [16]
	Costs and benefits	CSRI [17]

were performed on calculated when the data were demonstrated to be normally distributed. Analysis by logarithmic tranformations was also carried out where appropriate.

The study was approved by the Gothenburg University Ethical Commmittee.

Results

During the period 1994–1998, 84 urban patients with schizophrenic disorders entered the study. A total of eight patients withdrew consent to be treated by the IC program before treatment began and therefore continued their ongoing RR program. Only one patient (in the RR program of the RCT trial) could not be assessed at two years. He was murdered at 13 months into the project. In this case the principle of carrying the last observation forward was applied.

Analysis by Intention-to-Treat. The significant findings were increased consumer satisfaction ($P = 0.036$) with Integrated Care as well as improved social function: WHO-DAS ($P = 0.045$) and GAF-Disability ($P = 0.028$), in comparison with best clinical practice. There was a significant trend (Wilcoxon $P = 0.03$) towards more social remissions in the patient subgroup treated according to the IC program than in those in the RR subgroup. No statistically significant differences between the two care programs were found in the domains of quality of life, impact on informal carers, side effects, symptoms and signs, distress, on carer stress. The mean number of days in hospital during the first year of study was 36 for the IC program and 27 for the RR program. The corresponding figures for the second year were 22 and 39, respectively. Although these outcomes may be of clinical importance, they were statistically nonsignificant.

Analysis by Attention-to-Content-of-Care. For the subgroups ($N = 25/33$) that participated at least one year in programs of care (for the IC program with at least 70% of program fidelity), the significant findings were WHO-DAS total scores ($P = 0.043$), GAF-Disability ($P = 0.008$), and consumer satisfaction by UKU-ConSat ($P = 0.014$), with all differences in favour of the IC program. In summary, the main clinical outcome was increased consumer satisfaction and significant improvements in social function.

Our Research II: A Computer Tool-Kit for Outcome Reporting

Introduction

An essential element for the monitoring and planning of mental health services is the provision of repeated patient-related outcomes [18].

Objectives. The objective was to develop and implement a computer-aided tool-kit for the continuous evaluation of mental health. The new technology tool-kit was intended to be applied for comparisons within and between programs, in research as well as in clinical practice (manuscript submitted).

Materials and Methods

A personal computer equipped with Windows NT 4.0 software was used. On the research computer, an application written in (Borland)/Corel Paradox 8.0 was installed and gradually refined over time. The application served three purposes: to collect and organize data from the independent raters, to collect and organize data from the case managers' contacts with patients, and to present patient data at the group, subgroup, and individual levels, with various time frames and with one or multiple outcome domains or by comparison groups. The data from the independent raters were originally collected on printed paper forms. To facilitate the transfer, a computerized form, similar to the paper form, was developed.

Results

The anatomy of the multilevel outreporting consists of three different formats: psychiatric temperature charts for display of the individual patient (Fig. 1) and aggregated outcomes (Fig. 2), bar graphs for display of subgroup outcomes (Fig. 3), and Qual Star graphics (Fig. 4). The Qual Star graphic contains eight rays, or axes, each denoting one domain of measure. This can be used at all levels (group, subgroup, individual). It is possible to drill down into the database details, for instance, from a global measure of symptom outcome to a specific symptom item of a rating

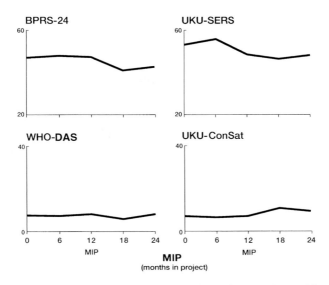

FIG. 1. Clinical care effectiveness. Two years of clinical care for 88 patients with schizophrenic disorders. Group out-reports representing the four domains "Symptoms and signs" (BPRS-24), "Side effects" (SSP-UKU-SERS), "Social function" (WHO-DAS) and "Consumer satisfaction" (UKU-ConSat)

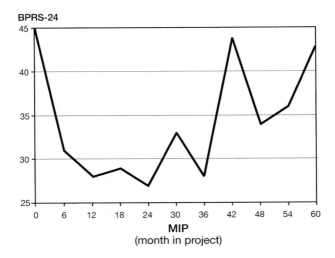

FIG. 2. Five-year course: single patient Brief Psychiatric Rating Scale (BPRS)-24

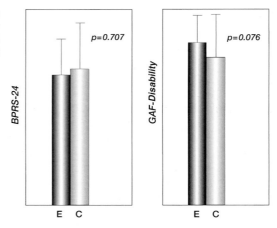

FIG. 3. Efficacy study. Total mean scores of BPRS-24, respectively GAF-Disability, for two compared Assertive Community Treatment programs. *E* and *C*

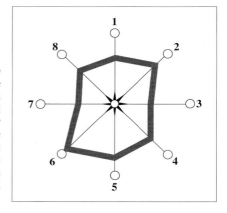

FIG. 4. One single patient in point estimate Quality Star graph. The domains of outcome are presented as a compass reading, beginning with north and proceeding clockwise. The centripetal circles represent 100% health as indicated by outcome measures, in the cost domain the average for patient group. Domains of outcome: 1 = Consumer satisfaction; 2 = Quality of life; 3 = Social function; 4 = Impact on informal carers; 5 = Costs; 6 = Side effects; 7 = Symptoms and signs; 8 = Distress

scale. The computer-aided outreport tool-kit is constructed to present a broad spectrum of outcomes, using eight domains of outcomes, as shown by the specific measurements.

Discussion and Conclusions

An essential element for the monitoring and planning of mental health services, based on empirical outcome data, is the provision of repeated dynamic outreporting of validated and consistent patient-related outcomes, on group and individual levels, with various time frames, and in one or multiple outcome domains. The time needed to obtain outreports from the data base, including graphs and preliminary statistical testings, is about five minutes. Our conclusion is that we have been successful in achieving a user-friendly and instant computer-aided tool-kit to be applied in research as well as in the everyday evaluation of mental health services practice, to maintain, monitor, and continuously improve the quality of services.

Main Discussion

One significant advantage was increased consumer satisfaction among patients in Integrated Care in comparison with best established community care [19]. The main clinical outcome was improvements in social function. This is similar to the outcomes of earlier studies of ACT in comparison with traditional and often hospital-based care [20], but differs from two recent studies in the United Kingdom, one quasi-experimental that compared sectors (PRiSM) and another RCT (the UK 700) [21] that compared case load sizes without finding any differences. Because we have access to process data, we carried out an attention-to-content-of-care approach. This suggests that one explanation for the different research findings might be anchored in the linking of new neurobehavioral findings to the psychosocial approaches implemented in the IC program. Overt dysfunctional symptoms are not necessarily a direct function of the basic impairment. Neuromodulation by optimal antipsychotic medication treatment might allow "new input" by various psychosocial ingredients in the programs to generate adaptive mechanisms that could compensate for deficits. Such treatment has even been thought to change cortical maps in the brain neocortex, according to the concept of neuroplasticity [22]. Treatment theory hypothesizes which ingredients of service practice are crucial for effectiveness. The IC program brings patients through a series of stages involving knowledge, involvement, attitude, and insight changes that are matched by a sequence of distinct intervention strategies promoting an enriched environment, resulting in impacts on neuroplasticity [23].

On the system levels, a major finding was that there were deficiencies in the mental health services in comparison with the current evidence base, such as a lack of 24-hour services and the fact that the ACT provider teams did not have control of admission or discharge from hospital. There were available alternatives to hospital care. No one was agency was responsible for the severely mentally ill. To put it if another way, for optimal outcomes the management and organization of the input system have to be congruent with the provider program [23,24]. Even if making changes in existing systems threatens to be a drawback, it is also an opportunity to create a new psychiatry.

In the ideal world, the decision-making settings for the implementation of evidence-based management and clinical practice for the severe mental ill (manuscript submitted) would contain the following seven steps (Table 3):

Decision-Making Setting 1. The tasks of governments are to introduce evidence-based psychiatric service decisions and to promote corresponding cooperation at various system levels.

Decision-Making Setting 2. The clinicians (in the provider team) have to make their decisons on which evidence-based program to implement, for instance, IC.

Decision-Making Setting 3. Provider teams are trained, and organizations are prepared through information and education.

TABLE 3. Decision-making settings of evidence-based mental health

Environmental and decision-making settings		Input	Process	Output
Society		Decision 7 Fighting stigma		
Individual	Patient and informal carers in social network			
	Clinicians in the provider team	Decision 2 Evidence-based programs to fit the need of the patients	Decision 4 The social network resource group	Decision 5 Clinical outcomes
System	Mental Health Services	Decision 3 I. Training of staff II. Preparing organizations		Decision 5 Incentives by clinical governance monitored by outcome and reviews
	National and regional politicians	Decision 1 To introduce evidence-based management		Decision 6 Decisions on system cooperating to create a "one-stop-station" for the patient

Decision-Making Setting 4. The case manager, the patient, and the psychiatrist should bring together the professionals and informal carers concerned into a social-network resource group for the individual patient. The resource group should be looked upon as a local social network "clan" for the individual patient [25]. The patient can then "play in his or her own recovery team", coached by the psychiatrist and the clinical case manager. In a supportive and informed microcosmos, the patient can be prepared for integration into the community, together with the people he or she knows and trusts. The patient and the clinical case manager screen all kinds of potential resource individuals in the patient's social network. The case manager and the patient together then initiate a first meeting of the resource group. A proposal for a personal growth plan is the main agenda for a series of decisions on how to achieve the patient's main personal goal—akin to setting up a theatre play. The personal-growth plan draft with its decisions is finalized by the patient, case manager, and psychiatrist together and then distributed to the members of the resource group. The resource group, including the case manager, meet regularly for follow-up, monitored by continuous outcome assessments by the patient, case manger, and independent assessors. The resource group acts as a kind of collaborative "one-stop-station" for acute and long-term management, with a continuous and integrated combination of medication and psychosocial treatment methods. Social and family support are also provided by the resource groups, as are the patient's needs for shelter and cover in crisis situations.

Decision-Making Setting 5. Clinical governance is introduced, with incentives for monitoring by indicators of quality and safety, such as outcomes and reviews based on clinical audits [19].

Decision-Making Setting 6. To create local "one responsible agencies" in order to make systems congruent with the program for clinical care, including guidelines, legal procedures, and budget.

Decision-Making Setting 7. We have now to combat healthy people's prejudiced attitudes in order to provide an environment in the community that is designed to help people who may be odd, but not mad.

Conclusions

The main research findings are that good clinical care for patients with schizophrenic disorders can be improved by introducing the ACT model program, Integrated Care. To promote putting effective services into practice, and achieving further improvements in outcome, structural changes in the delivery systems of services in harmony with the provider program have to be introduced.

Acknowledgments. We are indebted to the NU ACT-team at the Sahlgrenska University Hospital. This Research was funded by grants from the Swedish Medical Research Council, the Faculty of Medicine of the University of Göteborg, Vårdalstiftelsen, the Swedish Schizophrenia Fellowship, Socialstyrelsens nationella och regionala stimulansbidrag, Königsska-Söderströmska sjukhemmet/Svenska Läkaresällskapet, CEFOS, and the Torsten och Ragnar Söderbergs Foundation.

References

1. Kane JM, McGlashan TH (1995) Lancet 346:820–825
2. Cancro R, Meyerson (1999) In: Maj M, Sartorius N (eds) WPA Series: Evidence and experience in psychiatry. Vol 2. Schizophrenia. John Wiley & Sons, Chichester
3. Malm U (1997) Neuroleptics in combination with psychosocial interventions in the rehabilitation of patients with schizophrenia. English laguage manuscript. A systematic Cochrane review. In: SBU (The Swedish Council on Technology in Health Care), Report No. 133, Behandling med neuroleptika. Vol 1. SBU, Stockholm, pp 133–151
4. Vendsborg P, Nordentoft M, Hvenegaard, et al (1999) Opsogende psykoseteam—Assertive Community Treatment. DSI Report 99.06, Copenhagen
5. Falloon IRH (1999) Optimal treatment for psychosis in an international multisite demonstration project. Psychiatr Serv 50:615–618
6. Malm U (1990) Group therapy. In: Herz MI, Keith SJ, Docherty JP (eds) Handbook of schizophrenia. Vol 4. Psychosocial treatment of schizophrenia. Elsevier, Amsterdam, pp 191–211
7. Guy W (1976) Early Clinical Drug Evaluation Unit (ECDEU). Publication No. 76-338. Rockville, National Institute of Mental Health
8. American Psychiatric Association (APA) (1994) Diagnostic and Statistical Manual of Mental Disorders (4th edn) (DSM-IV). Washington, DC, APA
9. Lukoff B, Neuchterlein KH, Ventura J (1986) Manual for the expanded Brief Psychiatric Rating Scale. Schizophrenia Bulletin 12:594–602

10. Bech P, Malt UF, Dencker SJ, et al (1993) Scales for assessment of diagnosis and severity of mental health disorders. Acta Psychiatr Scand 87(Suppl 372):55–56
11. Jablensky A, Schwartz R, Tomov T (1980) WHO collaborative study of impairments and disabilities associated with schizophrenic disorders. A preliminary communication—objectives and methods. Acta Psychiatrica Scandinavica 62:152–163
12. Ahlfors UG, Lewander T, Lindström E, et al (2001) Assessment of patient satisfaction with psychiatric care. Development and clinical evaluation of a brief consumer satisfaction scale (UKU-ConSat). Nordic Journal of Psychiatry (in press)
13. Tarrier N, Wittkowski A, Kinney C, et al (1999) Durability of the effects of cognitive-behavioural therapy in the treatment of chronic schizophrenia: 12-month follow-up. Br J Psychiatry 174:500–504
14. Skantze K, Malm U, Dencker SJ, et al (1992) Comparison of quality of life to standard of living in schizophrenic outpatients. Br J Psychiatry 161:797–801
15. Sullivan M, Karlsson J, Ware JE (1994) SF-36 (Swedish manual and interpretation guide). Boston, Medical Outcomes Trust
16. Goldberg DP (1972) The detection of non-psychotic psychiatric illness by means of a questionnaire. Maudsley Monographs. Oxford, Oxford University Press
17. Knapp MRJ, Beecham JK, Koutsogeorgopoulou V, et al (1994) Service use and costs of home-based versus hospital-based care for people with serious mental illness. Br J Psychiatry 165:195–203
18. Marks I (1998) Overcoming obstacles to routine outcome measurement. Br J Psychiatry 173:281–286
19. Malm U, Lewander T (2002) Consumer satisfaction in schizophrenia. A 2-year randomized controlled study of two community-based treatment programs. Nordic Journal of Psychiatry (in press)
20. Marshall M, Bond G, Stein LI, et al (1999) PRiSM Psychosis study. Br J Psychiatry 175:501–503
21. Burns T, Creed F, Fahy T, et al (1999) Intensive versus standard case management for severe psychotic illness: a randomised trial. Lancet 353:2185–2189
22. Spitzer M (1998) The mind within the net. MIT Press, Cambridge, Mass
23. Hargreaves WAQ, Shumway M, Hu TW, et al (1998) Cost-outcome methods for mental health. Academic Press, London
24. Thornicroft G, Tansella M (1999) The mental health matrix. Cambridge University Press, Cambridge, England
25. Malm U (1999) "Clanning" for schizophrenia. In: Maj M, Sartorius N (eds) WPA Series: Evidence and experience in psychiatry. Vol 2 Schizophrenia. John Wiley & Sons, Chichester

Early Psychosis Intervention in Routine Service Environments: Implications for Case Management and Service Evaluation

STANLEY V. CATTS[1,3], MARYANNE O'DONNELL[1,2],
ELIZABETH A. SPENCER[3], KATHERINE D. STEWART[2],
MATTHEW OVENS[3], MEGAN STILL[3], and MIRIAM C. PROBERTS[1]

Summary. Although there are a number of demonstration early psychosis intervention (EPI) programs, comprehensive procedures for implementing EPI in routine community service environments have not been published. The present study describes the introduction and evaluation of a specialized EPI program in a routine Australian urban mental health service. The program was supported by enhancement funding for 18 months (December 1995 to June 1997) and consisted of four full-time staff and two quarter-time consultant psychiatrists who worked in an Assertive Community Treatment team framework. Of 161 referrals, 149 were assessed and 70 clients were actively treated. Clients showed statistically significant short-term (3–6 months) improvements on all outcome instruments. Detection and retention rates for the specialized EPI program appeared to be better than those for an adjacent service that used a case-manager-implemented EPI protocol but without additional resources or dedicated staff. Preliminary results of a medium-term (3–4 years) follow-up indicated that the social, but not the vocational, function of clients was greatly improved. The authors concluded that the appropriate level of specialized treatment and evaluation required for early psychosis intervention is only possible if models of specialized case management are used and there is a long-term commitment by the mental health service to support early psychosis intervention as a specialized function. Recommendations for the successful introduction and evaluation of early psychosis intervention are discussed.

Key words. Early psychosis intervention, Case management, Evaluation, Mental health services, Consumer participation

[1] School of Psychiatry, University of New South Wales, Sydney, NSW, 2052, Australia
[2] Psychiatric Unit, Eastern Suburbs Mental Health Program, The Prince of Wales Hospital, High Street, Randwick, NSW, 2031, Australia
[3] Liverpool Mental Health Service, Don Everett Building, Liverpool Hospital, PO Box 103, Liverpool, NSW, 2170, Australia

Introduction

Australasian clinicians have made a worthy contribution to the development of new approaches to the management of psychotic illness. The discovery of lithium [1], the first replication studies demonstrating the effectiveness of the Program of Assertive Community Treatment teams (PACT) model of community service specifically with schizophrenia [2,3], the pioneering work in psychosocial intervention [4] and models of primary care [5], and the development of demonstration Early Psychosis Intervention (EPI) programs [6,7] are but some of the highlights. Not surprisingly, Australian mental health services are among the most community-focused in the world, and rates of inpatient psychiatric service use are relatively low and continue to decrease. Case management is the backbone of community mental health service delivery [8]. Health service initiatives have been reinforced by government-sponsored initiatives to foster consumer participation, reduce stigma, and encourage primary care models of service delivery [9]. Government-funded pharmaceutical benefits schemes have enabled the early and low-cost availability of the new atypical neuroleptic agents.

Having worked so hard to develop what some think are world leading mental health services, many Australian clinicians must have been disappointed by the results of the Study of Low Prevalence (Psychotic) Disorders (SLPPD) [10], a component of the Australian National Survey of Mental Health and Wellbeing [11]. In the study, a 1-month census was undertaken in four urban catchment areas to identify people aged 18 to 64 years who were in active contact with a mental health service and met the screening criteria for psychosis. Of the 3800 people who screened positive for psychosis, a representative sample of patients ($n = 980$) was interviewed. Fifty-two percent of the interviewed group were diagnosed as having *Diagnostic and Statistical Manual of Mental Disorders*, 3rd edition, revised (DSM-III-R) Schizophrenia. The most disturbing findings from the study concerned the levels of disability detected in the interviewed patients. Despite being in treatment, the majority of patients suffered active psychotic symptoms, 85% were dependent on government welfare, only 10% were in full-time employment, and less than 2% were rated as having good psychosocial function.

What could explain the devastating disability evident in treated patients with psychotic illness? There are only three broad categories of explanation: treatment is ineffective, mental health services are not applying treatments competently, or patients with psychosis are unwilling to comply with treatments offered. There is now robust evidence that a broad range of pharmacological [12], psychological [13], family [14], and supportive employment [15–17] strategies are effective interventions for reducing symptoms and improving function in schizophrenia. Therefore, the highly interrelated domains of service competence and patient compliance seem to be the likely areas of weakness in routine service delivery environments [18,19].

Two bodies of research are particularly relevant to exploring Australian mental health service competence. One convincingly confirms the value of service delivery programs using multidisciplinary Assertive Community Treatment teams (ACT) [20]. Importantly, the same literature has demonstrated that brokerage or clinical models of case management that involve high case loads (more than 25 per case manager) have no effect on improving the symptoms and function of psychotic patients [20,

21]. The other body of literature demonstrates that the longer neuroleptic treatment is delayed after the onset of psychotic illness, the worse are the short-term [22] and long-term [23,24] outcomes. Concordant with this research are studies showing that with each relapse of psychosis, the chance of full recovery diminishes [25]. In terms of judging the degree of implementation of effective service models, the Early Psychosis Prevention and Intervention Centre (EPPIC) [6] represents a gold standard demonstration service for EPI, as does the PACT program [26] for ACTs.

Hence, in considering the effectiveness of Australian mental health services, it must be noted that ACT models of case management have been rarely implemented in routine service delivery environments. The vast majority of community mental health services support models of case management characterized by case loads greater than 30 patients per worker, which are known to be ineffective in improving patient outcomes [20, 21]. In terms of EPI, only rudimentary elements of the EPPIC Program have recently been implemented in a limited number of community services, and the duration of initially untreated psychosis in Australia is no shorter than in other countries [6]. The present paper describes a pilot project called the Early Psychosis Outreach Community Health (EPOCH) Program. This program was funded with the aim of stimulating the development of EPI in routine community mental health services in New South Wales. Its implementation and evaluation are presented. A number of recommendations concerning future attempts to implement EPI will be discussed.

The EPOCH Program

Program Description

The EPOCH Program was administered by one of the four sector services, the Eastern Suburbs Mental Health Service (ES-MHS) of the South Eastern (formally Eastern) Sydney Area Health Service (SESAHS). In 1996 the ES-MHS had a catchment population of 224541 people, who were mainly of middle-class socioeconomic background. At this time, the ES-MHS was in the early stages of integrating hospital and community services. The community service relied on a hybrid case management model that used both clinical and brokerage procedures and was characterized by caseloads in excess of 35 clients per worker. Limited backup was available from three specialist teams: an extended-hours team, an intensive case management team, and a rehabilitation team. The EPOCH Program started in December 1995 and closed in June 1997. It consisted of four full-time clinical staff members (senior registrar, clinical psychologist, family therapist, and occupational therapist) and a part-time secretary/research assistant. Two consultant psychiatrists devoted 10 hr per week each to the program. Office-based services were located in the basement of a psychiatric facility. Community outreach was facilitated by the purchase of two cars and mobile phones.

It was decided that EPOCH should function separately from other service components, though in a well-coordinated manner. It was considered desirable to stream young early-psychosis patients away from more severely disturbed patients with advanced psychotic illness. Incorporating the program into the routine case management team did not fit with the hybrid (but mainly brokerage-crisis intervention) case management model of that team. EPOCH proposed to use an ACT model and, a discipline-specific training and clinical practice approach to care, rather than a generalist case management model. Also, a separate team structure allowed the fostering of a team philosophy and the undertaking of developmental activities, usually done by trial and error, in a supportive atmosphere. This was important because clinical procedures for implementing EPI in routine service delivery settings had not been published at that time, although the rationale and principles of EPI had been well articulated by McGorry and colleagues [7]. Finally, a dedicated program intake provided the opportunity to assess barriers to seeking specialist referral by young people and to design procedures that were "user friendly" to referring agents, especially general practitioners and school counselors.

The EPOCH Program operated from 9 a.m. to 5 p.m. on weekdays, although after-hours appointments and family groups were arranged according to need. The program entry criteria were young people between the ages of 15 and 25 years living within the catchment area who were within 2 years after the onset of a psychotic illness (including the prodromal period). The last criterion was not always satisfactory, because it is often difficult to define the onset of the prodromal period. When there was doubt, clients were accepted if they had a psychotic illness and were within 12 months of their first service registration. The program emphasized assertive outreach, rapid response time, and intensive case and family work. A key worker who was responsible for program engagement and collecting outcome data was appointed for each client. The therapeutic role of staff members was fostered, and whenever possible specialized intervention was carried out by the person with the most appropriate discipline-specific skills and training.

Emergency out-of-hours contacts were provided by the ES-MHS Extended Hours Team (EHT), with whom EPOCH maintained close liaison. Capacity to carry out acute home-based [27] care was developed. EPOCH clients were admitted directly under the care of inpatient teams supervised by the EPOCH consultants. EPOCH staff attended the inpatient unit to facilitate admission formalities and support EPOCH clients during their stay in the hospital.

Service promotion and referring agent education were undertaken, including educational seminars for potential referrers, linkage with the shared care program for general practitioners (GPs), and encouragement of referrer contact with EPOCH medical personnel. Specific engagement procedures were supported, including acceptance of direct referrals; quick response time to referrals (less than 24 hr for outpatients); rapid multidisciplinary assertive community outreach for early assessment and home-based care; cotherapist assessment and treatment, with one or more staff flexibly dedicated to client work and another staff member for family/carer work; staff training in psychotherapeutic engagement strategies; and intensive follow-up procedures for clients judged to be at risk for treatment noncompliance or premature termination of contact. Broad-based team support for clients was fostered, which necessitated a well-developed staff meeting process. Full-team client review meetings that included the two psychiatrists were held three times weekly.

EPOCH was linked with two important service components. First, liaison meetings were conducted with representatives of the ES-MHS Drug and Alcohol Services. Because of the prevalence of substance abuse, it was concluded that EPOCH staff should provide drug and alcohol psychoeducation to clients and that the EPOCH psychologist should provide motivational counseling [28], rather than referring clients to the Drug and Alcohol Service. Second, a clinical attachment of a consultant from the ES-MHS Child and Adolescent Services was arranged for cosupervision of clients between the ages of 15 and 17.

Consumer collaboration was a focus of the EPOCH Program. After consultation with a professional consumer representative and a consumer organization leader, and feedback from a focus group of EPOCH clients, a novel partnership model of consumer and carer collaboration was implemented. Key to its success was the formation of separate forums for EPOCH clients, and their carers. EPOCH clients did not want their meetings to include carers, and they did not want to sit on a management meeting. Two semi-independent groups were established, one for clients and one for carers. Each group was composed of interested EPOCH primary or secondary consumers; a resource person who was a non-EPOCH primary or secondary consumer with negotiating, advocacy, and lobbying skills and access to the resources of other primary or secondary consumer groups; and a facilitator who was an EPOCH staff member with a program-reporting, group process-supporting, and mental health policy and procedures advisory role. The program psychologist fulfilled the role of client group facilitator, and the family therapist fulfilled the role of the carer group facilitator. Both facilitators were members of the program management meeting and could effectively act as spokespersons for the consumer groups, while providing immediate feedback on management's response to issues raised by consumers. The semi-independence of the consumer groups not only allowed consumers to effectively apply influence on program management, but also facilitated promotion of their concerns in a professional manner to the wider community or higher levels of the health service unencumbered by the bureaucratic constraints that apply to staff.

One of the most vexing issues for the EPOCH Program was to settle on a method of evaluation. Although a randomized, controlled trial (RCT) testing the effectiveness of early psychosis intervention had not been published, it was not feasible for the EPOCH Program to undertake such a study. There are strong ethical arguments against delaying effective treatment once a psychotic illness is clearly present. Alternatively, an RCT of specialized versus standard management is feasible in a routine service environment. However, this too was beyond the resources of EPOCH. A barrier to an RCT was the limited life of the program. Before a formal evaluation could commence, it was necessary to develop by trial and error the arrangements and procedures to support specialized EPI suitable for use in routine service delivery settings.

Despite the limitations of the approach, a decision was ultimately taken to compare detection and retention rates and client outcomes of our specialized EPOCH Program with those of an adjacent sector service that used early intervention strategies implemented by generalist case managers using a manualized protocol. The adjacent sector used no additional resources or supported dedicated staff, and only the very limited specialist backup of a family psychoeducation program and a rehabilitation team was available to assist in the implementation of EPI. The choice of outcome instruments was made easier, because a review of outcome measures for use in routine mental health service situations had recently been published [29]. The aim was to collect demographic and clinical data on the EPOCH clients and to assess levels of symptoms, distress, and function at baseline and again 3 to 6 months after program entry. Equivalent data on first service contact patients with psychosis in the same age range were to be collected in the adjacent comparison sector within an identical time period.

Specific Interventions

Medical Management

Psychiatric assessment was performed by the senior registrar (E.A.S.), who also arranged physical examinations and medical investigations. All patients with psychotic symptoms were offered neuroleptic medication. In outpatients, the dose was increased slowly to the lowest dose that produced a response according to a protocol (Catts, 1998; available on request from the senior author). During the life of the program, the atypical neuroleptics, risperidone and olanzapine, were beginning to be used in Australia. Initially, low-dose typical neuroleptics (haloperidol, less than 5 mg, or trifluoperazine, less than 10 mg) were used. However, these medications were found to cause significant extrapyramidal side effects in younger clients. As soon as the atypical neuroleptics were freely available, all new patients were switched to these agents (risperidone, up to 4 mg, and olanzapine, up to 15 mg). Clients with multiple risk factors for noncompliance (diminished insight, substance abuse, poor engagement, and risk of harm to others) were given low-dose injectable depot neuroleptics (zuclopenthixol decanoate at a starting dose of 25 mg weekly), if necessary, as involuntary treatment. Neuroleptic treatment for acute psychotic illness was routinely supplemented with benzodiazepine medication (diazepam, 5–40 mg daily). Depressive or manic features in an illness that was not primarily an affective disorder, which did not improve as the psychosis improved, were assertively treated with supplementary antidepressant (sertraline) or mood-stabilizing medication. Treatment resistance was diagnosed early, and clozapine was considered after two failed trials of neuroleptic medication of at least 12 weeks' duration each at optimal doses.

Psychological and Family Interventions

Supportive psychotherapeutic approaches were mainly used with both clients and family/carers. Two members of the staff were experienced in psychotherapy: the psychologist (K.D.S.) and the family therapist (M.O.), both being strongly influenced by solution-focused [30], competency-based [31], narrative [32], and strategic [33] frameworks. The psychologist also had a background in drug and alcohol services and was skilled in motivational interviewing [28] and treatment-matching [34] techniques. Structured cognitive-behavioral therapy (CBT) was not used with clients, although CBT techniques were used informally. Structured family psychoeducation was not used with family/carers, although elements of this approach were incorporated into a family education model [35,36]. A series of eight weekly support and education groups was held for carers only (not clients). These groups consisted mainly of multiple families who were encouraged to form a network for ongoing mutual support and advocacy.

Occupational Therapy

The EPOCH Program included a full-time occupational therapist (M.S.), who provided specialist individual and group assessments and interventions. Assessments utilized a client-centered [37] framework supplemented by the Perceive; Recall; Plan; Perform system of task analysis [38]. In the absence of a strong research footing for guiding occupational early psychosis interventions, the occupational therapist took a flexible approach to supporting role function, especially with adolescent clients. Decisions about time for school return, duration of initial school attendance, transfer to a specialized educational facility, or commencement of vocational training or placement were made on a case-by-case basis. Younger clients who found verbal therapies least helpful were often the most attracted to the real-world functional approaches of the occupational therapist. Productivity roles (vocational, scholastic, or leisure-based) seemed of the highest importance to EPOCH clients, and as it turned out, these roles may have been the most vulnerable to the impact of early-onset psychotic illness.

Evaluation Procedures and Instruments

Data Collection and Instrumentation

Demographic information and personal history, including illicit substance use, were obtained by file audit. Diagnostic assessment was based on all sources of information available, and rating was performed by using a checklist for the *Diagnostic and Statistical Manual of Mental Disorders*, 4th edition (DSM-IV) and the *International Classification of Diseases*, 10th revision (ICD-10). The Health of the Nation Outcome Scales (HoNOS) [39], the Life Skills Profile (LSP) [40], and the Depression, Anxiety, and Stress Scale (DASS) [41] were used at baseline and 3 to 6 months after program entry to assess levels of symptoms, distress, and function in EPOCH clients. Family/carer function was measured by using the Experience of Caregiving Inventory (ECI) [42], but these data will be reported elsewhere.

A carer-report questionnaire called "When Did the Difficulties Begin" was designed to estimate the time of illness onset based on probes reported by Beiser and colleagues [43]. The validity of this informant-report questionnaire was not tested prior to use in the EPOCH Program evaluation, and in fact it was found to provide data highly discordant with clinician ratings. Therefore, these data are not reported.

An 11-point checklist of reasons for a patient's ceasing to attend the service was developed to define premature treatment dropout (E. Spencer, unpublished dissertation, 1998). Use of this checklist with file audit was associated with high interrater reliability. The same checklist was used to determine premature dropout according to the judgment of the case manager or key worker. The two procedures were in good agreement when medical records were satisfactory.

In the medium-term follow-up, selected questions from the Demography and Social Functioning Module of the Diagnostic Interview for Psychosis (DIP) [44] were used to rate current social function on the Social and Occupational Functioning Assessment Scale (SOFAS) [45] and to determine occupational status.

Short-Term Evaluation Procedures

To test the feasibility of the evaluation procedures in routine clinical practice, EPOCH key workers were asked to be responsible for collecting data on their clients. Within 1 week of acceptance to the program, subjects were asked to complete the DASS, usually while the key worker was present. The key worker had to complete the HoNOS and the LSP. These measures were repeated after the client had been in treatment 3 to 6 months, usually at an outpatient review. A research assistant tabulated the data and reminded the key worker if data were due and not collected.

Across-Program Evaluation Procedures

A series of meetings between the EPOCH Program medical staff and the senior service managers of the comparison sector resulted in approval for the EPOCH senior registrar to seek the cooperation of the local case management staff to prospectively collect data on a sample of first-contact clients from their sector. A series of meetings with case managers occurred with senior management present. Agreement was obtained that for EPI clients, case managers would complete the HoNOS and the LSP (which was current practice in the sector), and would also ask the client to complete the DASS and the primary carer to complete the "When Did the Difficulties Begin" questionnaire, the LSP, and the ECI. These ratings were intended to be collected prospectively at baseline and 3 to 6 months later. However, before these procedures commenced, staff shortages resulted in the temporary cessation of all evaluation procedures in the adjacent sector, preventing a prospective two-time point comparison from occurring.

As an alternative, a retrospective comparison was made between the detection, retention, and client outcome of the EPOCH Program and the adjacent sector. Clients from the EPOCH Program or the adjacent sector service were included in the evaluation if they registered with their respective service for the first time between the dates of January 1, 1996, and April 1, 1997; were between the ages of 15 and 25 at the time of index registration; had an ICD-10 diagnosis of a psychotic disorder; did not have a neurological disease or a moderate or severe learning disability; and were within 12 months of their first mental health provider contact for treatment of a psychotic illness. All EPOCH Program files were reviewed by the senior registrar, and those cases that met the above criteria were included in the EPOCH comparison group. For the comparison sector, clients between the ages of 15 and 25 who had registered within the relevant period were identified from a computerized database called CRISP. All files identified this way were reviewed by the senior registrar, and cases with an ICD-10 diagnosis of psychotic illness that met the criteria were included in the comparison service group.

Simultaneously with the EPOCH Program collection of the 3- to 6-month client outcome data, case managers in the adjacent comparison sector attended teaching sessions explaining the nature of the assessment instruments they had agreed to encourage their clients and carers in the evaluation to complete. The questionnaire forms were distributed to case managers, who were asked to approach personally their comparison clients and their carers. The client simply had to complete the DASS, and the primary carer had to complete the ECI, the LSP, and the "When Did the Difficulties Begin?" questionnaire. EPOCH primary carers were asked to complete these three questionnaires when they were participating in the 3- to 6-month outcome assessment. Clients and their carers were instructed to complete the questionnaires (with or without the assistance of the case manager) and mail or hand them back to their case managers.

Medium-Term (3 to 4 Years) Follow-Up Evaluation Procedures

The consultant psychiatrists who had been attached to the EPOCH Program (M.O'D. and S.V.C.) identified and interviewed ex-EPOCH Program clients currently living in the ES-MHS catchment area who were still receiving treatment in April 2000.

Results

Description of EPOCH Clients

During the entire period of operation of EPOCH (December 1995 to June 1997), 161 patients were referred and 149 were assessed. Nonassessed patients were either uncontactable or refused assessment. At least five of these nonassessed referrals were probable cases of psychosis who did not appear to warrant involuntary assessment. Sixty-seven of the assessed clients did not meet program entry criteria. Most of these cases were diagnosed as having personality disorder (cluster B). All clients assessed who were not accepted into the program were in need of psychiatric care and were linked to alternative services. In the first six months of the program, general practitioners referred less than 5% of clients, and in the last 6 months of the program, GPs referred nearly 20% of clients.

Of the 70 clients accepted into the program, 44 (63%) were males. The mean age was 19.6 years (SD = 2.5). Most were living with their families (74%). Thirty clients (43%) were referred during their first psychiatric admission to the hospital, and another 9 (13%) had previously been admitted to the hospital for treatment of psychosis. Only 23 (33%) had had no previous contact with a mental health service provider. At program entry only a provisional diagnosis was made, and some delay in formulating a final diagnosis was permitted. The final DSM-IV diagnoses for EPOCH clients were as follows: schizophrenia, 42% ($n = 29$); psychosis, not otherwise specified, 29% ($n = 18$); schizoaffective disorder, 9% ($n = 6$); schizophreniform disorder, 7% ($n = 5$); bipolar disorder, 7% ($n = 5$); brief psychosis, 1% ($n = 1$); and major depressive disorder with psychosis, 1% ($n = 1$). Five patients (7%) were rated as "at risk mental states" [46], but none of these were treated for psychotic illness during the life of the program. Significantly, 38 (54%) met the criteria for substance abuse, most in relation to cannabis abuse (44%, $n = 31$). File audit revealed that regular illicit drug use (more than single-occasion experimentation) in the year before program entry occurred in at least 80% of the 70 clients accepted into the program.

Medication Usage

All patients with psychotic symptoms were strongly encouraged to take neuroleptic medication. At the commencement of the program, use of typical neuroleptics was standard clinical practice in Australia. The EPOCH Program prescribing practice changed over time as the atypical agents became freely available. The decision to prescribe typical or atypical agents was determined by the availability of atypical agents (the preferred option) rather than the clinical state of the client, except in the case of depot neuroleptic or clozapine. In fact, 26% ($n = 18$) received typical agents at some point in their treatment; 51% ($n = 36$) received atypical agents, of whom 11% were treated with clozapine ($n = 8$); and 10% ($n = 7$) received injectable depot neuroleptics.

Hospital Admissions and Critical Incidents

In the period that the EPOCH Program was operational, 34% ($n = 24$) of clients required hospital admission at least once. Critical incidents included self-harm ($n =$

4), harm to others ($n = 5$), unplanned pregnancy ($n = 1$), exclusion from home ($n = 2$), marital separation ($n = 3$), and police contact and arrest ($n = 1$). There were no suicides.

Short-Term Outcome of EPOCH Clients

A formal outcome evaluation was carried out on all clients with a psychotic illness assessed by the EPOCH Program between the dates of April 1, 1996, and January 1, 1997. In that period 29 new clients with psychotic illness were seen. Complete sets of baseline and follow-up (3–6 months after program entry) data were collected on 21 of these clients. The reasons for failing to collect full data on eight clients were program related (i.e., not due to client refusal). The demographic and clinical characteristics of these eight clients were no different from those for whom complete data were available.

Baseline and Short-Term Outcome HoNOS Scores

The baseline and short-term outcome HoNOS scores are illustrated in Fig. 1A. Compared with the total HoNOS score at baseline (mean, 15.3), the total HoNOS score at 3 to 6 months (mean, 4.5) showed significant improvement ($t = 7.35$, df $= 20$, $p < 0.000$). This difference represents a 70% improvement in total HoNOS scores, reflecting a change in client status from moderately to mildly impaired (the maximum HoNOS impairment score is 48). All subscale scores showed significant improvement, including the psychotic symptoms subscale ($p < 0.002$).

Baseline and Short-Term Outcome LSP Scores

The baseline and short-term outcome LSP scores are illustrated in Fig. 1B. Compared with the total LSP scores at baseline (mean, 121.8), the total LSP scores at 3 to 6 months (mean, 142.2) showed significant improvement ($t = 5.61$, df $= 20$, $p < 0.001$). This difference represents a 17% improvement in total LSP scores, reflecting a change in client functional status from mild disability to almost no disability (the maximum score on the LSP is 156, indicating no problems with life skills).

Baseline and Short-Term Outcome DASS Scores

The baseline and short-term outcome DASS scores are illustrated in Fig. 1C. Compared with the mean DASS Anxiety score at baseline (mean, 13.3), the mean DASS Anxiety score at 3 to 6 months (mean, 7.7) showed significant improvement ($t = 2.54$, df $= 23$, $p < 0.018$). Compared with the mean DASS Stress score at baseline (mean, 18.3), the mean DASS Stress score at 3 to 6 months (mean, 10.3) showed significant improvement ($t = 3.47$, df $= 23$, $p < 0.002$) Compared with the mean DASS Depression score at baseline (mean, 16.4), the mean DASS Depression score at 3 to 6 months (mean, 14.8) did not show significant improvement ($p > 0.05$). These results indicate that the DASS Stress score changed from moderately severe to normal, the Anxiety score changed from moderately severe to mild, and the Depression score remained in the moderately severe range.

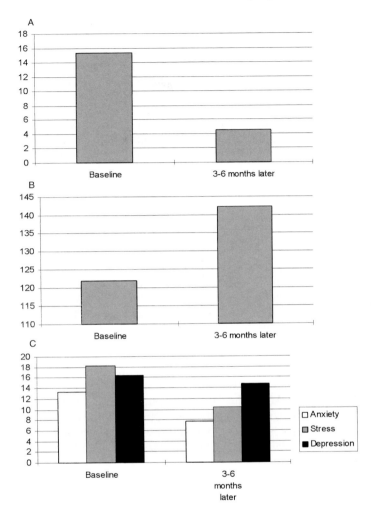

FIG. 1. Baseline and short-term outcomes of the EPOCH Program clients. **A** Mean baseline and 3- to 6-month outcome HoNOS scores. Score change $p < 0.001$; possible score range, 0–48. **B** Mean baseline and 3- to 6-month outcome LSP scores. Score change $p < 0.001$; possible score range, 0–156. **C** Mean baseline and 3- to 6-month outcome DASS scores. Anxiety score change $p < 0.02$; stress score change $p < 0.002$; depression score change $p > 0.05$. *EPOCH*, Early Psychosis Outreach Community Health; *HoNOS*, Health of the Nation Outcome Scales; *LSP*, Life Skills Profile; *DASS*, Depression, Anxiety, and Stress Scale

Comparison of the EPOCH Program with an Adjacent Sector Service

Comparison clients were those who met the previously listed criteria, including age between 15 and 25; index registration between January 1, 1996, and April 1, 1997; and an ICD-10 diagnosis of psychotic illness. The files of the EPOCH Program clients were easily identified, because all medical records were kept separately on the one site. A total of 56 EPOCH clients met the inclusion criteria. For the purposes of comparison with the adjacent sector, clients not registered with the ES-MHS were excluded. This identified 44 EPOCH clients ascertained from the ES-MHS catchment area. Of the 242 clients identified in the computer database of the adjacent comparison service in the above age range who registered between the above dates, 71 had a diagnosis of psychotic illness recorded, 66 had a nonpsychotic diagnosis recorded, and 105 had no diagnosis recorded. An exhaustive file-finding and review procedure of the clients with a database diagnosis of psychosis identified 13 clients who met the inclusion criteria. Of the clients with no diagnosis on the database, five met the criteria. Of the clients with a nonpsychotic diagnosis, none met the inclusion criteria. The files of 16 clients could not be found.

As a result of these case-finding procedures, 44 clients formed the EPOCH group and 18 clients formed the comparison sector group. The comparison sector group contained significantly ($p < 0.05$) more males (88% versus 63%) and was significantly ($p < 0.0001$) older (mean, 22.3 versus 19.4 years) than the EPOCH group. The number of clients with a previous psychiatric hospitalization before index registration (EPOCH, 57%; comparison sector, 71%) and the number living with their families at registration (EPOCH, 77%; comparison sector, 88%) were not significantly different. In terms of medication and hospital use, the number of clients who were prescribed atypical neuroleptics (EPOCH, 57%; comparison sector, 44%) and the number requiring hospital admission during the data collection period (EPOCH, 38%; comparison sector, 41%) were not significantly different. Apparently, the only difference in prescribing practice related to the use of clozapine, since no clients were prescribed clozapine in the comparison sector and eight (11%) of the EPOCH clients were taking clozapine.

To assess the impact of the EPOCH Program on the rate of detection of clients with early psychosis, the number of new cases ($n = 44$) identified by EPOCH in the ES-MHS (with a total catchment population of 224541) was compared with the equivalent number of new cases ($n = 18$) identified by the adjacent comparison sector (with a total catchment population of 207420) in the same time period. Based on the frequency of index cases among the clients whose files were audited in the comparison sector, it was estimated that about one case was missed (1.28, to be precise) because files could not be found and audited. Therefore, the number of cases detected in the comparison sector was adjusted from 18 to 19. In 1996 there were 28878 people between the ages of 15 and 24 years living in the comparison sector and 36292 same-aged people living in the ES-MHS. After adjustment for differences in the size of the catchment population, the equivalent numbers of cases identified were 44 for the EPOCH Program (in the ES-MHS) and 24 for the comparison sector service.

The comparison of cross-sectional outcomes across services using questionnaires met with mixed success. Questionnaires were returned by 41 of the 51 EPOCH clients (75%) to whom they were given, compared with 5 of the 17 (29%) clients in the comparison sector. This return rate was significantly different in the two groups ($p <$ 0.0007). Most of the EPOCH client nonresponders had been transferred to an out-of-area service and were difficult to follow up, whereas most of the comparison sector clients had refused to cooperate, although they were in current treatment with the comparison service. Questionnaires were returned by 33 of the 38 (total sample) EPOCH primary carers (87%) to whom they were given, compared with 4 of the 17 (24%) carers in the comparison sector. This too was a significantly different response rate. As a result of the failure to collect adequate questionnaire-assessed outcome data in the comparison sector, differences in outcome could not be investigated.

Spencer (unpublished dissertation, 1998) developed procedures to evaluate retention rate by assessing premature treatment dropout according to file audit and case manager judgment. These two methods were highly concordant when file notes were complete. Case managers in the comparison sector service judged that 6 (35%) of their comparison clients had prematurely terminated treatment, whereas EPOCH key workers judged that 5 (9%) of their clients were treatment dropouts. These significant differences ($p < 0.007$) in rates of premature dropout were validated by independent file audit.

Medium-Term (3–4 Years) Outcome of EPOCH Clients

Twenty clients were identified and interviewed in April 2000 who were living in the ES-MHS catchment area and still receiving treatment. All clients had a diagnosis of either schizophrenia (65%) or schizoaffective disorder (35%). All were prescribed atypical neuroleptics. Comorbid substance abuse was evident in three clients (15%). SOFAS social function ratings are presented in Fig. 2. These ratings are compared with

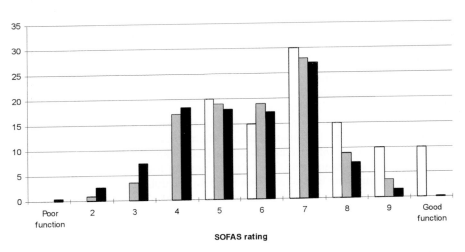

FIG. 2. Medium-term functional outcome (3–4 years posttreatment) of EPOCH Program clients. ☐ EPOCH, clients; ▨ ASLPPD, 18–24 years; ■ ASLPPD, all age groups. ASLPPD data from Jablensky et al. [10]. *EPOCH*, Early Psychosis Outreach Community Health; *ASLPPD*, Australian Study of Low Prevalence (Psychotic) Disorders

SOFAS ratings obtained in the Australian Study of Low Prevalence (Psychotic) Disorders (ASLPPD), using results from the total national sample ($n = 980$) and results from the subset of the sample between the ages of 15 and 24 years. As can be seen in Fig. 2, no EPOCH clients had a SOFAS rating below 50%, whereas 29% of the total ASLPPD sample and 22% of the ASLPPD sample aged between 18 and 24 years had a SOFAS rating below 50%. Further evidence of the general "shift to the right" to better function of the EPOCH group is the high percentage of EPOCH clients with SOFAS ratings of 80% and above (35%), compared with the proportions of the total ASLPPD sample (9%) and the ASLPPD sample aged between 18 and 24 years (13%) in the same range of high functioning. According to the same criteria for rating employment status as those used in the ASLPPD, only 30% of the EPOCH clients were rated as participating in full-time competitive employment or study, whereas the equivalent figure for the total ASLPPD sample was 10%. Consistent with the employment outcome for EPOCH clients were their rates of welfare dependency. Seventy percent of EPOCH clients were dependent on government or family welfare support, compared with an 85% rate of dependency on government welfare in the total ASLPPD sample.

Discussion

The description of the establishment of the EPOCH Program indicates that it is possible to implement specialized early psychosis programs in routine mental health service delivery environments, but apparently only with supplementary resources. The authors conclude that the success of the Program relied on the combination of an ACT service model with specialized case management, and ensuring coordination with other components of the community and hospital services. The EPOCH Program received on average about 10 referrals per month, with a trend for the number to increase toward the close of the program, suggesting the program was building a favorable profile. Only 70 of the 149 assessed clients met program entry criteria. The demographic and diagnostic characteristics of the accepted EPOCH clients were unremarkable, considering their age range. The overrepresentation of the diagnosis Psychosis: Not Otherwise Specified (29%) presumably simply reflects diagnostic caution. The high case identification rate was associated with a high assessment load. This was not considered inefficient, because all clients assessed were in need of psychiatric care, and the program acted as an effective pathway to care for a group of young people who are difficult to engage. The 67 clients who were assessed and referred away were not followed up. Therefore, it is not known whether any developed a psychotic illness subsequently. The fact that none of the cases classified as having an "at risk" mental state who were followed up for the duration of the program were rediagnosed with a psychotic illness suggests that the diagnostic accuracy of the assessment procedure was satisfactory.

The high prevalence of comorbid substance use disorder (54%) underlines the importance of EPI staff training in the management of substance disorder. Organizational integration of mental health and substance use programs does not seem to yield better results than ACT alone in clients with longstanding schizophrenic disorder and substance disorder [47]. Therefore, it is of great interest to determine whether assertive action early in psychotic illness will make a greater difference. To achieve success in patients with substance disorder with early psychosis, specialist assessment skills are required. Failure to detect other types of comorbidity in the younger substance-abusing client, such as attention deficit and conduct and personality disorders [48,49], will militate against effective intervention. Availability of biochemical monitoring of substance use may be an advantage [50,51]. The difficulty of working with these clients is emphasized by evidence that younger clients are less ready to cease drug use than are older clients [52]. Highly skilled interventions [53,54], including treatment matching [34] and motivational counseling skills, are essential. Effective pharmacological management of the psychotic illness and recognition of treatment resistance as a cause of persistent substance abuse are imperative [55].

The prevalence of illicit substance use (at least 80%, mainly cannabis) in EPOCH clients during the year before program entry appears to be in excess of the equivalent rate in a representative sample of Australian teenagers attending school. Lynskey and colleagues [56] found that 18% of 17-year-olds attending school reported using cannabis on 10 or more occasions in the past year. Although this figure may be a slight underestimate of use in a total sample in that age group, the majority of those included in the national sample would not have reached threshold for substance abuse, unlike most of the EPOCH clients. Of course, some would argue that any illicit substance use in early adolescence is abuse, given the evidence that it interferes with normal cognitive, emotional, and social development [57]. In either case, the apparently strong association of substance use and psychosis in EPOCH clients indicates the urgent need for additional research into the etiological connection between the two disorders.

Qualitative evaluation of the EPOCH program model of consumer collaboration was very positive. Although a partnership model was used that did not involve consumer participation in management processes, consumers and carers reported high levels of satisfaction with it. There is a danger of tokenism or domination of consumers in management settings [58], particularly with younger clients. The partnership model used was based on documented consumer feedback [59–61] that responsive and respectful service providers who want to enter a genuinely collaborative relationship with consumers are more important than program ownership. The authors concluded that consumer participation is essential to successful early psychosis intervention, but they agree with others that careful analysis of processes and desired outcomes is important [62,63].

Turning to the major findings, the evaluation showed that the total HoNOS scores for the symptoms and impairment of EPOCH clients improved by 70% within 6 months of active treatment. This result indicates that the HoNOS is sufficiently sensitive to detect clinical change in clients with early psychosis. However, baseline scores for EPOCH clients were relatively low. Considering the obvious seriousness of their condition at baseline, this suggests that other rating scales with more psychotic symptom items, such as the Brief Psychiatric Rating Scale [64], may be more appropriate in this client group. The total LSP scores of EPOCH clients improved by 17% after 3 to 6 months of treatment, indicating that this scale is able to detect significant functional change in this group of clients. Once again, the very low levels of dysfunction detected at baseline, when most EPOCH clients were experiencing psychotic symptoms and relatively severe disability, suggests that the LSP may not be suitable in this service setting.

Self-report DASS Anxiety and Stress subscale scores at baseline improved significantly within 3 to 6 months of treatment, whereas the DASS Depression subscale score did not. These results suggest that the DASS is a useful scale for clients with early psychosis, especially in the light of its ability to discriminate between depression and anxiety, and its brevity. However, we found that clients needed considerable clinician assistance at baseline to complete this self-report questionnaire, and therefore we do not recommend it for routine use for clients with early psychosis. Informal use of the DASS with carers was much more practicable, and perhaps this scale could be used routinely with this group. Significantly, the unimproved DASS depression ratings were concordant with clinical impressions of persistence of depression in the EPOCH clients, and are a reminder of the ongoing need to monitor for depression and suicide risk well after psychotic symptoms have improved.

Within-program evaluation procedures require comment, in the light of the failure to collect almost 30% of the outcome data on EPOCH clients. This was of particular concern because the data collection period was relatively brief (about 12 months), evaluation was a key program objective, and research assistance was provided. From observation, it was evident that most EPOCH staff perceived evaluation data collection as a "research" activity and gave it lower priority than "clinical" activity. Also, negative attitudes were expressed about the content of virtually all the scales proposed, and consensus about the instruments to be used took some months to achieve. Baseline data collection was seen as especially difficult because it was time-consuming with acutely psychotic clients, and the staff perceived form-filling as a hindrance to the process of initial engagement with clients and carers. If these barriers are evident in projects with specific evaluation agendas, they indicate the requirement for even more specific strategies to embed evaluation procedures into such projects and routine service delivery in a clinically meaningful way.

The EPOCH Program was faced with the common dilemma in service effectiveness research when a randomized, controlled trial is not possible, that of attempting to compare its program processes and client outcomes with those of a suitable comparison service. Whatever way this is done, whether by comparison with a historic cohort exposed to a different type or level of service or by comparison with a parallel, apparently different type of service, there are well-documented methodological limitations, particularly related to program fidelity and across-program diffusion [65,66] and controlling for nonprogram treatment effects and sample differences across cohorts [6]. In addition, EPOCH found that there were other types of problems in attempting to implement such a comparison that ultimately contributed to the failure to collect outcome data in the comparison service. These included staff shortages, (understandable) staff lack of interest, and difficulties with record keeping. Some degree of negative feeling across the staff of comparison programs would seem inevitable, because it is inherent to the process that one program is perceived as an inferior control and the other program is perceived as having additional expertise or resources. Discussions about the null hypothesis have no weight in an overworked and under-resourced comparison service.

Even where the EPOCH Program was successful in its across-service evaluation, the results are difficult to interpret. As compared with a service implementing protocol-guided EPI without additional resources or a specialist program, the EPOCH Program identified almost twice as many clients with early psychosis (44 versus 24) within the same specified period (16 months). In comparison with EPOCH clients, the early psychosis clients of the alternative service were significantly more likely to be male and older. The clients of the two services had had a similar number of hospital admissions before their index service registration. Premature treatment dropout affected significantly more comparison service clients than EPOCH clients (35% versus 9%). Finally, significantly more EPOCH clients (75% versus 29%) and their primary carers (87% versus 24%) were willing to cooperate with outcome evaluation, as compared with their counterparts in the comparison service. These results suggest that adding additional specialist resources to routine service delivery environments for the treatment of young people with early psychosis materially improves case detection rates, client retention rates, and client and carer engagement if cooperating with evaluation procedures is considered a proxy for engagement. However, these results could simply reflect the ineffective case management employed in the comparison sector, where caseloads were typically in excess of 35 clients. Or it could reflect the unsustainable enthusiasm for a new program. There is no evidence that the differences can be attributed to identification of EPOCH clients earlier in the course of their illness. Unfortunately, the measure of illness onset assessed retrospectively by primary carer report on a questionnaire was suspected to be invalid. However, the fact that the number of hospitalizations prior to index service registration was the same across the clients in the two comparison programs suggests that although EPOCH clients were younger, they were at similar stages in the course of their illness. Supporting this conclusion is the finding that most EPOCH clients were referred after they had been identified by other components of the ES-MHS, although a trend was emerging towards the end of the program for direct referral of clients by GPs and school counselors. In summary, the authors do not recommend evaluation procedures involving direct parallel program comparisons along the lines that the EPOCH program used, especially when staff attached to one service coordinate the evaluation of the comparison service.

The 3- to 4-year follow-up of EPOCH clients at this stage has provided interesting preliminary data on a subset of clients who have continued to be treated within the ES-MHS. The diagnostic outcomes indicate that our program did not reduce the prevalence of schizophrenia but may have reduced comorbid substance abuse. Simply using the SOFAS demonstrated a clear trend for ex-EPOCH Program clients to have better psychosocial function than an equivalent sample of individuals with psychosis from the ASLPPD (see Fig. 2). This apparently improved functional outcome did not translate into better vocational outcomes or lower rates of government or family welfare dependence for our EPOCH Program clients. A possible reason for the poor vocational outcomes may have been related to the general negative effect on client outcomes of premature withdrawal from the early intervention program [67]. This may have particularly affected the outcome of school-aged clients, who may have had to make their transition to competitive employment after program closure. The general rate of youth unemployment in Sydney was low in 2000 and therefore was probably not responsible for the outcome. Also, the poor vocational outcomes are probably not related to inadequate implementation of early psychosis procedures, because the medium-term vocational outcomes of clients of the demonstration program, EPPIC in Melbourne, are no better [68]. The authors have concluded that the most likely reasons for the poor return to competitive employment by the EPOCH clients are the same ones that may explain the very low rates of work participation in the ASLPPD sample, namely, the failure to use effective vocational rehabilitation strategies, such as those used in specialized programs for accelerated re-entry to supported employment [15–17], and social skills training [69], as well as the lack of affirmative workplace legislation for the mentally disabled in Australia.

Conclusions

So what are the general conclusions that can be drawn from the EPOCH Program experience? First, there is no doubt that early psychosis intervention can be implemented in routine mental health service environments. Second, findings were made that support the effectiveness of EPI in routine service delivery settings. The preliminary nature of these results is acknowledged (especially given that no correction was made for multiple comparisons), and they require confirmation by independent replication. Nonetheless, the findings are internally consistent and are in accord with a growing body of clinical research. Third, there are certain minimum service requirements for lasting success. Some simply relate to good management. The support of service team leaders must be secured, and the model of the existing organizational structure, models of service delivery, and clinical practice must be specified. Good linkage must be forged between a proposed EPI program and existing crisis assessment and extended-hours teams, and drug and alcohol and inpatient services. Of course, securing the long-term (at least 5 years) commitment of the service director to EPI services is essential. The first 2 years will be occupied by learning "how to do it," training staff, making service adjustments, and developing a highly structured intervention and evaluation protocol. Importantly, the design of the program must be outcome focused to facilitate specification of desired outcomes and their measurement. The following 2 years will be needed to run the protocol without varying it, so that the evaluation can occur. This will allow the results to be considered by management within the life of the program. The authors recommend that comparisons of closely related parallel programs be avoided, and instead suggest that a benchmarking process be used, as illustrated in the comparison of EPOCH client SOFAS scores with those of the ASLPPD sample.

One of the first practical steps in implementing EPI is to perform a service audit of all first registrations of clients with psychosis, their pathways to care, and the care they presently receive. This will provide a baseline to compare the effect of a proposed EPI program. Next, a flag for new EPI clients must be specified to enable an urgent notification system of all new first registrations. If it has not already been done, a senior clinician should be identified to lead and maintain the service focus on EPI, proposed changes in practice and service arrangements should be workshopped with service staff, and the model of consumer participation should be specified. Whenever possible, data items that provide clinically relevant information should be chosen, if it is expected that busy health workers will be asked to do the extra work involved in collecting evaluation data. Process indicators are valuable [57]. However, clinical pathway analyses have more utility in evaluating EPI. If rating scales are to be used, data from them should be rapidly fed back to clinicians via reports generated with score plots of normative and expected data ranges, much the same as pathology services provide to clinicians.

Implementing all of the above will not guarantee successful EPI. Even in the case of the EPOCH Program, it is unclear whether EPI was achieved, given the evidence that the program did not treat clients earlier in the course of their illness. What the authors believe is that EPOCH provided some of the elements of what today constitutes quality care for young people with psychotic illness. To achieve this, staff must be trained in specialized skills and supported to work in an effective ACT model of service provision. Generalist case management, whether it be based on a clinical or a brokerage model, does not fit into the future of the management of psychosis disorder. This is simply because there are an ever-increasing number of effective specialist approaches, many of them described in this volume, that now can be applied to schizophrenia. Specialization in general medicine was necessary to achieve the revolutionary improvements in outcome. We take for granted that specialized teams will deliver specialized treatment for virtually all serious conditions, such as burns, cardiac disorders, or children's cancer. Schizophrenia is the most costly disorder of all to achieve outcome improvement (Andrews G, personal communication, 2000). The only way to improve the standard of care and reduce this cost is by incorporating the many recent innovations in treatment. To implement EPI programs effectively, new models of case management [70], and evaluation processes, particularly clinical pathways analysis [71,72], will be required. This can only be done by specialist training and specialist service delivery.

Acknowledgments. The clients and carers of the EPOCH Program are gratefully thanked for their collaboration and insight into early psychosis intervention. The assistance of the staff of the South Eastern Sydney Area Health Service is acknowledged. Access to the data from the Australian Study of Low Prevalence (Psychotic) Disorders is gratefully acknowledged, as is the work of the Technical Advisory and Low Prevalence Disorder Study Groups in collecting these data.

References

1. Cade JFJ (1949) Lithium salts in the treatment of psychotic excitement. Med J Aust 2:349–352
2. Hoult J, Reynolds I, Charbonneau-Powis M, et al (1983) Psychiatric hospital versus community treatment: the results of a randomised trial. Aust NZ J Psychiat 17:160–167
3. Hoult J, Reynolds I, Charbonneau-Powis M, et al (1981) A controlled study of psychiatric hospital versus community treatment—the effect on relatives. Aust NZ J Psychiat 15:323–328
4. Falloon IRH, Fadden G (1995) Integrated mental health care. Cambridge University Press, Cambridge
5. Falloon IRH (1992) Early intervention for first episodes of schizophrenia: a preliminary report. Psychiatry 55:4–15
6. McGorry PD, Edwards J, Mihalopoulos C, et al (1996) EPPIC: an evolving system of early detection and optimal management. Schizophr Bull 22:305–326
7. McGorry PD, Jackson HJ (1999) The recognition and management of early psychosis. A preventive approach. Cambridge University Press, Cambridge
8. Rosen A (1994) Case management: the cornerstone of comprehensive local mental health services. In: Mental health—future directions. Proceedings from the AHA Mental Health Seminar. Australian Hospital Association, Sydney, pp 47–63

9. Australian Health Ministers (1992) National Mental Health Plan. Australian Government Publishing Service, Canberra

10. Jablensky A, McGrath J, Herrman H, et al (1999) National Survey of Mental Health and Wellbeing. People living with psychotic illness: an Australian study 1997–98. An overview. Commonwealth of Australia, Canberra

11. Australian Bureau of Statistics (1997) Mental health and wellbeing: profile of adults. Australian Government Publishing Service, Canberra

12. Fleischhacker WW (2000) Pharmacological treatment of schizophrenia. In: Maj M, Sartorius N (eds) Schizophrenia, vol 2. John Wiley & Sons, Chichester, UK, pp 75–146

13. Garety PA, Fowler D, Kuipers E (2000) Cognitive-behavioral therapy for medication-resistant symptoms. Schizophr Bull 26:73–86

14. Birchwood M, Spencer E (2000) Psychotherapies for schizophrenia. In: Maj M, Sartorius N (eds) Schizophrenia, vol 2. John Wiley & Sons, Chichester, UK, pp 147–241

15. Lehman AF (1995) Vocational rehabilitation in schizophrenia. Schizophr Bull 21:645–656

16. Drake RE, Becker DR, Biesanz JC, et al (1996) Day treatment versus supported employment for persons with severe mental illness: a replication study. Psychiat Serv 47:1125–1127

17. Barton R (1999) Psychosocial rehabilitation services in community support systems: a review of outcomes and policy recommendations. Psychiat Serv 50:525–534

18. Lehman AF (2000) Commentary: what happens to psychosocial treatment on the way to the clinic. Schizophr Bull 26:137–139

19. Andrews G, Teesson M (1994) Smart versus dumb treatment: services for mental disorders. Curr Opin Psychiat 7:181–185

20. Mueser KT, Bond GR, Drake RE, et al (1998) Models of community care for severe mental illness: a review of research on case management. Schizophr Bull 24:37–74

21. Marshall M, Gray A, Lockwood A, et al (1996) Case management for people with severe mental disorders. In: Case management for severe mental disorders. Module of the Cochrane Database of Systematic Reviews. Cochrane Collaboration, Oxford

22. Bottlender R, Strauss A, Möller H-J (2000) Impact of duration of symptoms prior to first hospitalization on acute outcome in 998 schizophrenic patients. Schizophr Res 44:145–150

23. McGorry PD, Krstev H, Harrigan S (2000) Early detection and treatment delay: implications for outcome in early psychosis. Curr Opin Psychiat 13:37–43

24. Scully PJ, Coakley G, Kinsella A, et al (1997) Psychopathology, executive (frontal) and general cognitive impairment in relation to duration of initially untreated versus subsequently treated psychosis in chronic schizophrenia. Psychol Med 27:1203–1310

25. Loebel AD, Lieberman JA, Alvir JM, et al (1992) Duration of psychosis and outcome in first-episode schizophrenia. Am J Psychiat 149:1183–1188

26. Stein LI, Test MA (1980) Alternative to mental hospital treatment: I Conceptual model, treatment program, clinical evaluation. Arch Gen Psychiat 37:392–397

27. Kulkarni J (1999) Home-based treatment of first-episode psychosis. In: McGorry PD, Jackson HJ (eds) The recognition and management of early psychosis. A preventive approach. Cambridge University Press, Cambridge, pp 206–225

28. Miller WR, Rollnick S (1991) Motivational interviewing: preparing people to change addictive behavior. Guilford Press, New York

29. Andrews G, Peters L, Teesson M (1994) The measurement of consumer outcomes in mental health: a report to the National Mental Health Information Strategy Committee. Clinical Research Unit for Anxiety Disorders, Sydney

30. Cade B, O'Hanlon WH (1993) A brief guide to brief therapy. Norton, New York

31. Rapp CA (1997) The strengths model. Case management with people suffering from severe and persistent mental illness. Oxford University Press, Oxford

32. White M, Epstein D (1990) Narrative means to therapeutic ends. Norton, New York
33. Madanes C (1981) Strategic family therapy. Jossey-Bass, San Francisco
34. Gastfriend DR, McLellan AT (1997) Treatment matching. Theoretical basis and practical implications. Med Clin North Am 81:945–966
35. Hatfield AB (1994) Family education: theory and practice. In: Hatfield AB (ed) Family interventions in mental illness. New Directions for Mental Health Service No. 62. Jossey-Bass, San Francisco
36. Solomon P (1996) Moving from psychoeducation to family education for families of adults with serious mental illness. Psychiat Serv 47:1364–1379
37. Law M, Baptiste S, Mills J (1995) Client-centred practice: what does it mean and does it make a difference? Can J Occup Ther 62:250–257
38. Chapparo C, Ranka J (1997) The Perceive; Recall; Plan; Perform (PRPP) system of task analysis. In: Chapparo C, Ranka J (eds) Occupational Performance Model (Australia) Monograph 1. Occupational Performance Network, Sydney
39. Wing J (1994) Health of the Nation Outcome Scales: HoNOS Field Trials. Royal College of Psychiatrists Research Unit, London
40. Rosen A, Parker G (1989) The Life Skills Profile: a measure assessing function and disability in schizophrenia. Schizophr Bull 15:325–337
41. Lovibond SH, Lovibond PF (1996) Manual for the Depression Anxiety Stress Scales. Psychology Foundation Monograph, Sydney
42. Szmukler GI, Burgess P, Herrman H, et al (1996) Caring for relatives with serious mental illness: the development of the Experience of Caregiving Inventory. Soc Psychiat Psychiatr Epidemiol 31:137–148
43. Beiser M, Erickson D, Fleming JA, et al (1993) Establishing the onset of psychotic illness. Am J Psychiat 150:1349–1354
44. Jablensky A (1997) Diagnostic Interview for Psychosis. University of Western Australia, Perth
45. Goldman HH, Skodol AE, Lave TR (1992) Revising Axis V for DSM-IV: a review of measures of social functioning. Am J Psychiat 149:1148–1156
46. Yung AR, McGorry PD, MacFarlane CA, et al (1996) Monitoring and care of young people at incipient risk of psychosis. Schizophr Bull 22:283–303
47. Drake RE, Mercer-McFadden C, Mueser KT, et al (1998) Review of integrated mental health and substance abuse treatment for patients with dual disorders. Schizophr Bull 24:589–608
48. Myles JS, Willner P (1999) Substance misuse and psychiatric comorbidity in children and adolescents. Curr Opin Psychiat 12:287–290
49. Van Horn DHA, Frank AF (1998) Substance-use situations and abstinence predictions in substance abusers with and without personality disorder. Am J Drug Alcohol Abuse 24:395–404
50. McPhilips MA, Kelly FJ, Barnes TRE, et al (1997) Detecting comorbid substance misuse among people with schizophrenia in the community: a study comparing the results of questionnaires with analysis of hair and urine. Schizophr Res 25:141–148
51. Claasen CA, Gilfillan S, Orsulak P, et al (1997) Substance use among patients with a psychotic disorder in a psychiatric emergency room. Psychiatr Serv 48:353–358
52. Melnick G, De Leon G, Hawke J, et al (1997) Motivation and readiness for therapeutic community treatment among adolescents and adult substance abusers. Am J Drug Alcohol Abuse 23:485–506
53. Bodes J, McCann UD (2000) Developments in the treatment of drug dependence. Curr Opin Psychiat 13:333–338
54. George TP, Krystal JH (2000) Comorbidity of psychiatric and substance abuse disorders. Curr Opinin Psychiat 13:327–331
55. Buckley PF (1998) Substance abuse in schizophrenia: a review. J Clin Psychol 59(Suppl 3):26–30

56. Lynskey M, White V, Hill D, et al (1999) Prevalence of illicit drug use among youth: results from the Australian School Students' Alcohol and Drugs Survey. Aust NZ J Public Health 23:519–524
57. Brook JS, Cohen P, Brook DW (1998) Longitudinal study of co-occurring psychiatric disorders and substance use. J Am Acad Child Adolesc Psychiat 37:322–330
58. Meagher J (1996) Partnership or pretence. Psychiatric Rehabilitation Association (PRA), Sydney
59. Epstein M, Shaw J (1997) Developing effective consumer participation in mental health services. The report of the Lemon Tree Learning Project. Victorian Mental Illness Awareness Council, Melbourne
60. Dulwich Centre Newsletter (1995) Speaking out . . . and being heard. Dulwich Centre Publications, Adelaide
61. Brown C, Kordas G, Reeves J (1993) Speaking up on mental health: creating a space for the consumer voice. Aust Disability Rev 4:47–58
62. Charles C, DeMaio S (1993) Lay participation in health care decision making: a conceptual framework. J Health Politics Policy Law 18:881–904
63. Sozomemou A, Mitchell P, Fitzgerald MH, et al (2000) Mental health consumer participation in a culturally diverse society, 2nd edn. Australian Transcultural Mental Health Network, Sydney, pp 21–58
64. Ventura J, Green MF, Shaner A, et al (1993) Training and quality assurance with the Brief Psychiatric Rating Scale: "the drift busters." Psychiatr Res 3:221–244 (plus appendices)
65. Marshall M, Bond G, Stein LI, et al (1999) PriSM Psychosis Study. Design limitations, questionable conclusions. Br J Psychiat 175:501–503
66. Sashidharan SP, Smyth M, Owen A (1999) PriSM Psychosis Study. Thro'a glass darkly: a distorted appraisal of community care. Br J Psychiat 175:504–507
67. Linzen D, Lenior M, De Haan L, et al (1998) Early intervention, untreated psychosis and the course of early schizophrenia. Br J Psychiat 172(Suppl 33):84–89
68. Henry L, McGorry P, Jackson H, et al (2000) What is the medium term course of first episode psychosis? Proceedings of the Second International Conference for Early Psychosis, p 32
69. Heinssen RK, Lieberman RP, Kopelowicz (2000) Psychosocial skills training for schizophrenia: lessons from the laboratory. Schizophr Bull 26:21–46
70. Edwards J, Cocks J, Bott J (2000) Preventive case management in first-episode psychosis. In: McGorry PD, Jackson HJ (eds) The Recognition and Management of Early Psychosis. Cambridge University Press, Cambridge, pp 308–337
71. Baker S, Mohr JW, et al (1996) Development and implementation of clinical pathways: Starter kit. London Health Sciences Centre. London: Ontario
72. Smith TE, Docherty JP (1998) Standards of care and clinical algorithms for treating schizophrenia. The Psychiatric Clinics of North America 21(1)

Part 9
Cognitive Remediation

Problem-Solving Skills and Sending Skills in Schizophrenia

Emi Ikebuchi

Summary. Schizophrenia is characterized by pervasive impairments of social skills. Thus, social skills training is thought to be an effective treatment to promote psychiatric rehabilitation. The present report reviewed our previous studies about components of social skills, factors influencing social skills, and predicting power of social skills over social functioning. A Japanese version of structured role-play test was devised, and by using the test we found three components of social skills in factor analysis: sending skills and social validity, problem-solving skills and goal attainment, and self-efficacy. Sending skills were at least partially based on early information-processing deficiency. Problem-solving skills were not directly related to elementary cognitive function ("molecular" stage of information processing), but might be based on more complex neuropsychological function and reflected by other factors, such as social learning. An association between some aspects of insight (compliance with treatment and recognition of mental illness) and sending skills was found, which might be mediated by neurocognitive deficits. Both sending skills and problem-solving skills contributed to global social functioning for almost five years. Improvement of problem-solving skills was achieved by 20 h of social skills training. Sending skills were strongly associated with negative symptoms in correlational analysis, and we thought that more time would be needed to improve them.

Key words. Schizophrenia, Cognitive-behavioral therapy, Social skills training, Problem-solving skills, Sending skills

Introduction

Schizophrenia is characterized by pervasive impairments across different areas of psychosocial functioning, including social relationships. Social skills are defined as the "ability to express both positive and negative feelings in the interpersonal context without suffering consequent loss of reinforcement. Such are demonstrated in a large variety of interpersonal context and the coordinated delivery of appropriate verbal

---

Department of Psychiatry, Teikyo University School of Medicine, 2-11-1 Kaga, Itabashi-ku, Tokyo 173-8606, Japan

and nonverbal responses. In addition, the socially skilled individual is attuned to the realities of the situation and is aware when he is likely to be reinforced for his efforts" [1]. Social disabilities are potent predictors of exacerbation of symptoms and rehospitalization [2], because social disabilities are a primary source of stress and prevent patients from developing supportive relationships.

Social skills are thought to include several components, as the definition of social skills above suggests. What are the components of social skills and how the components relate to each other are important issues in the development of technologies for improving social skills. It is also important to use precise measuring methods to evaluate each component of social skills. The role-play test is one of the most widely used behavioral measures of social skills [3,4]. In a series of studies, the feasibility, reliability, and validity of the role play-test were verified [5–8].

In addition, many factors may influence usage and learning of social skills. However, little is definitively known regarding which factors compromise social skills in schizophrenia. Persons with schizophrenia show deficits across a broad range of cognitive domains, and their deficits in social skills are thought to be caused by cognitive dysfunction [9]. Psychiatric symptoms are also known to be limiting factors for the acquisition of social skills. Mueser et al. [10,11] reported that patients with enduring thought disorder displayed limited maintenance of acquired social skills. The factors influencing social skills as well as cognitive deficits and psychiatric symptoms should be researched further.

The present report deals with our previous research on components of social skills, factors influencing social skills, and the power of social skills to predict social functioning.

What Are the Components of Social Skills?

The Japanese version of the structured role-play test was devised and its reliability and validity were verified [12,13]. By using the role-play test, we found three components of social skills, and the relationships among the components were analyzed [14].

During the role-play test, the subjects initially viewed a videotaped scene of social interaction. The subjects were then asked what they thought about the problems presented in the scene and the social goal of the scene, to assess their information-receiving and -processing skills. After questioning, the subjects were required to perform a role play with one of the testers. One man and one woman acted as testers to assess the subject's interaction with persons of both sexes. The role plays were recorded on videotape for subsequent evaluation of sending skills by raters who did not have any information on the individual subjects. After the role play, a tester questioned each subject to appraise his or her information-processing skills and self-efficacy. The role-play test consisted of 12 scenes. Four scenes were used to assess the ability to express negative feelings, three were for positive feelings, three were for initiating conversation, and two were for making a compromise. The test was used to evaluate 15 parameters (Table 1). Three parameters were assessed through questioning before and after the role play: social perception, making decisions, and self-efficacy. Ten parameters were assessed via videotaped role plays.

TABLE 1. Inter-rater reliability of the role-play test (ANOVA-ICC)

Items assessed using videotaped role plays

1. Eye contact	0.94
2. Facial expression	0.92
3. Emotional expression	0.79
4. Voice volume	0.85
5. Fluency	0.46
6. Voice tone	0.92
7. Duration	0.76
8. Meshing	0.92
9. Clarity of message	0.93
10. Validity	0.67
11. Goal attainment	0.83
12. Global assessment	0.87

Items assessed through questioning

13. Social perception	0.73
14. Making decisions	0.73

Self-assessment report
15. Self-efficacy

TABLE 2. Correlation between the total score on the role-play test and other psychiatric rating scales (Pearson's correlation coefficient)

Scale	Correlation
Scale for the Assessment of Negative Symptoms	−0.83*
Brief Psychiatric Rating Scale (NIMH version)	−0.49*
Global Assessment of Functioning	0.51*
Global assessment of social skills assessed in the group interaction	0.69*
Interaction number of sociogram in the group at the day-treatment center	0.42*
Social rank in the group at the day-treatment center	0.64*

* $P = 0.01$

Inter-rater reliability was calculated by analysis of variance intraclass correlation coefficients (ANOVA-ICC) [12,13,15]. Two raters independently assessed 12 subjects. The ANOVA-ICC of 14 parameters ranged from 0.94 (eye contact) to 0.67 (social validity); this range was considered sufficient to insure inter-rater reliability (Table 1). However, the ANOVA-ICC of item 5 (fluency) was 0.46, therefore this item was not used any more. Test-retest reliability was calculated by using Pearson's correlation coefficient between total scores of the role-play test with nine-week intervals. The Pearson's coefficient was 0.51, a statistically significant level ($P < 0.01$).

Correlation analysis was performed to verify the validity of the role-play test [12,13]. The subjects were 30 outpatients diagnosed with schizophrenia (DSM-III-R [13a]). Seventeen were men. Their mean age was 26 years (range, 18–37). The Pearson's correlation coefficients between the total score of the role-play test and other psychiatric rating scales were shown in Table 2. The criterion-related

TABLE 3. Factor analysis on 13 items of the role-play test (principal factor method, varimax rotation)

Variables	Factors (eigenvalue)		
	1 (7.27)	2 (2.19)	3 (1.17)
1. Eye contact	0.88	0.15	0.13
2. Facial expression	0.89	0.13	0.05
3. Emotional expression	0.92	0.14	0.05
4. Voice volume	0.56	0.02	0.65
5. Voice tone	0.84	0.21	0.31
6. Duration	0.88	−0.02	0.21
7. Meshing	0.86	−0.02	−0.17
8. Clarity of message	0.91	0.13	0.07
9. Validity	0.82	0.50	0.00
10. Goal attainment	0.38	0.77	0.05
11. Social perception	0.23	0.87	0.09
12. Making decisions	−0.17	0.88	0.15
13. Self-efficacy	−0.05	0.20	0.88
Percent of variables explained (Total 82%)	56%	17%	9%

validity was verified by significant correlations between the role-play test and other scales.

To analyze components of social skills, 43 persons diagnosed with schizophrenia (DSM-III) were assessed through the role-play test [14]. In factor analysis, three factors with eigenvalues of more than 1 were found (Table 3). Factor 1 consisted of sending skills and social validity. Factor 2 consisted of problem-solving skills and goal attainment. Factor 3 was self-efficacy. Social skills consist mainly of two parts: sending skills related to social validity of behavior, and problem-solving skills related to goal attainment of social interaction.

Neurocognitive Function and Social Skills

The relationships between components of social skills and neurocognitive function were analyzed by using auditory event-related potential for Study 1 [16], and the Continuous Performance Test (CPT) and the Span of Apprehension Test for Study 2 [17]. Sending skills were found to have a significant relationship with the early stage of information processing.

Study 1

Eleven men and nine women who were patients in the Teikyo University Hospital participated in the study. All subjects met DSM-IIIR criteria for schizophrenia. None of the patients exhibited acute psychotic symptoms. All were receiving neuroleptic medications averaging 326 mg chlorpromazine equivalents per day.

We calculated three scores by using several parameters of the role-play test. These scores are sending skills score (summation of each score of facial expression, emotional expression, and voice tone), problem-solving skills score (summation of each score of goal attainment and social perception), and total score of social skills. The Brief Psychiatric Rating Scale (BPRS, Beck version) was used to assess psychiatric symptoms. Each subject's level of cognitive functioning was rated with WAIS-R and an ERP task, a standard auditory oddball design was adopted, in which subjects listened to a series of binaural 1 KHz (frequent) and 2 KHz (target) tones. The tones were of 100 msec duration with rise and fall time of 10 ms duration, presented every 1.7 s, with target tones occurring randomly with a 0.2 probability. Target tones were presented 40 times, and nontarget tones were done 160 times. Electroencephalograms were recorded from the Fz, Cz, Pz, T3, and T4 regions. N1 was identified as the largest negative peak at Fz betwen 50 and 150 msec, N2 as the largest negative peak at Cz between 150 and 280 msec, and P3 as the largest positive peak at Pz between 250 and 500 msec for target tones. The peak latency and amplitude of N1, N2, and P3 were measured at Fz, Cz, and Pz, respectively. The subject's level of social functioning was rated by the Global Assessment of Functioning (GAF) Scale after an interview.

PIQ showed a significant correlation with problem-solving skills score (0.46, Spearman's rank order correlation coefficient) and total skills score (0.49). N1 amplitude showed a significant correlation with sending skills score (0.51) and total score (0.51). Multiple regression analysis was performed (Table 4). Independent variables were clinical indices including the dosage of medication, psychiatric symptoms, the levels of cognitive and social functioning. A stepwise procedure was followed, and only independent variables that met the 0.15 significance level were utilized for multiple regression analysis. The sending skills score was significantly associated with N1A, which

TABLE 4. Multiple regression analysis (Study 1)

Sending-skills score; independent variables—N1A, age of onset
    Variables that met the 0.15 significance level for entry into the model were N1A and age of onset
    Significance level of the model is 0.00 (D.f. 2,14; $F = 9.97$)
    Multiple correlation coefficient: 0.76
    Partial regression coefficients: age of onset—0.57, N1A—0.51

Problem-solving skills score; independent variables—BPRS score, PIQ, age
    Variables that met the 0.15 significance level for entry into the model were BPRS score, PIQ, and age
    Significance level of the model is 0.00 (D.f. 3,16; $F = 7.50$)
    Multiple correlation coefficient: 0.76
    Partial correlation coefficients: BPRS score—0.54, PIQ—0.45, age—0.31

Total score; independent variables—age of onset, N1A, N1L, and HR
    Variables that met the 0.15 significance level for entry into the model were N1A, age of onset, N1L, and HR
    Significance level of the model is 0.00 (D.f. 4,12; $F = 9.49$)
    Multiple correlation coefficient: 0.87
    Partial correlation coefficients: age of onset—0.59, N1A—0.53, N1L—0.25, HR—0.25

Stepwise procedure: dependent variables were sending-skills score, problem-solving skills score, and total score. Independent variables were selected if they met the 0.15 significance level in the multiple regression model
BPRS, the Brief Psychiatric Rating Scale

accounted for 26% of the variance, and age of onset accounted for 29%. The problem-solving skils score was significantly associated with the BPRS score, which accounted for 22% of the variance; PIQ accounted for 21% and age accounted for 10%. Total score was significantly associated with age of onset, which accounted for 31% of the variance, N1A accounted for 32%, N1 latency accounted for 12%, and hit rate accounted for 0.1%.

Study 2

The subjects were 22 men and 6 women who met the DSM-IV criteria for schizophrenia. All subjects were attending a rehabilitation program at the day treatment centers of the two hospitals. All were receiving neuroleptic medication, averaging 396 mg chlorpromazine equivalents per day. The DS-CPT (UCLA CPT computer program version 7.01, Nuechterlein and Asarnow, unpublished manual) was presented on an IBM-PC with a 14-inch NEC KM152 color monitor. The subjects were instructed to press a response button whenever they saw the target stimulus "0." The target was presented for 33 msec at 1-sec intervals for all trials. The numbers were degraded to a standardized degree by reversing the black/white setting of 40% of randomly selected pixels. The subjects were given 160 practice trials followed by 480 experimental trials, presented in 6 blocks of 80. The target "0" appeared in a quasi-random sequence, in 20 out of every 80 trials. Five indices—reaction time (RT), hit rate (HR), false alarm rate (the rate of commission errors of all trials, FAR), A', and β'—were calculated via 480 trials of CPT. A' is a nonparametric signal detection index of sensitivity (the ability to discriminate targets from nontargets). The SPAN (UCLA SPAN computer program, version 4.0, Nuechterlein and Asarnow, unpublished manual) is a measure of the capacity of visual information processing. The devices used were the same as those for CPT. The subjects were instructed to press a certain response button whenever they saw the target stimulus "T" and another button when they saw "F." The duration of stimulus presentation was 83 ms for all trials. Three alphabets (T or F plus two nontargets) were presented at the same time in SPAN3, and 12 alphabets (T or F plus 11 nontargets), arranged within a 4×4 matrix, were presented in SPAN12. The subjects were given 20 practice trials followed by 128 experimental trials. The target stimulus "T" or "F" appeared in a quasi-random sequence in 64 out of 128 trials.

The sending skills score was significantly correlated with CPT-FAR ($-0.51, P = 0.01$) and CPT-β' (0.43, $P = 0.03$). Social perception was a significantly correlated with SPAN3-RT ($-0.51, P = 0.01$) , and the social validity of interactions with CPT-FAR ($-0.44, P = 0.02$) and CPT-β' (0.59, $P = 0.01$). In multiple regression analysis (Table 5), the dependent variables included five social skill scores and the GAF score. Independent variables included clinical indices, dosage of medication, psychiatric symptoms, and the level of cognitive functioning. The sending-skills score was significantly associated with the total number of months of hospitalization and CPT-FAR. Social validity of interactions was significantly associated with CPT-β' and the total number of months of hospitalization.

Our tentative conclusion from Study 1 and Study 2 is that sending skills are at least partially based on deficiencies in early information processing, such as automatic discriminating processes or selective attention, reflected in N1A. Information-receiving

TABLE 5. Multiple regression analysis predicting social skills and social functioning from cognitive scores and other variables (Study 2)

Independent variable	Dependent variable that met the 0.15 significance level for entry into the model	Partial R^2	F	R^2	F
Sending skills	Total months of hospitalization	0.21	5.36 (P = 0.03)		
	CPT-FAR	0.21	6.77 (P = 0.02)	0.42	0.80 (P = 0.01)
Social perception[a]	—	—	—	—	—
Decision making[a]	—	—	—	—	—
Goal attainment	Decreased level of CPT-β′ during 6 block	0.11	3.05 (P = 0.09)		
	Duration of illness	0.12	3.46 (P = 0.07)	0.23	3.42 (P = 0.05)
Social validity of interaction	CPT-β′	0.33	9.96 (P = 0.01)		
	Total months of hospitalization	0.23	10.14 (P = 0.01)	0.56	12.33 (P = 0.01)

CPT, the Continuous Performance Test; FAR, False Alarm Rate
[a] No variable met the 0.15 significance level for entry into the model

and -processing skills are not directly related to elementary cognitive function ("molecular" stage of information processing), as assessed by analyzing, for example, the ERP P300 component, but are based on more complex neuropsychological functions and are reflected by other factors such as social learning.

The Contribution of Social Skills to Insight

The relationship between insight and components of social skills was analyzed in Study 4 [18]. Schizophrenia has been noted to exist between a patient's perception of the condition and the objective deficiency, which is referred to as lack of insight. Impaired insight was the most frequently encountered symptom, occurring in 97% of the sample population [19]. McEvoy et al. [20,21] found that insight was independent of global psychopathology and relatively unchanged despite clinical improvement. Lack of insight has often been emphasized in determining the prognosis [22].

Thirty-one subjects diagnosed with schizophrenia (ICD-10) were assessed. All were inpatients. Their mean age was 46.8 ± 10.9 (SD) years, and the ages ranged from 27 to 67 years. The mean number of previous hospital admissions was 4.3 ± 3.3 (range, 1–14). The mean duration of the current admission was 47.3 ± 26.1 months (range, 1–164). The mean duration of full-time education was 12.1 ± 2.8 years (range, 6–16).

Three measures were used to assess different aspects of insight. The first was an item from the Positive and Negative Syndrome Scale (PANSS) (G12), in which a psychiatrist objectively evaluated the lack of judgment and insight through a semi-structured interview. This evaluation depended on the psychiatrist's assessment. The psychiatrist estimated the extent to which each subject could recognize his or her previous and present psychiatric illness and symptoms and the need for psychiatric treatment, according to a 7-point scale ranging from 1 (good insight) to 7 (complete denial of previous or present illness). Another measure was the Schedule for Assessment of Insight (SAI) [23], which consists of three subscales: treatment compliance on a scale of 0 to 4, recognition of mental illness on a scale of 0 to 6, and relabeling of psychotic phenomena on a scale of 0 to 4. A high score on each subscale meant good insight. The third measure was the Rating of Medication Influences (ROMI) Scale [24], which consists of 26 items divided into two subscales: subjective reasons for taking medication and disadvantages of taking medication. The evaluation of ROMI depended on the subjective recognition of the reasons for taking or not taking medication during a structured interview.

According to the factor analysis, the scores for insight factors 1, 2, and 3 were calculated, which consisted of a linear combination of three measures of insight (G12 item from PANSS, 3 subscales of SAI, and 2 subscales of ROMI), which were converted to standardized scores, and the coefficient of each measure was determined by the factor-loading score. The factor 1 score was thought to present compliance with treatment and recognition of mental illness. The factor 2 score was the attitude towards medication. The factor 3 score was relabelling of psychotic symptoms. In the multiple regression analysis, the dependent variables consisted of the three insight factors. The independent variables included demographic and clinical indices: age, onset of illness, number of previous admissions, duration of illness, total years of education, and scores from four clinical measures (PANSS, REHAB, the role-play test, and the 21-item questionnaire). Insight factor 1 was significantly associated with the PANSS positive syndrome score (partial $R^2 = 0.20$), REHAB social behavior score (0.11), sending-skills score (0.09), and age (0.07); the coefficient of determination was 0.47. This result shows the association between some extent of insight (compliance with treatment and recognition of mental illness) and sending skills, which might be mediated by neuro-cognitive deficits. Macpherson et al. [25] speculated that cognitive impairment underlies the patients' inability to learn about his or her illness. Until now, however, no research has clearly shown evidence that neurocognitive deficit has the main role in the development of lack of insight. The coefficients of determination of insight factors 1 and 3 in multiple regression analysis were not very high, so there remains some room to explain lack of insight by other models.

The Relationship with Global Social Functioning

Two cohort studies were analyzed to assess the relationship between components of social skills and global social functioning.

The Global Assessment of Functioning (GAF) score was significantly correlated with problem-solving skills (the Spearman rank correlation coefficient was 0.52) in Study 1. Forty-one outpatients diagnosed with schizophrenia (DSM-IIIR) were evaluated by the structured role-play test and the GAF at the same time as the role-play test (GAF0), one year later (GAF1), and five years later (GAF5) (unpublished data).

The total social skills score was significantly correlated with GAF0 (Spearman rank correlation coefficient, 0.32, $P = 0.04$), GAF1 (0.43, $P = 0.01$), and GAF5 (0.53, $P = 0.05$). The sending-skills score was significantly correlated only with GAF1 (0.32, $P = 0.05$). The problem-solving skills score was significantly correlated with GAF5 (0.53, $P = 0.04$). Thus both the sending skills- and the problem-solving-skills scores contributed to global social functioning for almost five years.

The Effects of Social-Skills Training on Components of Social Skills

The purpose of Study 5 [26] was to verify the directive effects of social skills training by using the role-play test with testers and raters who were independent of the therapeutic team for social skills training. We tested eight subjects with schizophrenia (DSM-III-R) who were receiving day treatment and who participated in 20 hours of social skills training. Seven controls were outpatients with schizophrenia (DSM-III-R). Both groups were tested two times with the same test batteries at six-month intervals. The results were as follows: there was significant improvement in 3 items of the role-play test, which were items for assessing problem-solving skills. Improvement in problem-solving skills was presumed to be achieved by social-skills training. Sending skills were strongly influenced by negative symptoms in correlational analysis, and we thought that more than 20 hours would be needed to improve sending skills.

Conclusions

We found three components of social skills in factor analysis: sending skills and social validity, problem-solving skills and goal attainment, and self-efficacy. The sending skills were at least partially based on early information-processing deficiency. Sending skills were associated with compliance with treatment and recognition of mental illness, an association that might be mediated by neurocognitive deficits. The intervention study found that sending skills were strongly influenced by negative symptoms, and more time would be needed to improve sending skills than problem-solving skills.

As compared with sending skills, problem-solving skills are not directly related to elementary cognitive function, but are based on more complex neuropsychological functions and are reflected by other factors such as social learning. Indeed, improvement in problem-solving skills was achieved by social skills training lasting for 20 hours. Thus, the short-term goal of social skills training must be to improve problem-solving skills in order to cope with individual problems of skills of independent living. The longer-term goal should include improving both sending skills and cognitive deficits, which might be limiting factors of social learning. Problem-solving skills are complicated cognitive processes that deeply depend on social situation. Therefore, further research is needed to define and assess problem-solving skills not only in experimental laboratories but also in clinical settings.

References

1. Bellack AS, Hersen M (eds) (1979) Research and practice in social skills training. Plenum, New York
2. McGlashan TH (1984) Long-term outcome of schizophrenia and affective disorder: 2. The Chestnut Lodge follow-up study. Arch Gen Psychiatry 41:586–601
3. Benton MK, Schroeder HE (1990) Social skills training with schizophrenics: a meta-analytic evaluation. J Consult Clin Psychol 58:741–747
4. Corrigan PW (1991) Social skills training in adult psychiatric populations: a meta-analysis. J Behav Ther Exp Psychiatry 22:203–210
5. Bellack AS (1983) Recurrent problems in the behavioral assessment of social skills. Behav Res Ther 21:29–41
6. Bellack AS, Morrison JT, Wixted JT, et al (1990) An analysis of social competence in schizophrenia. Br J Psychiatry 156:809–818
7. Bellack AS, Morrison RL, Mueser KT, et al (1990) Role play for assessing the social competence of psychiatric patients. Psychological Assessment: A Journal of Consulting and Clinical Psychology 2:248–255
8. Mueser KT, Bellack AS, Douglas MS, et al (1991) Prevalence and stability of social skill deficits in schizophrenia. Schizophr Res 5:167–176
9. Penn DL, Mueser KM, Spaulding W, et al (1995) Information processing and social competence in chronic schizophrenia. Schizophr Bull 21:269–281
10. Mueser KT, Bellack AS, Douglas MS, et al (1991) Prediction of social skill acquisition in schizophrenic and major affective disorder patients from memory and symptomatology. Psychiatry Res 37:281–196
11. Mueser KT, Kosmidis MH, Sayers MD (1992) Symptomatology and the prediction of social skills acquisition in schizophrenia. Schizophr Res 8:59–68
12. Ikebuchi E, Miyauchi M, Anzai N, et al (1994) Assessment of social disability of patients suffering from chronic mental illness with the role play test. Psychiat Neurol Japon 96:157–173
13. Ikebuchi E, Anzai N (1995) Effect of the medication management module evaluated using the role play test. Psychiatry Clin Neurosci 49:151–156
13a. Diagnostic and statistical manual of mental disorders, 3rd edn-rev (1987) American Psychiatric Association, Washington, DC
14. Ikebuchi E, Satoh K, Katsuyo H (1999) Analysis on the structure of social skills of persons with schizophrenia (in Japanese) Psychiatr Disorder Rehabil 3:150–156
15. Bartko JJ, Carpenter WT (1976) On the methods and theory of reliability. J Nerv Ment Dis 163:307–317
16. Ikebuchi E, Nakagome K, Tsugawa R, et al (1996) What influences social skills in patients with schizophrenia? Preliminary study using the role play test, WAIS-R and event-related potential. Schizoph Res 22:143–150
17. Ikebuchi E, Nakagome K, Takahashi N, et al (1999) How do early stages of information processing influence social skills in patients with schizophrenia? Schizophr Res 35:252–262
18. Ikebuchi E, Anzai N, Yoneda S, et al (in press) What predict insight in schizophrenia. Jpn Bull Soc Psychiatry
19. World Health Organization (1973) Report of the International Pilot Study of Schizophrenia. Vol 1. WHO, Geneva
20. McEvoy JP, Freter S, Everett G, et al (1989) Insight and the clinical outcome of schizophrenic patients. J Nerv Ment Dis 177:48–51
21. Heinrichs DW, Cohen BP, Carpenter WT (1985) Early insight and the management of schizophrenic decompensation. J Nerv Ment Dis 173:133–138
22. Cuesta MJ, Peralta V (1994) Lack of insight in schizophrenia Schizophr Bull 20:359–361

23. David AS, Buchanan A, Reed A, et al (1992) The assessment of insight in psychosis. Br J Psychiatry 161:599–602
24. Weiden P, Rapkin B, Mott T, et al (1994) Rating of Medication Influences (ROMI) Scale in schizophrenia. Schizophr Bull 20:297–307
25. Macpherson R, Jerrom B, Hughes A (1996) Relationship between insight, educational background and cognition in schizophrenia. Br J Psychiatry 168:718–722
26. Ikebuchi E, Kazuyuki N, Tsugawa R, et al (1996) Effects of social skills training on disabilities of schizophrenia. Jpn J Psychiatr Treatment 11:627–638

Cognitive Impairment, Symptoms, Social Functioning, and Vocational Rehabilitation in Schizophrenia

KIM T. MUESER

Summary. This study evaluated whether cognitive impairment, negative symptoms, positive symptoms (all measured with the Positive and Negative Syndrome Scale), and social adjustment (measured with the Social Adjustment Scale) predicted work outcomes over two years in 134 unemployed patients with schizophrenia or schizoaffective disorder who were randomly assigned to participate in one of three vocational rehabilitation programs: Individual Placement and Support (IPS, a supported employment model), psychiatric rehabilitation center (PSR), and standard services (Standard). Cognitive impairment predicted worse outcomes (hours worked and wags) in the PSR group, and negative symptoms predicted work outcomes for both the PSR and the IPS programs. There were no predictors of work outcome in the Standard group. The results suggest that cognitive impairments may interfere with response to social learning-based interventions, but not responses to supported employment.

Key words. Schizophrenia, Cognitive impairment, Vocational rehabilitation, Supported employment, Symtomatology

Cognitive impairment is widely accepted as an important characteristic of schizophrenia that is independent or semi-independent of negative and positive symptoms [1,2]. Although deficits in cognitive functioning are common in schizophrenia, their functional significance remains a topic of hot debate. Ample evidence indicates that cognitive impairment is related to poor social and vocational functioning [3–8]. However, cognitive impairment is also moderately correlated with the severity of negative symptoms [9–11], and negative symptoms are related to social and vocational functioning [1,12]. Thus, the unique contribution of cognitive impairment to social and vocational functioning remains unclear and may depend upon the specific type of impairment (e.g., attention vs. executive functions) and the nature of the role (e.g., interpersonal relationships vs. work task performance) [5,13].

A related question that has been the focus of much recent research concerns the relationship between cognitive impairment and response to psychiatric rehabilitation.

Departments of Psychiatry and Community and Family Medicine, Dartmouth Medical School, New Hampshire-Dartmouth Psychiatric Research Center, Main Building, 105 Pleasant St., Concord, NH 03301, USA

Most work in this area has examined cognitive functioning and social skills training, with the evidence indicating that more severe cognitive impairments are related to a lower rate of skill acquisition (Green et al., 2000). There has been less work examining other approaches to psychiatric rehabilitation, including vocational rehabilitation.

Mueser et al. [14] failed to find an association between disorganization on the Brief Psychiatric Rating Scale [15,16] and competitive employment outcomes over 18 months in a mixed sample (40% schizophrenia-spectrum) of patients participating in a study of supported employment compared with group skills training. In contrast, two other studies using different cognitive measures and studying different approaches to vocational rehabilitation reported significant associations. Hoffman and Kupper [17] reported that conceptual disorganization on the Positive and Negative Syndrome Scale (PANSS) [18] predicted work outcome in patients with schizophrenia over 18 months in a traditional vocational rehabilitation program including skills training, sheltered work, job coaches, and competitive work. Lysaker et al. [19,20], in a study of a work program for schizophrenia including paid work and group support, reported that performance on the Wisconsin Card Sorting Test (WCST) at baseline predicted improvements in both social skills and work performance at 12 weeks.

Inconsistencies in the relationships between cognitive functioning and response to vocational rehabilitation may be related to the different programs studied. Some programs used skills training (the group skills training program in Mueser et al. [14] and Hoffman and Kupper's [17] program), whereas others did not (the supported employment program in Mueser et al. [14] and Lysaker's program). No study evaluated whether cognitive impairment predicted work in patients participating only in a supported employment program. The relationship between cognitive impairment and benefit from supported employment is particularly important, because the preponderance of evidence indicates that this approach is more successful at improving work outcomes than skills training and other approaches to vocational rehabilitation [21,22].

This study examined the relationships between cognitive impairment, other symptoms, and social adjustment as predictors of response to vocational rehabilitation in a large cohort of patients with schizophrenia who were randomly assigned to one of three programs: Individual Placement and Support (a supported employment model), a psychiatric rehabilitation center, or standard services.

Methods

The study was conducted at the Capitol Region Mental Health Center (CRMHC) in Hartford, Connecticut. All patients were receiving public mental health services and were receiving standard care for severe mental illness, including medication, case management, housing assistance, and access to psychiatric rehabilitation programs.

Patients

The study participants were 134 patients with schizophrenia or schizoaffective disorder. These patients are a subset of a total of 204 patients with severe mental illness who were participants in the study. Patients were excluded from this report if they

TABLE 1. Demographic and clinical characteristics

Characteristic	Value
Age (mean)	36.72
Sex—no. (%)	
Male	96 (72)
Female	38 (28)
Ethnicity—no. (%)	
American Indian/Alaskan	1 (1)
African American	67 (50)
Hispanic	36 (27)
White	23 (17)
Other	7 (5)
Marital status—no. (%)	
Never married	104 (78)
Married	30 (22)
Education—no. (%)	
Did not complete high school	72 (54)
Completed high school	62 (46)
Diagnosis—no. (%)	
Schizophrenia	95 (71)
Schizoaffective disorder	39 (29)

did not have a diagnosis of schizophrenia or schizoaffective disorder, or if they had not completed the two years of the study by February 2000. Criteria for participation included not currently employed in competitive work (defined by the US Department of Labor), interest in competitive employment, and attendance at two research introduction groups designed to inform patients about the study. The demographic characteristics of the sample are summarized in Table 1.

Vocational Programs

Following completion of the baseline assessment, patients were randomly assigned to one of three vocational programs for two years: Individual Placement and Support (IPS) ($n = 44$), a psychiatric rehabilitation center (PSR) ($n = 44$), or standard services ($n = 46$).

Individual Placement and Support

IPS [23] is a model of supported employment that de-emphasizes extensive prevocational assessment and focuses on helping patients find competitive jobs based on their own preferences in integrated work settings. Once a patient has found a job, the employment specialist provides support to help him or her succeed on the job, either off-site or on-site, and is available to the employer (if the patient has consented) to address work-related issues. In the IPS model, each patient is assigned one employment specialist. The employment specialist functions as a member of the patient's treatment team in order to integrate psychiatric and vocational services. The IPS program was created at CRMHC for this study.

Psychiatric Rehabilitation Center

The PSR model was based on a transitional work model conducted at a psychiatric rehabilitation program separate from the mental health center [24]. Patients first became "members" of the PSR and participated in work training crews at the program (e.g., janitorial, computer training). Then, patients worked in transitional jobs in the community to gain work experience. Last, patients secured their own jobs with the help and support of PSR staff.

Standard Services

These patients were provided access to any other of the vocational rehabilitation programs available to patients receiving services at CRMHC. Almost all patients in Standard received services from one of two different programs, both which were at a different location than CRMHC. The first program provided supported employment services in a manner similar to IPS, except that employment specialists did not function as members of patients' treatment teams and had infrequent contact with the team. The second program obtained contracts to provide services for companies (e.g., janitorial) and then employed patients to fulfill these contracts, while providing ongoing job training and supervision.

Measures

At baseline, prior work history was determined, including the number of paid jobs the patient worked and the number of months worked over the past two years. Information on work, including jobs, wages, and hours worked, was obtained weekly for all patients over the two years through brief interviews with patients and vocational staff. Psychiatric symptoms were assessed with the Positive and Negative Syndrome Scale (PANSS) [18] at baseline and every six months for two years. For this report, three scales were formed: positive symptoms, negative symptoms, and cognitive impairment. Social functioning was assessed with the Social-Leisure subscale of the Social Adjustment Scale-II [25].

Results

The analyses are divided into two parts. First, the three vocational rehabilitation programs were compared on competitive work outcome, and demographic characteristics were examined to determine whether they predicted work. Second, analyses were conducted to determine whether symptoms or social functioning were correlated with prior work history and, within each of the three vocational programs, predicted work outcomes.

Demographic Predictors of Work and Vocational Program Outcomes

Throughout the two-year study, 54% of the patients worked competitively at some point. Chi-square analyses and t-tests were computed to compare patients who worked with those who did not on demographic characteristics (age, sex, ethnicity, marital status, and education) and diagnosis (schizophrenia or schizoaffective). None of these differences was significant.

To evaluate whether the three programs differed in competitive work outcomes, we performed a chi-square analysis comparing the cumulative proportion of patients who worked in each program over the two years. This result was significant (chi-square = 9.03, df = 2, $P < 0.01$): patients in IPS were most likely to work (71%), followed by Standard (52%), followed by PSR (39%).

Correlates of Prior Work and Predictors of Future Work

Correlations were computed between number of jobs worked and months worked over the past two years, and symptoms, cognitive functioning, and social adjustment at baseline. One-tailed significance tests were used to test the hypotheses that worse symptoms or functioning would be associated with poorer work history. Two correlations were significant at $P < 0.05$: patients with more negative symptoms worked significantly fewer months ($r = -0.21, P < 0.01$), and poorer social adjustment was related to fewer jobs over the past two years ($r = -0.16, P < 0.05$). There was a trend for cognitive impairment to be related to fewer months worked ($r = -0.12, P < 0.1$).

Analyses were conducted to evaluate whether positive symptoms (PANSS), negative symptoms (PANSS), cognitive impairment (PANSS), or social adjustment (SAS-II) were predictive of work. Because the vocational programs differed in their approach to rehabilitation, separate analyses were conducted for each program. Three vocational outcomes were examined: whether patients worked competitively (yes/no), cumulative wages earned, and cumulative hours worked. The results were analyzed by t-tests (worked or did not work) and correlations (wages, hours). One-tailed significance tests were used to test the hypotheses that greater cognitive or social impairment or more severe symptoms predicted poorer work outcomes.

Regarding competitive work, patients who worked in IPS had better social adjustment at baseline than patients who did not work [$t(40) = 2.07, P < 0.03$] but did not differ in cognitive impairment, positive symptoms, or negative symptoms. For PSR, patients who worked also had better social adjustment at baseline [$t(40) = 1.71, P < 0.05$]. In addition, patients who worked had less severe positive symptoms [$t(42) = 1.66, P < 0.05$] but did not differ in negative symptoms or cognitive impairment. For Standard, there were no differences at baseline in symptoms, cognitive impairment, or social functioning between patients who worked and those who did not.

Because some patients worked very small amounts of time, a somewhat different picture arose from examination of predictors of hours worked and wages earned. Correlations between baseline symptoms, cognitive impairment, and social functioning, and wages earned and hours worked over the two years are presented in Table 2. Cognitive impairment predicted work outcomes for the PSR program but not for IPS or Standard. Higher negative symptoms predicted work in both the IPS and PSR programs, but not Standard. Neither positive symptoms nor social adjustment significantly ($P < 0.05$) predicted work outcomes in any of the programs.

TABLE 2. Correlations between baseline symptoms, cognitive impairment, social adjustment, and future work within three vocational programs[a]

Variable	IPS (N = 44)		PSR (N = 44)		Standard (N = 46)	
	Wages	Hours	Wages	Hours	Wages	Hours
Positive symptoms	−.18	−.18	−.13	−.12	−.10	−.02
Negative symptoms	−.27**	−.27**	−.25**	−.23*	−.16	−.05
Cognitive impairment	−.16	−.16	−.28**	−.25**	−.12	−.03
Social adjustment	−.23*	−.23*	−.19	−.16	−.05	−.17

* $P < 0.10$; ** $P < 0.05$; one-tailed significance tests
[a] High scores on all measures reflect more severe symptoms, cognitive impairment, and worse social functioning

Discussion

The relatively high rates of competitive work for patients in the IPS program are consistent with two other controlled studies of IPS [22]. Previous research on IPS has included patients who were either white or African American. The present findings suggest that IPS may also be effective for Hispanic patients.

Work history was most strongly related to severity of negative symptoms, in line with other research [1,12]. Social adjustment was also related to work history, in line with prior research [26]. Somewhat surprisingly, cognitive impairment was not significantly related to prior work history, although there was a trend in this direction.

Analyses of symptoms, cognitive impairment, and social adjustment as predictors of work within each vocational program revealed an interesting pattern. For IPS, negative symptoms at baseline predicted work, whereas positive symptoms, cognitive impairment, and social adjustment did not. For PSR, negative symptoms also predicted work, but cognitive impairment was an even stronger predictor. For Standard, there were no significant predictors of work.

The different pattern of predictors may reflect the different nature of the vocational programs. The IPS model is based on the premise that work outcomes are best optimized by finding a good "fit" between a patient's strengths and interests and the workplace. Effort in this model focuses mainly on matching patients to suitable work settings and providing follow-along supports to facilitate job retention. IPS is not a learning-based program, and for that reason cognitive impairment may have not been related to outcomes. The PSR model, on the other hand, relies more heavily on training of job skills early in the program, and may place a greater premium on cognitive functioning. Negative symptoms may impede response to either program as they reflect core motivational deficits to participate in rehabilitation. Interestingly, among patients in the Standard group there were no consistent predictors of work. This may reflect the fact that this group was a hybrid of two different programs, one a supported employment approach and the other involving supervised work-for-contract.

The findings have several potentially important implications for cognitive predictors of vocational rehabilitation. Cognitive functioning predicts response to learning-based rehabilitation programs but appears to be unrelated to benefit from supported employment programs, such as IPS. The results suggest that the limitations imposed by cognitive deficits may interfere with response to some, but not other, rehabilitation programs. Bellack [27] has suggested that an alternative to cognitive rehabilitation in schizophrenia may be to teach patients compensatory strategies for managing their cognitive impairments. IPS may provide such a strategy for cognitively impaired patients by identifying appropriate work in supportive environments and providing ongoing supports to maximize success on the job. The positive outcomes of IPS compared with other, more learning-oriented, vocational rehabilitation programs [28] suggest that supported employment may be a more viable model for improving work outcomes in patients with schizophrenia, especially those patients with the most severe cognitive deficits.

Acknowledgments. This publication was made possible by cooperative agreement UD7 SM51818 from the U.S. Department of Health and Human Services (DHHS) Substance Abuse and Mental Health Services Administration (SAMHSA) Center for Mental Health Services (CMHS) as part of the Employment Intervention Demonstration Program (EIDP). Its contents are solely the responsibility of the author and do not necessarily represent the official views of the DHHS, SAMHSA, CMHS, or other EIDP collaborating partners.

References

1. Liddle PF (1987) The symptoms of chronic schizophrenia: a re-examination of the positive-negative dichotomy. Br J Psychiatry 151:145–151
2. Mueser KT, Drake RE, Bond GR (1997) Recent advances in psychiatric rehabilitation for patients with severe mental illness. Harvard Rev Psychiatry 5:123–137
3. Bartels SJ, Mueser KT, Miles KM (1997) A comparative study of elderly patients with schizophrenia and bipolar disorder in nursing homes and the community. Schizophr Res 27:181–190
4. Breier A, Schreiber J, Dyer J, et al (1991) National Institute of Mental Health longitudinal study of chronic schizophrenia. Arch Gen Psychiatry 43:239–246
5. Brekke JS, Raine A, Ansel M, et al (1997) Neuropsychological and psychophysiological correlates of psychosocial functioning in schizophrenia. Schizophr Bull 23:19–28
6. Jaeger J, Douglas E (1992) Neuropsychiatric rehabilitation for persistent mental illness. Psychiatr Q 63:71–93
7. Penn DL, Mueser KT, Spaulding W (1996) Information processing, social skill, and gender in schizophrenia. Psychiatry Res 59:213–220
8. Spaulding WD, Reed D, Elting D, et al (1997) Cognitive changes in the course of rehabilitation. In: Brenner HD, Boeker W, Genner R (eds) Towards a comprehensive therapy for schizophrenia. Hofgrefe-Huber, Seattle, pp 106–117
9. Davidson L, McGlashan TH (1997) The varied outcomes of schizophrenia. Can J Psychiatry 42:34–43
10. McCreadie RG, Connolly MA, Williamson DJ, et al (1994) The Nithsdale Schizophrenia Surveys. XII. "Neurodevelopmental" schizophrenia: a search for clinical correlates and putative aetiological factors. Br J Psychiatry 165:340–346
11. Roy MA, DeVriendt X (1995) Positive and negative symptoms in schizophrenia: a current overview. Can J Psychiatry 39:407–414
12. Sayers SL, Curran PJ, Mueser KT (1996) Factor structure and construct validity of the Scale for the Assessment of Negative Symptoms. Psychol Assessment 8:269–280
13. Ikebucki E, Nakagome K, Tugawa R, et al (1996) What influences social skills in patients with schizophrenia? Preliminary study using the role play test, WAIS-R and event-related potential. Schizophr Res 22:143–150

14. Mueser KT, Penn DL, Blanchard JJ, et al (1997) Affect recognition in schizophrenia: a synthesis of findings across three studies. Psychiatry Interpers Biol Proc 60:301–308

15. Overall JE, Gorham DR (1962) The Brief Psychiatric Rating Scale. Psychol Rep 10:799–812

16. Woerner MG, Mannuzza S, Kane JM (1988) Anchoring the BPRS: an aid to improved reliability. Psychopharmacol Bull 24:112–117

17. Hoffman H, Kupper Z (1997) Relationships between social competence, psychopathology and work performance and their predictive value for vocational rehabilitation of schizophrenic outpatients. Schizophr Res 23:69–79

18. Kay SR, Opler LA, Fiszbein A (1987) The Positive and Negative Syndrome Scale (PANSS) for schizophrenia. Schizophr Bull 13:261–276

19. Lysaker PH, Bell MD, Zito WS, et al (1995) Social skills at work: deficits and predictors of improvement in schizophrenia. J Nerv Ment Dis 183:688–692

20. Lysaker P, Bell M (1995) Work rehabilitation and improvements in insight in schizophrenia. J Nerv Ment Dis 183:103–107

21. Bond GR, Drake RE, Mueser KT, et al (1997) An update on supported employment for people with severe mental illness. Psychiatr Serv 48:335–346

22. Drake RE, Becker DR, Clark RE, et al (1999) Research on the individual placement and support model of supported employment. Psychiatr Q 70:627–633

23. Becker DR, Drake RE (1994) Individual Placement and Support: a community mental health center approach to vocational rehabilitation. Commun Ment Health J 45:487–489

24. Beard JH, Propst RN, Malamud TJ (1982) The Fountain House model of rehabilitation. Psychosoc Rehabil J 5:47–53

25. Schooler N, Hogarty G, Weissman M (1979) Social Adjustment Scale II (SAS-II). In: Hargreaves WA, Atkisson CC, Sorenson JE (eds) Resource materials for Community Mental Health Program Evaluations. Rockville, Md, USA, pp 290–303

26. Mueser KT, Salyers MP, Mueser PR (2001) A prospective analysis of work in schizophrenia. Schizophr Bull 27:281–296

27. Bellack AS (1992) Cognitive rehabilitation for schizophrenia: Is it possible? Is it necessary? Schizophr Bull 18:43–50

28. Bond GR (1992) Vocational rehabilitation. In: Liberman RP (ed) Handbook of psychiatric rehabilitation. Macmillan, New York, pp 244–275

Understanding the Outcome Findings of Cognitive-Behavioral Therapy for Psychosis: A Cognitive Model and Its Clinical Implications

David Fowler, Philippa Garety, and Elizabeth Kuipers

Summary. There is now strong evidence that cognitive-behavioral therapy provides an effective new treatment for people with schizophrenia spectrum disorders (which will be referred to throughout this chapter as psychosis). In this chapter, we first briefly review evidence for the effectiveness of cognitive-behavioral therapy (see also Tarrier et al. this volume). Next we describe our findings concerning the association between the outcome of cognitive-behavioral therapy and the presence of cognitive deficits and predictors of outcome. Finally we describe a new integrative cognitive model of the development and maintenance of psychotic episodes and discuss its implications for clinical understanding and the development of hypotheses concerning the mode of action of cognitive-behavioral therapy for psychosis.

Key words. Cognitive-behavioral, Cognitive, Therapy, Deficits, Model

A Brief Description of Cognitive-Behavioral Therapy for Psychosis

Unlike other psychological interventions used with people with psychosis, such as social skills training or cognitive remediation approaches, cognitive-behavioral therapy takes as its central focus the subjective experiences of psychosis (i.e., the symptoms) and the person's attempts to understand them. Our approach to cognitive-behavioral therapy for people with psychosis is described in detail in our treatment manual [1], in other papers [2–4], and in case descriptions [2,3]. Although there are some differences of emphasis, there is agreement concerning the goals and main methods of therapy with others (see Tarrier et al., this volume) [5,6]. Indeed, there has been a fruitful cross-fertilization of ideas. The principal aim of cognitive-behavioral therapy for medication-resistant psychosis is to reduce the distress and interference with functioning caused by the psychotic symptoms. The thoughts, beliefs, and images experienced by people are the core material with which cognitive-behavioral therapists work. The approach draws extensively on the wider cognitive-behavioral therapy tradition initiated by Beck and colleagues. In terms of style, the

University of East Anglia, Norwich NR4 7TJ, UK

therapist works collaboratively, setting agendas and agreeing on therapy goals, and takes an actively enquiring stance towards the clients' accounts of their experiences. Therapy involves first building a good working therapeutic relationship with the patient, then undertaking detailed assessment of the way thoughts, feelings, and experiences arise in relation to events and moods, thinking biases, and how the individual responds or acts in reaction to such feelings or thoughts. The therapist first seeks to understand presenting problems in terms of an individualized formulation informed by the cognitive model and then seeks to offer an alternative explanation of the person's difficulties based on this formulation. This provides the basis for further discussions about the nature of the person's difficulties and leads to a process of identifying specific appraisals, thoughts, and beliefs and reviewing evidence for these. The cognitive-behavioral therapist also seeks to encourage a more adaptive behavioral response to the predicament of psychosis by the use of activity scheduling and advice on coping strategies. The standard cognitive therapy approach is modified to address effectively the particular problems of psychosis. A more flexible and individualized strategy is used to take account of challenges associated with establishing a therapeutic relationship which are specific to this client group and the typical complexity and severity of the problems presented [1].

The Efficacy of Cognitive-Behavioral Therapy in Psychosis

Three large randomized controlled trials enrolling people with medication-resistant psychosis have recently been completed [7–11]. A Cochrane systematic review of cognitive-behavioral therapy for psychosis [12] includes the three studies mentioned above together with two other studies of cognitive-behavioral therapy with acute inpatients [13–15]. Overall, this review concludes that there is good evidence from controlled trials that cognitive-behavioral therapy is effective in terms of psychotic symptom reduction, and encouraging evidence that it may contribute to relapse reduction. The current evidence can be regarded as substantive, since trials undertaken independently by different research groups are producing similar findings. This is a relatively small data base from which to draw conclusions, but further evidence is accumulating rapidly. Supportive results from other recent trials are now emerging both from within the United Kingdom and elsewhere (Tarrier et al., Roncone et al., and Falloon et al., this volume) [16].

The Presence of Cognitive Deficits Is Not Associated With Poorer Outcome of Cognitive-Behavioral Therapy: Indeed, It May Be Associated With Better Outcome

Understanding prognostic factors that may be associated with outcome is important. It has long been established that many people who have psychotic symptoms show impairment on a range of tasks assessing cognitive functioning and that such deficits show strong associations with impairment in social abilities and social functioning (Roder et al., Liberman, and Mueser, this volume) [17]. Given these findings in the pre-

liminary stages of the development of cognitive-behavioral therapy, we initially hypothesized that the presence of cognitive deficits in general cognitive functioning (IQ),
memory, and planning might be associated with the outcome of cognitive-behavioral
therapy. Specifically, we predicted that those individuals who showed severe impairments in cognitive functioning might be unlikely to be able to respond to cognitive-
behavioral therapy. We undertook a preliminary investigation of these hypotheses
while undertaking our first trial [18]. We describe the results of this study in detail for
the first time below. We will also summarize findings from a subsequent study [19].

The assessments of symptoms used in the context of our pilot trial [4] included the
Brief Psychiatric Rating Scale and individualized personal questionnaires to assess
the conviction, preoccupation, and distress associated with delusions. We also assessed patients at intake using a neuropsychological test battery. This included tests
of current IQ (estimated from five subtests of the WAIS using a weighted formula),
the National Adult Reading Test [20], immediate and delayed recall of a short story
[21], immediate and delayed and cued recall of an array of pictures [22], cognitive
estimation [23], and verbal fluency FAS [24]. In addition, we included a probabilistic
reasoning task [25]. These tests were completed on 16 patients (11 treated cases, 5
controls). The sample as a whole showed expected impairments. Eight patients had a
significant discrepancy between predicted and obtained IQ scores. Four patients had
memory impairments. Seven patients gave extremely bizarre guesses on cognitive
estimates. One patient had impaired verbal fluency. Six patients showed evidence of
rapid, overconfident, or over-responsive reasoning. The small sample size meant that
the study had insufficient power to test hypotheses about associations between deficits
and outcome. However, it was surprising to find that there were no indications at all
of associations between deficits and the outcome of therapy. Furthermore, some of
the individuals who showed clear cognitive deficits (including low IQ and memory
problems, and cognitive estimates) also showed clinically significant improvements
in therapy.

An example of a case of an individual who responded well to cognitive therapy
despite having severe cognitive impairment is that of a 40-year-old man ((A.B.),
treated by D.F) who presented with paranoid beliefs that he had been set up by colleagues at work and this involved him in accusations of arson and murder. He had
held these beliefs continuously for over 10 years, with occasional hospital admissions.
He had a current IQ of below 70. He also showed clear deficits on probabilistic reasoning tasks and cognitive estimation, limited delayed and cued recall of pictures, and
very limited immediate and delayed recall of a story. At the start of therapy, A.B. had
been completely convinced and preoccupied with beliefs about the setup (to the extent
that he had repeatedly got into trouble with the police for pestering them about
making an enquiry into potential threats against him). At the end of therapy, A.B.
reported to the assessor that he thought it was 50–50 whether it was all in his head or
not. A.B. also said that he no longer felt paranoid and that he felt a lot better after
therapy. The assessor recorded that A.B. said, "I can see now how I exaggerated what
happened to me and it made me ill, thinking I was set up all over the place." The measures confirmed this qualitative impression of change. From the initial to the post-
treatment assessment, the personal questionnaire measures showed his delusional
belief conviction dropping from 5 (maximum) to 3 (moderate). His preoccupation
dropped from 5 to 2 and his distress from 5 to 2. A year later he had lost all his delusions and was still well. Although this was a preliminary study, it appeared to suggest,

contrary to hypothesis, that the presence of low IQ, memory impairment, and reasoning impairment was not necessarily associated with poor outcome from cognitive-behavioral therapy.

Building on this study, we set out to investigate further the association between cognitive deficits and the outcome of cognitive-behavioral therapy in the context of a randomized, controlled trial with sixty participants (see Garety et al. [19] for a full report). This time we used the Quick Test [26] as an estimate of current IQ. As in the previous study, we also used the NART [20] the cognitive estimates test [23], the verbal fluency test [24], and a test of probabilistic reasoning [25]. The current IQ and the other cognitive functioning variables (probabilistic reasoning and verbal fluency) showed no association with outcome. Furthermore, when trends were detected, they were interestingly in the direction of a tendency for greater impairment to be associated with better outcome. The findings from the cognitive estimation task were of particular interest in this regard. What was found (contrary to what we had expected) was that a higher number of bizarre errors on this task (normally regarded as a marker of cognitive impairment) were associated with better outcome from cognitive-behavioral therapy. Our general conclusion from this study was that high IQ, or intact cognitive functioning, is clearly not required for cognitive-behavioral therapy to be effective. Indeed, as in the previous study, we observed that even individuals with quite severe impairments can do quite well. The findings suggesting that the presence of impairment (particularly on the cognitive estimates task) was associated with better outcome are intriguing. One interpretation may be that in some people cognitive impairment may lead to biases in reasoning, such as making bizarre guesses or over-rapid and overconfident social judgments. This may lead to errors in judgment and thus delusions. However, the same cognitive impairments may also be associated with a tendency to alter judgments with limited further information [19,27] and therefore a susceptibility to altering beliefs when alternative suggestions or interpretations are offered by a therapist. Although this is highly speculative, it would be consistent with the hypothesis that cognitive-behavioral therapy helps to provide compensatory methods that assist in re-evaluating beliefs for those people whose cognitive biases may tend to lead to delusions.

Predictors of Outcome

In our study on predictors of outcome [19], we found that a positive response to cognitive therapy was predicted by four variables: whether or not individuals could acknowledge that another view of the delusion may be possible at the beginning of therapy (as identified by the MADS [28] "possibility of being mistaken" question), where reporting a possibility of being mistaken was associated with better outcome; the cognitive estimates test (as described above), where a higher error score predicts good outcome; the number of admissions in five years, where having more admissions was associated with better outcome; and insight, where better insight correlated with better outcome. The findings of this study offer intriguing pointers to understanding treatment response to cognitive-behavioral therapy. The MADS finding confirmed our hypothesis, based on earlier work by Chadwick and Lowe [29] and Sharp et al. [30], that a flexibility in delusions, as measured by admitting of the possibility of an alternative view of the delusion, would predict a good response. However, although this finding was present in 50% of patients and predicted better outcome at the end of treatment, the prediction did not hold as strongly at nine-month post-therapy follow-up [8]. At this stage, we found that those participants who admitted the possibility that they might be mistaken responded more quickly and to a greater extent to therapy than the others, but that the others appeared to benefit in the end, albeit to a lesser extent, from the therapy. It seems that a more rapid and quicker response to cognitive therapy may occur when people with psychosis have a chink of insight. However, persistence with cognitive-behavioral therapy over nine months can lead to clinically significant gains, even among those who started with limited insight and do not show a rapid response. This observation (that slower responders who do not have good prognostic features make gains at follow-up that are not neccesarily apparent at the end of treatment) also provides support for the use of longer-term approaches to therapy that take place over at least a nine-month period, especially when working with more resistant patients.

Toward an Integrative Framework

Although evidence for the efficacy of cognitive-behavioral therapy is consolidating rapidly, our understanding of the mode of action of this therapy is still at a preliminary stage. Further research is needed into what may be the processes of change associated with cognitive-behavioral therapy and into predictors of outcome. Next we outline a cognitive model of the formation and maintenance of psychosis. This model can serve both as a basis for clinical formulations undertaken by cognitive therapists and as a source of testable hypotheses about the mode of action of therapy (see also [52,53]).

A Cognitive Model of the Development of the Symptoms of Acute Psychosis

Our cognitive model assumes that the symptoms of acute psychosis develop over time, as represented in Fig. 1. This model is consistent with vulnerability-stress models (e.g., Strauss and Carpenter [31]). Psychosis is assumed to arise in the context of a vulnerable predisposition (of bio-psycho-social origin), and triggers to the onset of psychosis are assumed to include factors such as life events and taking street drugs. There may be different types of vulnerability, triggers, and stresses for different cases. The cognitive perspective puts particular emphasis on the way in which different vulnerability factors interact with, and shape the evolution of, premorbid beliefs about the self and others. It is assumed that it is cognitive vulnerability in interaction with evolving beliefs and triggering factors that leads to psychosis. Complex psychotic symptoms, such as delusions and hallucinations, can be regarded as thoughts, beliefs, emotional reactions, and behaviors. The cognitive model implies that by careful assessment it may be possible to trace the evolution of such cognitions from their formation as premorbid beliefs. Subsequent beliefs about self, others, and psychosis are then assumed to be shaped by appraisals of previous stressful events, anomalies of experience and early psychotic symptoms, early and subsequent experiences during

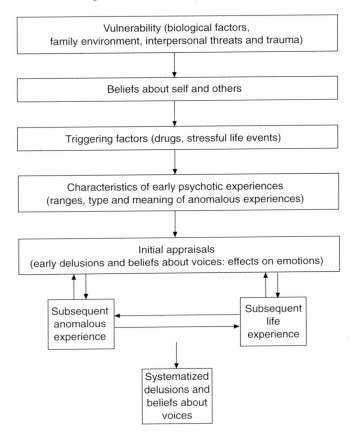

FIG. 1. Development history of delusions and beliefs about voices

psychotic episodes and hospitalization, current life experiences, stresses, and psychotic experiences.

This model can provide a basis for therapists to understand the presenting problems of their patients in terms of an individualized formulation. Such formulations aim to summarize the factors associated with an individual's personal vulnerability to psychosis and can form the basis for customized cognitive interventions [1]. A basic assumption of a cognitive perspective on psychosis is that the content of voices, paranoia, and delusions may be intelligible in terms of the person's life history and circumstances. The model clearly defines two central processes of cognitive-behavioral therapy: first, attempting to make sense of the person's experiences in the context of his or her life experiences and how these shaped his or her beliefs and behavior (developing a formulation); and second, discussing the nature of the person's predicament and different interpretations of experiences (sharing and discussing the formulation). Strategies that are specific to cognitive-behavioral therapy are offering an alternative understanding based on the cognitive model, attempting to foster alternative interpretations of specific belief and appraisals, and attempting to promote alternative behavioral and emotional reactions to psychosis.

The cognitive model can provide a clear hypothesis to account for what is perhaps the most important specific clinical effect of cognitive-behavioral therapy. Randomized, controlled trials have consistently shown that gains in terms of symptom reduction that occur as a consequence of cognitive-behavioral therapy tend to be maintained, and occasionally improve further after the period of active intervention [8,10,11]. Although symptom improvement has also been observed as a consequence of many other therapies (see systematic review by Motjaibi et al. [32]), such gains are not maintained. In direct comparisons between cognitive-behavioral therapy and supportive therapy, cognitive-behavioral therapy shows considerably better outcomes in terms of the degree of clinically significant change at follow-up [10,11]. Potentially the specific effect of cognitive-behavioral therapy arises as the patient learns new ways of thinking about psychosis, new ways of compensating for cognitive biases, and new behavioral reactions. The effect of such learning may be that the person learns a more adaptive response to triggering events. Application of such new responses may stop the vicious cycles that can potentially lead to the maintenance of psychotic symptoms and thereby relapse (see below). Such learning has the potential to produce specific effects that are maintained when the therapist is no longer present.

The Maintenance of Psychosis

A better understanding of the processes of cognitive-behavioral therapy emerges from a consideration of the factors associated with the maintenance as well as the development of psychosis. From a cognitive perspective, the maintenance of clinical problems with psychosis may be characterized as people becoming "stuck in psychosis" or "locked into a vicious cycle." Such cycles can explain how triggering factors, such as the experience of anomalous experiences or threatening life events, can eventually lead to episodes of acute psychosis. Such episodes may be characterized by extreme levels of conviction and preoccupation with beliefs, an increase in the severity and frequency of anomalies of experience and hallucinations, and the association of psychosis with severe emotional and behavioral reactions. Consistently with other theorists [33–35], we propose that a critical feature leading to the vicious cycle characterized as becoming "stuck in psychosis" may be the way in which individuals appraise and then develop attributions or beliefs about psychotic experiences. The association of an affective response with specific attributions which suggest that anomalous experiences represent either an external interpersonal threat ("Everyone is against me") or a personally meaningful external event ("God is talking to me") may determine whether or not triggering factors lead to the maintenance of psychosis. This model is represented in Fig. 2. The numbers in parentheses below refer to the numbers in Fig. 2.

Triggers

The model implies that there may be two types of trigger to psychosis: (1) the occurrence of anomalies of experience and (2) the occurrence of stressful life events (or events which lead to the accessing of threatening memories or emotional responses). Often these may co-occur.

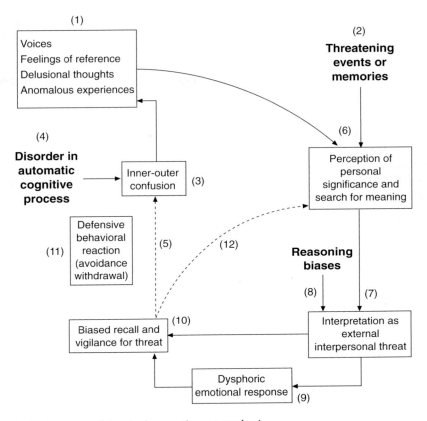

FIG. 2. Maintenance of threatening reactions to psychosis

The Origins of Anomalous Experiences

(3) Source-monitoring problems (inner/outer confusion). The model assumes that there is a final common pathway that underpins the experience of many different types of anomalous psychotic experience (hallucinations, delusional experiences, experiences of thought disorder). This final common pathway may be described as confusion in distinguishing between experience that is internally generated (e.g., thoughts, memories, hopes, and fears) and experience that is externally generated (e.g. sensations and perceptions of events in the world). Cognitive confusion of this type has been described variously by other theorists as a problem in reality monitoring [36], self-monitoring [37,38], metacognition [39], source monitoring [35], or more recently autonoetic agnosia [40]. Research indicates that there may be two routes to such confusion.

(4) Neurocognitive deficits and source memory problems. Source-monitoring problems may be associated with impairments to basic or automatic cognitive

processes (or cognitive deficits). The presence of such cognitive deficits has been commonly observed among people with psychosis and is most often assumed to reflect the underlying biological vulnerability to psychosis (see Frith [39] and Hemsley [38]. Such proposals are also consistent with contemporary models of brain function [39,41]. Specific support for the idea that source-monitoring reflects a type of neurocognitive deficit that can be described as autonoetic agnosia derives from a recent study [40]. This showed that although source-monitoring problems can be independent of general deficit, they are often associated with general memory problems; that people with psychosis tend to show general rather than specific difficulties in distinguishing the sources of information; and that such deficits are not necessarily associated with specific psychotic symptoms [40].

(5) Cognitive biases and source-monitoring problems. Unlike cognitive deficits, cognitive biases are assumed to be shaped by psychological processes such as beliefs and expectations and by variations in environmental stimulation. Experimental evidence for the role of cognitive bias and source monitoring in hallucinations is provided by Bentall et al. [42] and by Morrison and Haddock [43]. There is also evidence that source-monitoring problems leading to anomalous experiences (hallucinations, perceptual oddities, déjà vu type experiences) can occur among people without clinical psychosis, particularly under conditions such as tiredness, high arousal, and in the context of ambiguous stimulation and information overload (see Bentall [36] and Morrison [35] for reviews).

The Importance of the Appraisal of Psychosis

Maher [33] has suggested that delusions may arise as attributions or explanations for threatening, ambiguous, or anomalous experiences. Our model is consistent with this idea but also takes account of reasoning and emotional biases that may influence such appraisals (see Garety and Freeman [44] for review of experimental evidence).

(6) Triggering events demand a search for explanation. The experience of anomalies of experience (deriving from source-monitoring problems) or threats from the world is likely to give rise to an initial appraisal (e.g., What is happening to me?) and demand a search for explanation. Attribution theorists have long suggested that such processes are an aspect of a normal reaction to the occurrence of anomalous experience and that similar processes may be involved in delusion formation [45]. For example, a common reaction to an anomalous experience such as déjà vu is a perception of salience and a initial feeling of personal significance, accompanied by a preliminary search for attribution: "What was the meaning of that?" However, in a typically adaptive reaction, such a search leads to a neutral explanation that tends to disregard the meaning, e.g., "It was just an anomaly."

(7) What may be critical to driving cycles of processing that characterize preoccupation with delusions and voices is the attribution that triggering experience represents a personally significant external event. This may be positively toned, e.g., "It's God talking to me, telling me I am the saviour" and accompanied by positive lift in mood (excitement, feeling of purpose). In many psychiatric patients, the attribution is negatively toned and infers a specific external interpersonal threat (e.g., "These experiences mean everyone is against me"). In such cases, the associated affect is

typically high levels of anxiety, suspiciousness, and fear. The emergence of these specific attributions for triggering events is likely to occur in the context of, and in association with, pre-existing beliefs about anomalies, self, and others and previously learned emotional responses to perceived threat (see Fig. 1). It is the occurrence of these specific attributions for triggering events that leads to preoccupation with a search for further meaning and a defensive response, and thereby give rise to reactions that can maintain psychosis. The point at which people with psychosis form specific delusional attributions and lose insight has been identified as a point of crucial catastrophic change in several careful prospective studies of the development of psychotic relapse from recovery states (see Birchwood et al. [46] for review).

(8) Reasoning biases. Research suggests that the emergence of the above attributions with strong conviction is not solely the product of normal attributional biases. There is clear evidence for the presence of reasoning biases among people with psychosis (see Garety and Freeman [44] for a detailed review of the empirical literature). This review concludes that people with delusions may be subject to biases that lead to over-rapid and overconfident judgments; that people with paranoia also tend to also have biases to seeking external and personal explanations for negative events; and that there is evidence that people with pychotic symptoms have problems in social judgment. There is also evidence that people with paranoia tend to have depressed mood and low self-esteem and show attention biases and recall biases similar to those found in depression (e.g., they tend to recall negative information) [47]. Both individually and collectively, cognitive processes of this type can assist individuals to select personally threatening external explanations for anomalous experience. They also provide a basis for understanding aspects of the form of delusional thinking, e.g., the extreme certainty with which beliefs are held, why alternative information is discounted, and why limited evidence may lead to extreme conviction. None of the above cognitive processes are universally found among all people with psychosis. However, this observed heterogeneity is consistent with the theories which suggest that the processes underpinning belief formation and attribution processes associated with delusions are multifactorial and may occur as a final common pathway of different underlying processes [27].

Consequences of Attributing Psychosis As an External Interpersonal Salient Event

(9) Emotional consequences (distress, anxiety, fear, suspiciousness) are associated with beliefs or appraisals about psychosis. Several recent studies have demonstrated that distress associated with hallucinations is associated with the person's beliefs about psychosis (in particular, whether the voice is regarded as malevolent) (e.g., Birchwood and Chadwick [48]). Distress in reaction to psychosis also appears to be consistent with ongoing mood, and may be associated with negative beliefs about self and about the meaning of psychosis [49]. In a recent study we have found that the person's attributions about the way they relate to voices and voices relate to them also appear to be associated with distress (Vaughan and Fowler, in preparation). Such beliefs about psychosis may arise as a consequence of the evolution of beliefs

described in Fig. 1 and are associated with premorbid beliefs about self and others and past reactions to threatening events, traumas, and stresses.

(10) Cognitive biases may consequently play a role in maintaining psychosis. Freeman and Garety [50] have shown that delusional distress is closely associated with internal focus associated with worrying about the delusion. Such worries may maintain distress, because an internal focus on threatening thoughts and images increases the likelihood of the occurrence of such images. Morrison [35] similarly has proposed that metacognitive processes similar to those which maintain intrusive thoughts may play a role in the maintenance of hallucinations. Baker and Morrison [51] provide evidence in support of these ideas.

(11) Safety behaviors. People with paranoia often adapt their behavior to avoid threat (e.g., they may become socially withdrawn). Although the short-term consequence of such behavior may be to reduce distress, the long-term consequence of such behavior may be to reinforce the belief that there is a threat. The effect of such behavior may therefore play a role in maintaining delusions in a similar manner to the role of safety behaviors in obsessional problems. One member of our group (Daniel Freeman) is currently undertaking empirical research in this area.

Consequences of the Vicious Cycle: The Maintenance of Psychosis

The outcome of the processing biases associated with being "stuck in psychosis" may be to reinforce delusional attributions and lead to an increase in triggering events. An increase in the occurrence of source-monitoring problems may occur via increasing cognitive bias in the context of increases in arousal and the accessing of beliefs and expectations of seeing an external threat when there is none. This may lead to further anomalous experience (5). The processing biases describe above would also lead to an increase in the frequency of intrusive thoughts, threatening memories or perception of threat in the world and thus reinforcing of a perception of threat (12). This would lead to a repetition of the cycle and thus maintenance of psychosis.

The Utility of the Model in Providing a Basis for New Clinical Insights and Predictions for Further Research

In general, the cognitive model implies a vulnerability to psychotic disorder of two types. A biological predisposition (which may become manifest as a breakdown in automatic neurocognitive processes and thereby anomalies of experience) and an emotional vulnerability (characterized by beliefs about self and others, appraisals, and emotional processing biases). However, we suggest that is the continuing attribution of psychotic experience as a personally significant external event which is assumed to be critical in maintaining the cycle. The model is consistent with existing findings. It provides a way of integrating what at present are diverse strands of research that are sometimes regarded as competing hypotheses. However, the model also implies clear and testable hypotheses concerning the way in which specific cognitive processes may be associated with either the maintenance of symptoms or change in terms of a reduction in conviction, preoccupation or distress with delusions, or frequency and severity of hallucinations and other anomalous experience. The model also provides a framework for developing hypotheses about the mode of action of cognitive-behavioral therapy concerning its role in directly altering attributions but also in ameliorating cognitive processing styles and behavior.

The model leads to new and nonobvious predictions about cognitive-behavioral techniques. For example, the teaching of certain types of coping strategy may worsen, not improve, psychosis if they lead to an increase in internal focus on psychosis. Certain types of behavioral advice may also worsen beliefs if they reinforce safety behavior. The effect of supportive listening and empathy may provide a "safe inter-personal context" in which the immediate search for signals of threat may be amelio-rated and may also have direct effects on reducing arousal. However, such effects would only last while the person is in contact with the safety figure. Conversely, an argu-mentative or pressurising style in therapy, perhaps used by an unsophisticated cogni-tive therapist, may lead to the patient's not feeling understood or confused or threatened. This can potentially access triggers in the therapy session. The accessing of vicious cycle in the session would lead to an internal focus and suspiciousness and possibly the therapist's being incorporated into the delusion. Persisting with ques-tioning may maintain or worsen delusions, but acknowledging the problem, recog-nizing and dealing with the specific threatening interpretation about the therapist, and possibly returning to an empathic style may stop the exacerbation of the vicious cycle.

Conclusion: The Further Development of Cognitive-Behavioral Therapy for Psychosis

Cognitive-behavioral therapy for psychosis is now a sophisticated treatment that pro-vides a practical link between clinical need, theory, and practice. The model described in this chapter may help to clarify what are the important processes of cognitive-behavioral and other therapies. Cognitive-behavioral therapy is not simply verbal challenge of delusions (all too often misunderstood as confronting patients). It is an approach that seeks first to understand the person's beliefs, experiences, and behav-iors and then to place them in the context of that individual's life history, current stresses, and beliefs. Linking a rationale to the use of specific techniques with a coher-ent theoretical model will allow to the further development of this therapy. Research evidence indicates that there is a specific benefit to the use of cognitive therapy tech-niques over and above the benefit of supportive psychotherapeutic help that may be common to several different types of therapy (although not all). The model implies that assisting people with psychosis to reject externalizing and threatening appraisals and, where possible, to adopt a less distressing alternative understanding of the nature of their difficulties may be crucial. The model also provides clear suggestions as to which types of appraisals, styles of thinking, and behaviors are associated with becom-ing "stuck in psychosis." This can potentially lead to the clearer identification of the characteristics of individuals who have poorer symptomatic outcomes and who may be unresponsive to therapy. Our group is in the planning a series of studies to be carried out in the context of further trials comparing cognitive-behavioral therapy with other therapies. In the course of this research, we intend to examine closely the processes of therapy. This may help to define specifically what kinds of interactions between patients and therapists lead to beneficial and deleterious effects. We also intend to carry out a further series of experimental studies testing hypotheses about the relation of cognitive processes to symptomatic outcomes. The field is expanding rapidly. The results of both explanatory and further efficacy trials are likely to move our understanding forward considerably over the next few years. This progress is exciting. Its success will be measured by the extent to which patients benefit.

References

1. Fowler DG, Garety P, Kuipers E (1995) Cognitive behavior therapy for psychosis: theory and practice. John Wiley and Sons, Chichester
2. Fowler DG, Garety P, Kuipers E (1998) Understanding the inexplicable: an individually formulated approach to cognitive therapy for delusions. In: Perris C, McGorry P (eds) Cognitive psychotherapy of psychotic disorders: handbook of theory and practice. John Wiley and Sons, Chichester
3. Fowler D, Garety P, Kuipers E (1998) Cognitive therapy for psychosis: formulation, treatment, and service implications J Ment Health 7:123–133
4. Garety P, Fowler D, Kuipers E (2000) Cognitive-behavioral therapy for medication resistant symptoms. Schizophr Bull 26:73–86
5. Kingdon DG, Turkington D (1994) Cognitive-behavioral therapy of schizophrenia. Lawrence Erlbaum, Hove
6. Chadwick P, Birchwood M, Trower P (1996) Cognitive therapy for delusions, voices and paranoia. Wiley Series in Clinical Psychology. John Wiley and Sons, Chichester
7. Kuipers E, Garety P, Fowler D, et al (1997) The London-East Anglia randomised controlled trial of cognitive-behavioral therapy for psychosis 1: Effects of the treatment phase. Br J Psychiatry 171:319–327
8. Kuipers E, Fowler D, Garety P, et al (1998) The London-East Anglia RCT of CBT for Psychosis III. Follow up and economic evaluation at 18 months. Br J Psychiatry 173:61–68
9. Tarrier N, Yusupoff L, Kinney C, et al (1998) Randomised controlled trial of intensive cognitive behavior therapy for patients with chronic schizophrenia. BMJ 317:303–307
10. Tarrier N, Wittkowski A, Kinney C, et al (1999) Durability of the effects of cognitive-behavioral therapy in the treatment of chronic schizophrenia: 12-month follow-up. Br J Psychiatry 1999:500–504
11. Sensky T, Turkington D, Kingdon D, et al (2000) A randomized controlled trial of cognitive-behavioral therapy for persistent symptoms in schizophrenia resistant to medication. Arch Gen Psychiatry 57:165–172
12. Jones C, Cormac I, Mota J, et al (1999) Cognitive behavior therapy for schizophrenia (Cochrane systematic review). The Cochrane Library, Issue 1, 1999. Update Software, Oxford
13. Drury V, Birchwood M, Cochrane R (1996) Cognitive therapy and recovery from acute psychosis: a controlled trial 1: Impact on psychotic symptoms. Br J Psychiatry 169:593–601
14. Kemp R, Hayward P, Applethwaite G, et al (1996) Compliance therapy in psychotic patients: a randomised controlled trial. BMJ 312:345–349
15. Kemp R, Kivor G, Everitt B, et al (1998) Randomised controlled trial of compliance therapy: 18 month follow up. Br J Psychiatry 172:413–419

16. Pinto A, La Pia S, Mennella R, et al (1999) Cognitive behavioral therapy and clozapine for clients with treatment refactory schizophrenia. Psychiatr Serv 50:901–904
17. Green MF, Kern RS, Braff DL, et al (2000) Neurocognitive deficits and functional outcome in schizophrenia: Are we measuring the "right stuff"? Schizophr Bull 26:119–136
18. Garety PA, Kuipers E, Fowler DG, et al (1994) Cognitive behavioral therapy for drug resistant psychosis. Br J Med Psychol 67:259–271
19. Garety P, Fowler D, Kuipers E, et al (1997) The London-East Anglia randomised controlled trial of cognitive behavioral therapy for psychosis II: Predictors of outcome. 171:420–426
20. Nelson HE (1982) The National Adult Reading Test. NFER-Nelson, Windsor
21. Wechsler F (1945) A standardised memory scale for clinical use. J Psychol 19:87–95
22. Williams M (1968) The measurement of memory in clinical practice. Br J Soc Clin Psychol 7:19–34
23. Shallice T, Evans ME (1978) The involvement of the frontal lobes in cognitive estimation. Cortex 14:294–303
24. Miller E (1984) Verbal fluency as a function of a measure of verbal intelligence and in relation to different types of cerebral pathology. Br J Clin Psychol 23:53–57
25. Garety PA, Hemsely DR, Wessely S (1991) Reasoning in deluded schizophrenic and paranoid patients: biases in performance on a probabilistic inference task. J Nerv Ment Dis 179:194–201
26. Ammons RB, Ammons CH (1962) Quick Test. Psychological Test Specialists, Missoula, MT, USA
27. Garety PA, Hemsley DR (1994) Delusions: investigations into the psychology of delusional reasoning. Oxford University Press, Oxford
28. Wessely S, Buchanan A, Reed A, Cutting J, Everitt B, Garety P, Taylor TJ (1993) Acting on delusions 1: Prevalence. Br J Psychiatry 163:69–76
29. Chadwick PDJ, Lowe CF (1994) A cognitive approach to measuring and modifying delusions. Behav Res Ther 32:355–367
30. Sharp HM, Fear CF, Williams MG, Healy D, Lowe CF, Yeadon H, Holden R (1996) Delusional phenomenology—Dimensions and change. Behav Res Ther 34:123–142
31. Strauss JS, Carpenter WT (1981) Schizophrenia. Plenum, New York
32. Mojtabai R, Nicholson RA, Carpenter BN (1998) Role of psychosocial treatment in the management of schizophrenia: A meta-analytic review of controlled outcome studies. Schizophr Bull 24:569–587
33. Maher BA (1988) Anomalous experience and delusional thinking: the logic of explanations. In: Oltmanns TF, Maher BA (eds) Delusional beliefs. John Wiley & Sons, New York, pp 15–33
34. Birchwood M (1996) Early intervention in psychosis. In: Haddock G, Slade P (eds) Cognitive-behavioral interventions with psychotic disorders. Routledge, London
35. Morrison A (1999) A cognitive analysis of the maintenance of auditory hallucinations: Are voices to schizophrenia what bodily sensations are to panic? Behav Cogn Psychother 26:289–302
36. Bentall RP (1990) The illusion of reality: a review and integration of psychological research on hallucinations. Psychol Bull 107:82–85
37. Hemsley DR (1993) A simple (or simplistic?) cognitive model for schizophrenia. Behav Res Ther 31:633–645
38. Hemsley D (1998) The disruption in the sense of self in schizophrenia: potential links with disturbances of information processing. Br J Med Psychol 1998:115–124
39. Frith CD (1992) The cognitive neuropsychology of schizophrenia. Lawrence Erlbaum Associates, Hove
40. Keefe RSE, Arnold MC, Bayen UJ, et al (1999) Source monitoring deficits in patients with schizophrenia: a multinomial modelling analysis. Psychol Med 29:903–914

41. Gray JA (1998) Integrating schizophrenia. Schizophr Bull 24:249–266
42. Bentall RP, Baker G, Havers S (1991) Reality monitoring and psychotic hallucinations. Br J Clin Psychol 30:213–222
43. Morrison AP, Haddock G, Tarrier N (1995) Intrusive thoughts and auditory hallucinations: a cognitive approach. Behav Cogn Psychother 23:265–280
44. Garety PA, Freeman D (1999) Cognitive approaches to delusions: a critical review of theories and evidence. Br J Clin Psychol 38(2):113–154
45. Johnson WG, Ross JM, Mastria MA (1977) Delusional behavior: an attributional analysis of development and modification. J Abnorm Psychol 86:421–426
46. Birchwood M, Macmillan F, Smith J (1994) Early intervention. In: Birchwood M, Tarrier N (eds) Psychological management of schizophrenia. John Wiley and Sons, Chichester
47. Bentall RP, Kinderman P (1998) Psychological processes and delusional beliefs: the implications for the treatment of paranoid states. In: Wykes T, Tarrier N (eds) Outcome and innovation in psychological treatment of schizophrenia. John Wiley and Sons, Chichester
48. Birchwood M, Chadwick P (1997) The omnipotence of voices: testing the validity of a cognitive model. Psychol Med 27:1345–1353
49. Close H, Garety P (1998) Cognitive assessment of voices: further developments in understanding the emotional impact of voices. Br J Clin Psychol 37:173–188
50. Freeman D, Garety PA (1999) Worry, worry processes and dimensions of delusions: an exploratory investigation of a role for anxiety processes in the maintenance of delusional distress. Behav Cognitive Psychother 27:47–62
51. Baker CA, Morrison AP (1998) Cognitive processes in auditory hallucinations: attributional biases and metacognition. Psychol Med 28:1199–1208
52. Fowler DG (2000) Psychological Formulation of Early Psychosis: A Cognitive Model. In: Birchwood M, Fowler D, Jackson C (eds) Early intervention in Psychosis: A guide to concepts, evidence and interventions. John Wiley and Sons, Chichester
53. Garety P, Kuipers E, Fowler D, Freeman D, Bebbington PE (2001) A cognitive model of the positive symptoms of psychosis. Psych Med 31:1–7

A New Cognitive Therapy for Auditory Hallucinations and Delusions: Development of a Guide for Psychotic Patients and Their Family Members

Seiichi Harada and Yuji Okazaki

Summary. We have developed a new cognitive therapy for auditory hallucinations and delusions, along with a guide intended to familiarize clients and their families with it. The title of the guide is "A Guide to Coping with Voices of Unknown Origin—10 Items Containing Useful Information on the Treatment of Voices of Unknown Origin." The guide consists of a preface, 10 chapters, and a postscript, and has the advantages of being easily understandable, quickly readable (in approximately 20 minutes), and full of accurate and useful information to assist clients in coping with psychotic symptoms. Psychiatrists can employ this guide as a teaching aid in psychoeducational therapy sessions for clients and their families. In this chapter, we introduce a portion of the guide, namely Chapters 1, 4, and 10. Next we show the results of a questionnaire administered to clients and their families as an index of the guide's efficacy.

Key words. Auditory hallucination, Delusion, Cognitive therapy, Guide for clients and their families

Introduction

We have developed a new cognitive therapy for auditory hallucinations and delusions, along with a guide intended to familiarize clients and their families with it. We published a report describing this therapy and published the accompanying guide in Japanese in 1997 [1,2]. Recently several cognitive therapies for auditory hallucinations and delusions have been developed, but as far as we know, our guide is among the first to describe the content of the cognitive therapy for auditory hallucinations and delusions for clients and their families.

The title of the guide is "A Guide to Coping with Voices of Unknown Origin—10 Items Containing Useful Information on the Treatment of Voices of Unknown Origin." The guide consists of a preface, 10 chapters, and a postscript. The titles of the 10 chapters are shown in Table 1.

Department of Psychiatry, Mie University Faculty of Medicine, 2-174 Edobashi, Tsu 514-8507, Japan

TABLE 1. Titles of the chapters in "A Guide to Coping with Voices of Unknown Origin"

1. Four factors that produce voices of unknown origin: anxiety, isolation, exhaustion, and insomnia
2. The psychiatric term "voices of unknown origin" (auditory hallucination) and their various types
3. The individual's own thoughts as the contents of the speech in auditory hallucinations
4. The negative influences auditory hallucinations have on a person (1): Hallucinations create inner conflicts and produce various types of misunderstandings. They might also incite the fear that a person's private experiences and thoughts are known publicly, or that one's thoughts and feelings are transmitted directly to specific others
5. The negative influences auditory hallucinations have on a person (2): Commonplace happenings by chance seem to be vitally concerned with a person
6. Essential methods for treating auditory hallucinations
7. Essential precautions in daily life to reduce auditory hallucinations
8. The effectiveness of medicine to treat auditory hallucinations
9. An accurate and useful understanding of auditory hallucinations to aid in to coping with them (The contents of the voices in auditory hallucinations are produced by an individual's own thoughts under the influence of the four factors. Neither the voices in auditory hallucinations nor the unknown strange person who produces the voices is real)
10. A constructive attitude toward the voices in auditory hallucinations (not to act on the voices and to try to disregard them)

We employ this guide as a teaching aid in psychoeducational therapy sessions for clients and their families. The guide has the advantage of being easily and quickly readable (in approximately 20 minutes), contains accurate and useful information to assist clients in coping with psychotic symptoms, and enables them to pursue appropriate assistance.

In this paper, we first describe a portion of the guide, namely chapters 1, 4, and 10. We then show the results of a questionnaire administered to clients and their families as an index of the guide's efficacy.

Contents of the Guide (Chapters 1, 4, and 10)

Chapter 1: Four Factors That Produce Voices of Unknown Origin: Anxiety, Isolation, Exhaustion, and Insomnia

When anxiety, isolation, exhaustion, and insomnia simultaneously exist in one's life over a period of time, one may hear voices of unknown origin. The experience of hearing voices of unknown origin under such conditions is not a rare phenomenon, but actually, a rather common one. For example, when being treated in a germ-free room or involved in a marine or mountain accident, a person may become very anxious, isolated, and exhausted.

As an example, let us consider patients with leukemia. Immunity is severely weakened in patients with leukemia both by the disease itself and by the drug treatment. Therefore, in some cases, patients have to be quarantined in a germ-free room for long periods to prevent lethal infections. While in the germ-free room, patients often experience at least one of the above four factors at the same time. That is to say, they might experience anxiety (e.g., "My disease is severe. Can I survive this?"), isolation (no one other than the patient himself can enter the room, as a rule), exhaustion (the patient may be completely exhausted both mentally and physically due not only to the disease itself but also to drug side effects, such as nausea and anemia), and insomnia (the patient would suffer from insomnia in a germ-free room due to anxiety, drug side effects, and lack of exercise). Even a patient who has never been mentally disturbed before the treatment may hear voices of unknown origin if the treatment in a germ-free room lasts for more than a week.

Another example of hearing strange voices can be found in notes written by victims of marine and mountain accidents. Those who have these accidents probably experience all four factors (anxiety, isolation, exhaustion, and insomnia) and, after a few days, might hear voices of a rescue party ("We have come here to save you") or pessimistic voices ("It's all over now"). Anyone may hear voices of unknown origin under conditions that produce some combination of the four factors.

Although the experience of hearing voices of unknown origin is not rare, it is true that the experience is rather dangerous to mental health. Those who hear voices of unknown origin may become mentally confused if they do not receive appropriate treatment. It is important to emphasize to these persons, however, that they should not be overly pessimistic regarding their condition, since recovery is fully possible with appropriate psychiatric treatment.

Because we have cited rather exceptional situations, such as treatment in a germ-free room or marine and mountain accidents, one might doubt whether there are situations simultaneously producing the four factors in daily life. In fact, there are many situations in which this may occur, for example, during important life events, such as an entrance examination, entrance into school, graduation from school, studying abroad, independence from family, falling in love, disappointed love, marriage, divorce, troubles in human relations, getting a job, transfer, promotion, change of job, unemployment, and so on. Anxiety, isolation, exhaustion, and insomnia may simultaneously arise under these situations for the following reasons: 1 one could become very busy and tired; 2 a radical changes in daily life would occur; 3 a person is often challenged by new work or encounters work that he or she is not good at; 4 a person would worry about various matters and would have to endure them; 5 one might have to take full responsibility for difficult situations.

To add to these matters, there are various stressful experiences in modern life. In general, the bonds between people tend to be weaker nowadays than in the past, as the nuclear family has become more common and human relations within communities have become increasingly estranged. Therefore, even in our daily life, we might experience situations that are in effect as extreme as treatment in a germ-free room or a marine or mountain accident, and that could produce the four factors.

It is well known that the first instance of hearing voices of unknown origin often occurs in youth, from the middle teens to the late twenties. The reason why young people are most likely to hear strange voices is that they have to confront and settle many critical issues that can produce anxiety, isolation, exhaustion, and insomnia. Young people have to complete many important tasks, such as taking entrance examinations and finding a job. They may have inferiority complexes regarding their looks, character, or school records. They may also have difficult love affairs or be disappointed in love. They may be shocked by their failures due to their lack of experience. They might be living on their own for the first time. Youth is one of the most dangerous periods because it can simultaneously produce the four risk factors for hearing voices of unknown origin. It is therefore especially important for young people and their families to have accurate information regarding this psychiatric condition.

Chapter 4: The Negative Influences Auditory Hallucinations Have on a Person

Hallucinations create inner conflicts and produce various types of misunderstandings. They might also incite the fear that a person's private experiences and thoughts are known publicly, or that one's thoughts and feelings are transmitted directly to specific others. Assuming that the voices in auditory hallucinations are real creates various types of misunderstandings and serious confusion, which in turn create pain and inconvenience in daily life. First, the person feels strange because he or she hears voices of unknown origin, although there is no one close by who is speaking. One might mistake the voices for telepathy, revelation, or radio waves.

People often hear someone saying bad things about them in auditory hallucinations, because in many cases, the contents of the voices express one's own feelings of regret or have to do with self-blame. Therefore, if one considers the voices in auditory hallucinations as real, one might grow irritable or become angry.

The contents of voices in auditory hallucinations are often absurd or illogical, as are dreams, which are also composed of one's own thoughts and frequently make little apparent sense. As a result, thinking the voices in auditory hallucinations are true might create gross misunderstandings. One might behave in a peculiar or even dangerous way because one might believe and obey the directions of the voices in auditory hallucinations.

In auditory hallucinations, one might hear many strangers, who actually exist, talking about one's private affairs, and if one thinks the voices are real, it is natural for one to consider that many people, including many total strangers, are actually talking about him or her, and that one's private affairs are known to the world.

As mentioned earlier, one might experience auditory hallucinations together with the real sounds of television or radio (functional hallucination), and if one takes the voices in functional hallucinations for real ones, the following gross misunderstandings would naturally arise. "My private affairs are broadcast on TV! (or on the radio!)." "The multiplex broadcast is on the air! The usual programs and the special programs are on the air at the same time! The special programs deal exclusively with my private affairs!" One might even go to the broadcast station and ask the staff to stop broadcasting programs revealing his or her private affairs.

However, in some cases, what the voices in auditory hallucinations say to the individual could be partially true, and one might perceive the voices reacting to changes in one's thinking instantly and accurately, since the voices are manufactured from the individual's own thoughts. One might also hear the voices at times that may be considered appropriate, again due to the voices' interior sources. In another case, as mentioned before, one might feel as if one was chatting with someone in auditory hallucinations, and the reason why one might feel so is the same, too. If one has these experiences and misunderstands them, one might experience the fear that his or her thoughts are revealed directly to the unknown person who participates in hallucinated conversations, and who in turn sees into the individual's mind to his or her pure thoughts.

When one experiences the fear that one is directly transmitting one's thoughts to unknown persons, it is natural for one to consider the reason why he or she is in such an extraordinary and terrible condition. One might construe the following reasons: "My mind is being tapped, or they must keep watch on me thoroughly and systematically." "They might read my emotions by telepathy or by supernatural power." "They might be using me as a subject for an experiment on human beings and might be operating a new machine that can read and interfere with my mind directly." In a case such as this, one might imagine a new machine that can control other people's brain waves.

If an individual fears that he or she is directly transmitting thoughts to others, he or she might be concerned that secret thoughts or feelings that should be concealed are accessible to others. For example, one might feel annoyed when he or she has a bad feeling toward a particular person or a secret affection for someone. In this case, one might feel annoyed and terribly confused because one thinks these secret feelings would be directly transmitted to such a person.

An individual would feel that one could never hide one's innermost feelings and private thoughts from unknown, unusual persons if the individual assumes that he or she is directly transmitting thoughts to others. It is understandable that living under such conditions would be very painful, and that one could never relax while in this state of mind. A recovered client said that it was a terrific pain for him to feel that he had been directly transmitting his thoughts and feelings to others and had been deeply disgraced in public. The fear that one might be unintentionally revealing one's self to others is one of the most serious and dangerous influences produced by auditory hallucinations.

Chapter 10: A Constructive Attitude Toward the Voices in Auditory Hallucinations (Not to Act on the Voices and to Try to Disregard Them)

In order to reduce the negative influences of the voices in auditory hallucinations, one would be better off not taking them seriously and trying to ignore them. If one can take this desirable attitude, both inner conflicts and misunderstandings produced by the voices would decrease. On the contrary, if one takes the contents of the voices in auditory hallucinations seriously, gets angry at them, or argues with the unknown strange person who produces the voices, inner conflicts and misunderstandings may increase, the frequency of hearing the voices may also increase, and the contents of the voices may escalate. Conflicts will often intensify if the persons concerned get angry and excited; on the other hand, conflicts will often be settled if the persons concerned keep their composure.

A client said, "If I stop thinking, I hear the voice saying, 'How unkind you are!' and then the voice stops." This phenomenon seems to be reasonable, because the voices in auditory hallucinations are produced by the person's own thoughts. Another client said, "When the voices appear, I try to ignore them and make it a rule to listen to my favorite music. Then the voices will disappear unnoticed." Another client said, "I try not to pay attention to the voices and ignore the directions of the voices. Then the voices will fade away." As is clear from these examples, if one has an accurate and useful understanding of the voices in auditory hallucinations and takes a desirable attitude toward them, the negative influences of auditory hallucinations will decrease considerably.

Though we have explained how to take a desirable attitude toward the voices in auditory hallucinations and how to cope with them (not to take the voices seriously and to ignore them), some readers may wonder whether they might mistake actual voices for the voices in auditory hallucinations and whether complications might occur due to this error. To reduce this worry, it may be useful for a person to take the voices seriously only on the following two occasions: when one can see the person who speaks, and the person is speaking directly to one's face (if a person has some business with another person, he or she would speak directly to the person's face in most cases); when some other person (e.g., a family member, a friend, or a member of the psychiatric staff) says he or she can also hear the voices.

Some readers may also wonder whether they may injure the unknown person's feelings by ignoring the voices. However, the voices in auditory hallucinations are produced by the person's own thoughts, and the unknown person who produces them is not real. Therefore, even if one ignores the voices, one never injures an existing person's feelings. If one can ignore the voices, one can ease one's own exhausted mind and brain and can take care of oneself.

In addition, some readers may think that they can know themselves better by taking the contents of the voices seriously and examining them thoroughly, since the voices are produced by their own thoughts. But this way of thinking is incorrect. Let us take a dream as an example. The contents of a dream are also made up of the person's own thoughts and feelings, and one neither takes the contents of a dream seriously nor examines them thoroughly. To do such a thing would be both ineffective and nonsensical. In the same way, one would be better off not taking the contents of the voices in auditory hallucinations seriously and ignoring them.

In some cases, the voices in auditory hallucinations will begin when one tries to hear what the unknown person will say on such an occasion. In other cases, the voices will begin when one speaks to the unknown person who produces them. (We could say that this phenomenon seems to be a particular type of inner dialogue in which the individual plays a double role.) It is advisable not to wait for the voice to appear, and not to speak to the unknown person.

TABLE 2. Results of a questionnaire to clients and their families

Q: Could you understand the contents of the guide?
A: "Understandable": More than 90% of both clients and families
Q: Did you find this guide useful?
A: "Found useful": 100% of both clients and families

Clients: $n = 50$; families: $n = 30$

It is important to understand and practice the following three behaviors: do not take the contents of the voices in auditory hallucinations seriously and try to ignore them; acquire some ways to cope with them; do not wait for the voice to appear, and do not speak to the unknown person.

Results of a Questionnaire

We administered a questionnaire to clients and their families as an index of the guide's efficacy. In this preliminary inquiry, we asked clients with schizophrenia and their families to respond to the items contained in the questionnaire on condition of it being returned without their signature and sent by mail. Fifty clients and 30 families were surveyed. One hundred percent of the questionnaires were returned.

Table 2 shows a portion of the results. More than 90% of the clients and their families responded positively to the item "The guide is understandable." All clients and their families agreed that "the guide is useful."

This survey was preliminary, and we cannot rely on these figures alone, but these results suggest the efficacy of our new cognitive therapy and the guide. We are going to carry our investigation forward to determine the efficacy and limitations of the therapy.

References

1. Harada S, Kikkawa T, Okazaki Y, et al (1997) A new cognitive and psychoeducational therapy for auditory hallucinations (1); A pamphlet for psychotic patients and their families about how to cope with auditory hallucinations (in Japanese). Seishin Igaku 39:363–370
2. Harada S, Okazaki Y, Kikkawa T, et al (1997) A new cognitive and psychoeducational therapy for auditory hallucinations (2); A practical method for using the pamphlet, and the results of a questionnaire to patients and their families concerning the pamphlet (in Japanese). Seishin Igaku 39:529–537

Treating Anxiety Disorders in Schizophrenia: How to Tailor Optimal Treatment in Clinical Practice

Marco Lussetti

Summary. In everyday clinical practice, when the patient's psychotic symptoms are reasonably under control, the clinician's challenge is to deal with concomitant psychopathology and psychosocial problems in the most appropriate way. Anxiety disorders can be diagnosed in up to 43% of patients with a diagnosis of schizophrenia and may considerably influence the quality of life of the patient and the carers and the prognosis of the psychotic disorder. A cognitive-behavioral approach based on psychoeducation and using the appropriate strategies (e.g., slow breathing and gradual exposure for panic disorder and agoraphobia, problem solving for general anxiety) can be sufficient to control the anxiety disorder without adding new medications. The clinical improvement of anxiety can lower the general level of stress and often leads to better control of the psychotic disorder and a decrease in disabilities, and can foster the collaborative alliance with the patient and the carers. A module on anxiety disorders for patients and their carers can be easily integrated into the clinical management of schizophrenia. Four clinical vignettes will illustrate specific issues, such as the diagnostic approach, integrating the intervention on anxiety with the treatment of schizophrenia, and "dosing" the approach to individual needs.

Key words. Schizophrenia, Anxiety disorders, Comorbidity, Cognitive-behavioral therapy, Integrated care

Introduction

Anxiety disorders are often associated with schizophrenia. Obsessive-compulsive disorders occur in 7.5% to 29.7% [1,2] and panic disorder occurs in 10.8% to 37% [2,3] of patients with schizophrenia. Anxiety disorders can worsen the prognosis of psychosis [4,5] and increase the risk of suicide and postpsychotic depression [6]. For the patient, the subjective feeling of anxiety may often be as important as the psychotic symptoms [7] and can require a similar therapeutic investment of resources [8]. Despite the extent of the problem and the availability of evidence-based effective treatments for anxiety disorders (see, for example, Roth and Fonagy [9]), there are

Centro di Salute Mentale, A.S.L. n. 9 di Grosseto, Via Cimabue 109, 58100 Grosseto, Italy surprisingly few articles in the literature on the treatment of anxiety disorders in schizophrenia.

Regarding panic disorder, for example, Sandberg and Siris [10] reached an improvement in panic and psychotic symptoms by adding alprazolam to fluphenazine. In a more recent paper, Arlow et al. [11] used a cognitive-behavioral approach to treat panic attacks in an open clinical trial on eight patients with a DSM-III diagnosis of schizophrenia and panic disorder. Anxiety disorders in schizophrenia are also receiving little attention in clinical practice: Cosoff and Hafner [1] found an overall prevalence of 43% for anxiety disorder in a cohort of 100 patients with a *Diagnostic and Statistical Manual of Mental Disorders*, 3rd edition, revised (DSM-III-R) diagnosis of schizophrenia or schizoaffective disorder, but "almost none of those with anxiety disorders were being treated for them." For Bermanzhohn [12], psychiatrists do not really listen to the patients they treat, and they see schizophrenics, rather than individuals affected by schizophrenia. This is partly due to a hierarchical system of classifying mental disorders linked with the tendency to treat only the acute (i.e., inpatient) phase of schizophrenia.

The new cognitive-behavioral approaches to schizophrenia help to fill the gap by promoting an individualized approach that is based on a shared model of illness [7]; it is problem-oriented and uses different therapeutic modules to address each patient's needs.

In Italy the old psychiatric system centered on asylums was questioned scientifically and politically in the 60s and 70s. In 1978 a law forbade new admissions to mental hospitals and promoted a pioneer policy of community care [13]. The big discrepancy between a rich experience in community practice and university psychiatric departments, which were mostly biologically or psychoanalytically oriented [14], has not promoted a proper codification in procedures and evaluation of such policies. On the other hand, psychiatrists and psychologists working in the community mental health services have been detached from new cognitive-behavioral therapies, which could have been a valuable technical support for the treatment of severe mental disorders in the community. Professor Pier Luigi Morosini at the Italian National Institute of Health, working in close collaboration with regional health authorities and single services, promoted several workshops on evidence-based treatments throughout the 90s, narrowing the distance between routine clinical practice and formal research. Practical manuals and psychoeducational materials have been translated into Italian as working guides for patients [15,16], and some of them have been published [17,18].

A new interest in how to treat associated syndromes has been promoted in the Italian context of intensive community care and long-term follow-up of psychotic patients. In this article, special attention is paid to a practical problem, how to "grade" the intervention according to the relative importance of psychotic and anxiety symptoms.

Treatment of Anxiety Disorders

Evaluation of Anxiety Symptoms

The first important step is to recognize the anxiety problems and to encourage the patient to describe his or her problems, using, if necessary, some simple probing questions that may help to elicit common anxiety symptoms. In this first exploratory phase, it is important to rule out the eventuality that anxiety is secondary to practical problems or to psychosis. Using active listening, that is, paying attention to what the patient says, showing interest in what he or she is saying, and asking clarifying questions [7,19], will help to sort out practical problems (for example, difficulties in reassuming a role of greater responsibility in his or her life) that are the base of the patient's anxiety. Clarifying the problem and working towards its resolution in a structured way (problem solving [19]) is usually the best way to help the patient in this case.

If the anxiety is not clearly caused by any life events, it is worth exploring any possible connection with the psychosis. A good starting point is to review with the patient and, whenever possible, with the persons closest to the patient (the support group) the patient's symptoms of psychosis and to ask if there is any relation with the anxiety symptoms previously described.

When anxiety does not seems to be correlated with life events or psychosis, a structured interview such as *Structured Clinical Interview for DSM-IV Axis I Disorders* (SCID)-I [20] is needed to properly assess the presence of anxiety disorders.

Specific Interventions

If anxiety is secondary to specific problems or to psychosis, the focus of intervention will be on resolution of the problems through problem analysis and problem solving or by reviewing the treatment of psychosis. Simple techniques, such as progressive muscle relaxation or slow breathing [15], may help the process, and in this case psychoeducation is rarely necessary. On the other hand, specific techniques are probably the best way to deal with primary anxiety symptoms or disorders. Whenever possible, the patient's support group should be included in the psychoeducational and therapeutic phase to assist the patient and to encourage adherence to treatment. The first step will be to help the patient to distinguish anxiety symptoms from stress or exacerbation of psychosis, using the Socratic method [7] and encouraging the patient and the support group to integrate the information offered by the clinician with their personal experience of the disorder. Clinical information should include a definition of the disorder, the mechanisms of symptom formation and maintenance, the main treatments, and how to prevent relapses after the end of the specific treatment [15]. Because the stress due to an anxiety disorder may trigger a psychotic exacerbation and vice versa, in discussing with the patient and the support group special attention should be paid to the connections of the two disorders in their own experience. An individual treatment plan is to be worked out for every patient, using evidence-based techniques to address specific problems when available. Even if there are interesting packages with comprehensive patients' manuals [15], these are rarely necessary, because often most of the cognitive-behavioral frame of treatment has been used already to deal with the psychosis. Furthermore, the treatment of psychosis is usually rather demanding for both the patient and the therapist, and additional efforts should be kept to the minimum.

Four short clinical vignettes will outline how to integrate specific interventions on different associations of anxiety and psychotic symptoms.

Illustrative Case Vignettes

First Case. Sue: Severe Delusions with Panic Attacks and Lower Back Pain due to Muscular Tension

Sue is 23 years old. She had been admitted to the psychiatric ward in the General Hospital with frightening delusions of being threatened by her family with black magic. The "proofs" are the chuckles and knowing looks which the other members of the family are exchanging among themselves. After she was discharged from the ward, a reduction of an excessively high dose of risperidone ameliorated a mild anxiety with akathisia. The treatment began with two sessions of psychoeducation on schizophrenia, which were followed by training of the whole family in communication skills [19]. Working on these skills helped Sue to challenge some of her misinterpretations, with an evident reduction of delusions. In a following session, Sue complained of bad lower back pain due to muscular tension. Progressive muscular relaxation [21] followed a brief explanation of the fight-flight response and of the connection between prolonged muscular tension and back pain. In this technique, all the principal groups of muscles are tensed and then relaxed. The exercise is done together with the rest of the family. Sue was invited to repeat the exercise at least once a day with the supervision of her sister, and each time she felt pain in her back. The following week, Sue suffered from an episode of acute anxiety not due to her delusions. The symptoms fulfilled the *Diagnostic and Statistical Manual of Mental Disorders*, 4th edition (DSM-IV) [22] criteria for panic attack. Treatment for this started by giving basic information about the role of hyperventilation and other factors in panic attacks. By the end of the session, slow breathing [15] was taught and practiced during the family meeting. The instructions are rather simple: "Breathe through the nose, using your belly . . . slowly . . . three seconds in . . . and three seconds out." Progressive muscular relaxation and slow breathing were done at home with the support of Sue's sister. At the beginning of each of the following sessions, these techniques were briefly reviewed with the clinician. No new panic attack was reported, and the back pain subsided. The treatment of psychosis was resumed in an atmosphere of improved optimism.

Second Case. Tom: Schizophrenia, Panic Disorder, and Obsessive-Compulsive Disorder

Tom is 34 years old. He had his first episode at 20 while serving in the army. In the last 12 months, he has had several admissions to the psychiatric ward, totaling more than 7 months of hospitalization. He believes that aliens are trying to kidnap him to steal a chip with military intelligence inside his brain. Following the integrated approach for schizophrenia with him and his family (psychoeducation, communication skill training, and problem solving [17]), he recovered from the psychotic symptoms and began to go out again with his friends. One night at the cinema, he felt that other people from the audience were watching him, had a panic attack, and felt obliged to rush home. In the same week he had two more panic attacks. The third attack came out of the blue, and he was frightened that he had lost all control of his anxiety. He took 100 drops of diazepam and phoned his psychiatrist to communicate his decision not to leave his house for the next 5 years. A crisis session was held at home with the family on the same day. Information on panic disorder was shared, and slow breathing and progressive muscular relaxation [16] were taught in the first two sessions. In 5 days, Tom reached some control over his panic and started to go out again. Using problem analysis [19], Tom recognized the main factors related to his phobia: being in a crowded place where it is difficult or embarrassing to escape; a dim light ("it is difficult to understand if the others are watching me"); being alone and not being able to rush home. He felt safer when he had some benzodiazepine with him and could thoroughly plan what to do in case of panic. With this information, a program of gradual exposure [15] was built up with the help of the family. With a friend, he started to watch people playing tennis, and within a couple of weeks he was again able to go to the cinema alone.

His rehabilitation program was interrupted again by obsessive-compulsive symptoms. Tom was afraid of becoming bald and spent most of the day controlling his hair in any reflective surface. He "saw" many "patches," which he tried to cover by continuously combing his hair. Information on the disorder was again shared with the family. Through the use of problem solving [19], Tom decided to limit looking at himself in the mirror to no more than three times a day. Anxiety dropped quickly, and for the second time the rehabilitation program could be resumed.

Third Case. Paola: Brief Psychotic Episode and Generalized Anxiety

Paola was admitted for the first time to the psychiatric ward of the General Hospital when she was 27 years old in a severe delusional state. She had lost her job a few months earlier, and she was more tense than usual. The psychotic symptoms abated quickly, and soon she refused any psychiatric follow-up. After one year, a few weeks before her marriage, her anxiety increased and she had a new psychotic episode: she was confused and afraid of being kidnapped by the police. With the help of the family, she was "hospitalized at home" [17]. In a few days, the psychotic symptoms waned. A model of the disorder was built with the patient [18]. She realized that she was a rather nervous person and that she began to feel anxious when she had problems she was not able to deal with. The anxiety grew, and in a few months, without any clear reason, she had a psychotic breakdown. The treatment plan was aimed to improve communication within her support group (her family and her future husband) and to train them in the six steps of problem solving [19]: to single out the goal or problem and describe it in a concrete operational way, to find five or six different solutions through brainstorming, to highlight the pros and cons of each solution, to choose the most functional solution, to devise a proper plan to carry it out, and to review the results. Paola and her support group started with simple tasks (household chores) to gradually arrive at dealing with the major changes in her life brought on by her marriage.

In building the vulnerability model of psychosis, a subjective stress scale has been devised [17]. The anchor points were chosen: 0 on the scale was how she felt last year when she was on holidays, 10 was the maximum of stress during the acute psychotic episode, and 5 was the stress she felt immediately after losing her job. Looking back on her experience, she noticed that more than two consecutive weeks with a score of over 5 or any stress rated 8 or above made a problem-solving session with her support group necessary.

Fourth Case. Ann: Panic Disorder with Agoraphobia, Obsessive-Compulsive Symptoms, Auditory Hallucinations, and Ideas of Reference

Ann came to the Community Center with her mother. At 22 years of age, she was suffering from panic disorder with severe agoraphobia: she was not able to leave her house unaccompanied. Before going out, she had to spend more than 2 hours to get herself ready. Two years earlier, she had dropped out of school. During the last week, she had the feeling that people on the street were watching her and criticizing her. On two or three occasions, when the tension was high, she heard a "voice" calling her. Furthermore, her relationship with her parents was very tense. Because she presented with more than one problem, after the assessment she decided to start working with the panic and agoraphobia problems. Ample time was given to psychoeducation and specific techniques (slow breathing, progressive muscular relaxation, gradual exposure, and cognitive restructuring) [15]. She asked the therapist not to involve her family. A friend was chosen instead for support. After three sessions, she was able to travel to the center by bus unaccompanied. Ann was able to use the techniques learned to overcome her agoraphobia for her compulsive symptoms. Hallucinations and the ideas of reference disappeared as the stress related to anxiety disorder was resolved. Ann improved her relationship with her parents and started studying again.

Conclusions

Treating schizophrenia is still a big challenge. There are two approaches: specialized programs, like the EPPIC unit in Melbourne [23], which mainly treats early psychosis; or organizations that treat all mental health problems. The one in Buckingham described by Ian Falloon [24] is an example of this. Apart from the various approaches discussed, the best treatment depends on a balance between two extremes: focusing on the illness but losing the person suffering from the illness, and being close to the sufferer on a human level but not applying the most efficient therapeutic tools available.

In everyday clinical practice, the psychiatrist is often asked to deal with problems that still lack scientific evidence. An example of this is anxiety disorders in schizophrenia. The method proposed in this article assumes a certain strategy. The treating clinician focuses on the patient and his or her support group, spending most of the time training and assisting them in their effort to communicate better and to solve their problems. When a more specific problem arises, the clinician will shift the focus to more technical resources, offering the patient and the support group information about the disorder and helping them to implement any valid treatment available for that specific problem. The patient will maintain a central role in setting priorities and deciding the program of treatment. Whenever possible, clinicians will make the most of resources already present in the patient and in the support group, and the introduction of new techniques will be kept to a minimum. In order to do this, it is advisable to use a unique frame of treatment for every disorder (see, for example, Falloon [25] and World Health Organization [26]) and to have materials prepared for different degrees of complexity. As illustrated in the vignettes, a symptom of anxiety will require a simpler intervention (and simpler educational materials) than full-blown anxiety disorder. Staff will need proper training in which they are taught to use simple techniques in a flexible way, respecting the patient and the support group. Furthermore, proper research should be carried out to test the clinical hypothesis proposed here.

References

1. Cosoff SJ, Hafner RJ (1998) The prevalence of comorbid anxiety in schizophrenia, schizoaffective disorder and bipolar disorder. Aust NZ J Psychiat 32:67–72
2. Bermanzhohn PC, Porto L, Siris SG (1997) Associated psychiatric syndromes (APS) in chronic schizophrenia: possible clinical significance. Paper presented at the XXVII Congress of the European Association for Behavioral and Cognitive Therapies, Venice, Italy, 24–27 September 1997
3. Argyle N (1990) Panic attacks in chronic schizophrenia. Br J Psychiat 157:430–433
4. Fenton WS, McGlashen TH (1986) The prognostic significance of obsessive-compulsive symptoms in schizophrenia. Am J Psychiat 143:437–441
5. Cassano GB, Pini S, Saettoni M, et al (1998) Occurrence and clinical correlates of psychiatric comorbidity in patients with psychotic disorders. J Clin Psychiat 59: 60–68
6. Siris SG, Mason SE, Shuwall MA (1993) Histories of substance abuse, panic and suicidal ideation in schizophrenic patients with histories of post-psychotic depressions. Prog Neuropsychopharmacol Biol Psychiat 17:609–617
7. Fowler DG, Garety P, Kuipers E (1995) Cognitive behaviour therapy for psychosis: psychotherapy for psychosis. Wiley, Chichester, UK
8. Falloon IRH, Boyd JL, McGill CW (1985) Clinical outcome: exacerbations, symptom patterns, and community tenure. In: Falloon IRH et al. Family management of schizophrenia. A study of clinical, social, family, and economic benefit. Johns Hopkins University Press, Baltimore and London
9. Roth A, Fonagy P (1996) What works for whom? A critical review of psychotherapy research. Guilford Press, New York
10. Sandberg L, Siris SG (1987) "Panic disorder" in schizophrenia. J Nerv Ment Dis 175:627–628
11. Arlow PB, Moran ME, Bermanzohn PC, et al (1997) Cognitive-behavioral treatment of panic attacks in chronic schizophrenia. J Psychother Pract Res 6:145–150
12. Bermanzohn PC, Porto L, Siris SG (1997) Schizophrenia and hierarchical diagnosis: a clinical study and some clinical implications. Paper presented at the XXVII Congress of the European Association for Behavioral and Cognitive Therapies, Venice, Italy, 24–27 September 1997
13. Ghirardelli R, Lussetti M (1993) Italy. In: Kemp DR (ed) International handbook on mental health policy. Greenwood Press, Westport, USA
14. Morosini PL (2000) Evaluation of psychological intervention in Italy. Keio J Med Suppl 2, 49:A32
15. Andrews G, Crino R, Hunt C, et al (1994) The treatment of anxiety disorders. Clinician's guide and patient manuals. Cambridge University Press, Cambridge, UK
16. Hunt C, Falloon IRH. What is anxiety? Mimeograph
17. Falloon, et al (1994) Intervento integrato in psichiatria. Erickson, Trento, Italy
18. Fowler D, Garety P, Kuipers E (1998) Terapia cognitivo-comportamentale delle psicosi. Teoria e pratica. Masson, Milan, Italy
19. Falloon IRH, Laporta M, Fadden G, et al (1993) Managing stress in families: cognitive and behavioral strategies for enhancing coping skills. Routledge, London

20. First MB, Spitzer RL, Gibbon M, et al (1997) Structured clinical interview for DSM-IV Axis I Disorders. Clinical version. Administration booklet. American Psychiatric Press, Washington, DC
21. Clark DM (1989) Anxiety states. Panic and generalized anxiety. In: Hawton K, Salkovskis PM, Kirk J et al (eds) Cognitive behaviour therapy for psychiatric problems. A practical guide. Oxford University Press, Oxford, UK
22. American Psychiatric Association (1994) Diagnostic and statistical manual of mental disorders, 4th edn. American Psychiatric Association, Washington, DC
23. Mc Gorry PD, Jackson HJ (1999) The recognition and management of early psychosis. A preventive approach. Cambridge University Press, Cambridge, UK
24. Falloon IRH, Fadden G (1993) Integrated mental health care. Cambridge University Press, Cambridge, UK
25. Falloon IRH (2000) Trattamento integrato per la salute mentale. Guida pratica per operatori e utenti. Parte seconda. Moduli educazionali. Ecomind Publications, Salerno, Italy
26. World Health Organization (1997) Management of mental disorders, 2nd edn. World Health Organization, Darlinghurst, NSW, Australia

Cognitive-Behavioral Treatment of Schizophrenia

NICHOLAS TARRIER, CHRISTINE BARROWCLOUGH,
and GILLIAN HADDOCK

Summary. This chapter aims to briefly summarize the background and evidence base for adjunct psychosocial treatments of schizophrenia, with special emphasis on the program of research carried out in Manchester. The research of family interventions and cognitive-behavioral therapy is outlined. It is concluded that there is good evidence for the efficacy of both family intervention and cognitive-behavioral therapy and that their use should become part of established practice in the management of patients suffering from schizophrenia.

Key words. Cognitive-behavior therapy, Coping, Schizophrenia, Non-drug treatment

Introduction

Since the early 1950s, neuroleptic medication has been the mainstay of treatment for schizophrenia, in terms of both symptom reduction and relapse prevention. However, such medication has numerous disadvantages, compliance is often poor, patients experience unpleasant side effects, residual and treatment-resistant symptoms are frequent, and relapse is common. In spite of the introduction of the atypical neuroleptics and the claims made for their advantages, the improved benefits conferred by these drugs must be viewed with caution [1].

The relative failure of drug treatment to achieve anything other than partial management of schizophrenia has resulted in the investigation of nondrug treatments as an adjunct to medication. There have been two major developments in this area, family interventions and individual cognitive-behavioral therapy. There have been developments and evaluations in both these areas from the Clinical Psychology Research Group in Manchester, and we shall largely restrict ourselves to an account of this research, although that does not signify that similar developments have not taken place elsewhere. We will mainly focus on developments in individual cognitive-behavioral therapy, because this is a newer development and in its application to schizophrenia has originated almost solely from the United Kingdom.

Academic Division of Clinical Psychology, School of Psychiatry and Behavioural Sciences, University of Manchester, Withington Hospital, Manchester M20 8LR, UK

Family Interventions

Background

Studies in the 1960s and 1970s carried out in the United Kingdom demonstrated that the quality of the home environment that schizophrenic patients returned to after hospitalization was important in determining clinical outcome [2,3]. This environment could be quantified by a measure of Expressed Emotion (EE) that was derived from measuring the amount of criticism, hostility, and marked over-involvement in an audiotaped interview with the patient's key relative. A relative and also a household could be classified as either high or low on EE, depending on whether threshold scores for these three dimensions were reached or not [4]. Subsequent relapse was found to be significantly related to returning to live with a high-EE relative. Over the years, numerous studies from different countries and cultures have replicated this association of high EE and poor subsequent outcome [5,6].

Efficacy Trials

Family interventions were based on the finding that EE was associated with outcome and were developed to reduce the ambient stress in the home environment through reducing EE. A number of family intervention programs were developed and evaluated. There are consistent results from well-conducted clinical trials that problem-oriented, usually behavioral family interventions reduce relapse rates in high-risk families [7–9]. In Manchester a behavioral family intervention was devised that included education about schizophrenia and its treatment, stress management for relatives, and family goal planning [10]. The results from a randomized, controlled trial indicated that relapse rates in high-risk families who received the behavioral family intervention were significantly reduced at the end of the nine months post-discharge intervention period compared with an appropriate control group [11]. Significant reductions in relapse rates remained demonstrable at two-year follow-up [12] and even at five- and eight-year follow-ups [13].

Effectiveness Trials

A further study investigated whether family intervention would be effective in a routine health service rather a than research setting in which patients and their relatives were recruited as outpatients irrespective of their EE status and treated by a psychologist in collaboration with other mental health staff. Patients and their carers were randomly allocated to the family intervention and treatment as usual or treatment as usual alone. Relapses in the family intervention group were significantly lower (24%) than in the control group (46%), indicating that family interventions were effective and could be delivered routinely as part of a standard clinical service.

Individual Cognitive-Behavioral Therapy

Background

The version of cognitive-behavioral therapy used to treat schizophrenia developed in Manchester has been based on developing the patient's ability to cope with his or her symptoms. This was initially based on the observation that the majority of patients who experienced persistent hallucinations and delusions made active attempts to cope with their symptoms with at least some success [14]. This observation was in accord with other reports [15–19]. It was reasoned that since many patients used coping strategies naturalistically, they would further benefit from systematic training in coping skills, combined with an awareness of the antecedents and context of their symptoms. Further research indicated that patients' beliefs about their symptoms and their appraisal were important in determining whether and how they coped [20].

The use of coping strategies to treat the symptoms of psychotic disorders has developed over the last 10 to 15 years. The origin of this approach has also been influenced by a number of other sources. First, the way people deal with aversive experience and events has long been of interest in general psychology, and there is an extensive literature on such coping mechanisms [21]. Central to the idea of coping is the process of appraisal, whereby the person evaluates a set of circumstances or experience as a problem and attempts to cope and subsequently evaluates the success or otherwise of these attempts. Similarly important has been the related concept of self-efficacy [22].

Second, it has long been recognized that the use of personal resources such as coping strategies is important in buffering against psychotic decompensation, leading to exacerbations or relapse of positive psychotic symptoms. For example, in the model of stress-vulnerability of psychosis of Nuechterlein et al. [23], coping and self-efficacy are cited as important personal protective factors.

Third has been the influence of theoretical positions that have developed to underpin cognitive-behavioral therapy. The seminal paper by Kanfer and Saslow [24] advanced the position that clinical problems could best be understood by a detailed analysis of the contextual circumstances, the applied behavioral analysis of the antecedents and consequences of the defined problem, rather than psychiatric classification into diagnostic groups. The use of behavioral analysis of positive psychotic symptoms was central to the development of a case formulation on which coping interventions were based [25]. With the development of cognitive models of other disorders, mainly anxiety and affective disorders, the understanding of cognitive mechanisms and the inclusion of these in behavioral analysis has been advanced [26].

Fourth is the work on self-regulation of Kanfer and Karoly and others [27], in which a target behavior is identified as undesirable or inappropriate and monitored with the purpose of implementing alternative learned responses through a process of self-regulation. This approach has also been shown to be effective with schizophrenic patients [16]. Clearly, there is considerable overlap between coping and self-regulation. Further, self-regulation and coping may improve executive functioning by increasing control over basic processes such as attention, response inhibition, and response initiation.

Cognitive-Behavioral Therapy in Chronically Ill Patients

The original impetus to the development of cognitive-behavioral therapy was the frequently encountered problem that patients suffering from chronic schizophrenia had residual psychotic symptoms that did not respond further to medication.

Cognitive-behavioral therapy was developed as an adjunct treatment to medication to see whether these unpleasant and distressing symptoms could be reduced. A number of case studies suggested that this was a feasible approach (see Haddock et al. [28] for a review), and a research program was instigated to investigate this issue.

Preliminary Studies

A small, randomized, open controlled trial compared Coping Strategy Enhancement, a treatment based on improving coping skills, with problem-solving training in medicated patients suffering persistent positive symptoms [29]. The results indicated that both Coping Strategy Enhancement and problem-solving resulted in a significant decrease in positive symptoms as compared with a waiting list control period. There was some evidence that Coping Strategy Enhancement was superior to problem-solving in reducing symptoms, especially delusions and anxiety. Hallucinations and depression showed less improvement. In some patients there was an increase in depressed mood associated with improvements in positive symptoms, although this was not statistically significant. Thus the effect of cognitive-behavioral therapy on some types of symptoms in schizophrenic patients was unclear. Changes in measures of coping skills and problem-solving skills were also examined. The coping skills group showed significant increases both in the number of positive coping skills used and in their efficacy, whereas the problem-solving group showed a decrease in these measures during treatment. Both groups showed significant improvements in problem-solving skills. Improvements in coping but not problem-solving were significantly related to decreases in psychotic symptoms during treatment [30].

Larger Randomized, Controlled Trials

A second study, which recruited a geographical cohort rather than a convenience sample, investigated whether a combination of Coping Strategy Enhancement, problem-solving, and relapse prevention, as an adjunct to routine care including neuroleptic medication, would be efficacious when compared with supportive counseling and routine care, and routine care alone. Supportive counseling was used to control for therapy contact and social interaction and the nonspecific factors of such contact and to provide general emotional support. An intention-to-treat analysis indicated that, even when refusers and drop-outs were included in the analysis, cognitive-behavioral therapy was superior to supportive counseling, which in turn was superior to routine care alone in reducing positive symptoms. The significant differences, however, were mainly between cognitive-behavioral therapy and routine care alone, and there were some improvements in patients receiving supportive counseling. Analysis by logistic regression indicated that the receipt of cognitive-behavioral therapy resulted in almost eight times (odds ratio, 7.88) the chance of showing a 50% reduction in positive symptoms compared with receiving routine care alone [31]. In evidence-based medicine, the benchmark with which to judge treatments is the number of patients needed to treat (NNT) [32]. This is the number of patients that are required to be treated to result in one more successful outcome than the control or comparison treatment. When an improvement of 50% or more in positive symptoms was used as the outcome at post-treatment, the NNT for CBT over routine care was 5, for CBT over supportive counseling it was 6, and for supportive counseling over routine care it was 25. An NNT of 5 and 6 is a very positive benefit in these terms [32].

A more detailed analysis of the changes in different symptoms in an analysis-to-protocol, that is of patients who completed the treatment program, demonstrated that both delusions and hallucinations responded to cognitive-behavioral therapy [33]. There were indications that delusions generally responded better to treatment and that patients who experienced hallucinations alone, without secondary delusions, did not respond at all. Delusions also responded significantly to supportive counseling but hallucinations did not. Patients suffering persecutory delusions showed greater symptomatology at pretreatment but a greater change over treatment. Negative symptoms and thought disorder also showed improvement with cognitive-behavioral therapy, although affective symptoms and social functioning did not. Depression showed a modest positive correlation with changes in positive symptoms, and there was no indication that patients became depressed with the loss of their positive symptoms.

An investigation was made of why patients drop out of treatment [34]. The most common reason given was that the patients did not perceive the treatment as suitable for their problems. Patients who dropped out of treatment were more likely to be male, unemployed and unskilled, single, with a low level of educational attainment, and with low premorbid IQ. They had a lengthy duration of illness, although at the time of discontinuation they were not necessarily severely ill and they were able to function at a reasonable level. They suffered both hallucinations and delusions and were likely to be depressed and moderately hopeless. They were as likely as not to be paranoid, although not necessarily suspicious of the therapist.

Follow-up at one year after the end of treatment showed that the differences between those receiving cognitive-behavioral therapy and supportive counseling had decreased, but those receiving routine care alone were significantly worse on both positive and negative symptoms [35]. At two-year follow-up, a significantly greater number of patients who received routine care alone now showed a deterioration from baseline of over 20% [36]. Patients who received routine care alone had higher relapse rates and a shorter time to relapse over the 27-month treatment and follow-up period, although these differences did not reach significance.

Two other UK trials of cognitive-behavioral therapy in chronic schizophrenia have reported similar results. The London-East Anglia trial compared patients receiving cognitive-behavioral therapy and routine care with those receiving routine care alone in a three-center study. Routine care consisted of maintenance medication and case management. Sixty patients were randomly allocated into the study and treated over a nine-month period, receiving a mean of 18.6 individual sessions. Assessments were independent but not blinded to treatment allocation. At post-treatment, patients who received cognitive-behavioral therapy showed significant symptomatic improvements compared with the control group [37], and these improvements were maintained at nine months [38].

A second trial from the London-Newcastle group compared a group receiving cognitive therapy with a befriending control group in a two-center study. All patients received routine care, including maintenance medication and case management. Ninety patients were recruited into the study and treated over a nine-month period, receiving a mean of 19 individual sessions. Assessments were independent and blinded to treatment allocation, and treatment quality was assured through independent rating of audiotaped therapy sessions. Analysis was carried out on an intention-to-treat basis. At post-treatment there were significant improvements in both positive and negative symptoms but no difference between the two treatment groups. At nine-month follow-up significant differences emerged between the treatment groups, with the cognitive therapy group showing maintained improvement while the befriending group did not [39].

Acute Schizophrenia

Preliminary Studies

Although treating chronic schizophrenic patients with cognitive-behavioral therapy poses difficulties, treating the acutely ill patient raises a completely different set of clinical challenges. The first indication that this might be possible was a report published by the Birmingham group [40,41]. Patients admitted to an acute psychiatric ward were randomly allocated to either a cognitive-behavioral therapy treatment consisting of individual sessions, group sessions, family sessions, and activity scheduling, or a control treatment of recreational activities matched for therapist time. The receiving group cognitive-behavioral therapy had a significantly shorter time to recovery of symptoms (between 25% and 50%) and a reduced time spent in hospital (approximately 50%) compared with the control group. However, the study was limited by a number of methodological weaknesses: the evaluation was not independent or blind; the cognitive-behavioral therapy treatment consisted of a number of different elements; and the control treatment did not control for a number of the nonspecific aspects of therapy. These were encouraging results but need to be interpreted cautiously. A preliminary study was carried out in Manchester for two reasons: to see whether cognitive-behavioral therapy would be clinically feasible with these acutely ill patients and to ascertain whether the results reported by Drury et al. could be replicated with a sample of similar size but with independent and blind assessment, using only individual cognitive-behavioral therapy, and controlling for the nonspecific effects of therapy [42]. Twenty-one acutely ill hospitalized schizophrenic patients experiencing a recent onset episode were randomly allocated to either cognitive-behavioral therapy or supportive counseling. Although there were no significant differences between the two groups at post-treatment or two-year follow-up, the number of relapses was lower and the time to relapse was delayed in the cognitive-behavioral therapy group.

The SoCRATES Trial

A large, multisite, randomized, controlled trial was carried out to investigate whether cognitive-behavioral therapy delivered early to recent-onset schizophrenic patients would speed recovery and improve outcome [43]. This was called the SoCRATES trial (Study of Cognitive ReAlignment Therapy in Early Schizophrenia) and was funded by the Medical Research Council, UK. Patients with first-episode or early-onset (second episode within two years) schizophrenia from 11 hospitals across three sites (Manchester, Liverpool, and Nottinghamshire) were recruited into the trial and randomly allocated to one of three treatments: cognitive-behavioral therapy and treatment as usual, supportive counseling and treatment as usual, or treatment as usual alone. Four hundred fifty-three patients were screened, of whom 370 met eligibility criteria and 318 gave written informed consent to participate in the study after 10 were judged incapable of giving informed consent and 42 declined to consent. The study had two main aims: to investigate whether cognitive-behavioral therapy speeded recovery during the treatment phase and to investigate whether cognitive-behavioral therapy reduced relapse over the 18-month follow-up phase. At the time of writing, the follow-ups are just being completed, so no answer can yet be given to the second question. The evidence suggests that the first aim was achieved. Over the 50-day treatment period, the mean weekly changes in delusion scores were significantly greater in the cognitive-behavioral therapy group than in the groups receiving counseling or treatment as usual alone, and the mean weekly change in auditory hallucination score was greater in the cognitive-behavioral therapy than in the counseling group [43].

Dual Diagnosis Patients

Many studies have shown that the rate of substance abuse in patients with severe mental illness is high; this co-morbidity is often referred to as "dual diagnosis." The indications are that substance misuse, even at quite low levels, is a risk factor for serious illness complications, including suicide, poor compliance with treatment, more inpatient stays, violence, and poorer overall prognosis [44]. There has been little methodologically rigorous work on treating these patients, although opinion abounds. In Manchester a randomized, controlled trial of a psychosocial intervention program compared with treatment as usual was carried out [45]. The intervention program integrated motivational interviewing, a psychological intervention used in the substance abuse field [46,47], with the individual cognitive-behavioral therapy and family intervention developed for use with psychosis. Particular attention was given to the successful integration of these three interventions into a cohesive and coherent treatment program with a focus on the role of substance use in the onset and maintenance of psychotic symptoms. Patient and relative dyads were recruited into the trial, and from the 66 eligible, 36 were randomly allocated to the two treatment groups. Patients receiving the psychosocial intervention program showed significant improvements in clinical and symptom outcome at the end of treatment and at the three-month follow-up and reduced substance use. There were also indications of reduced carer burden in the relatives of this group [45].

Conclusions

There is accumulating evidence that psychosocial treatments have a beneficial effect on clinical outcomes, at least in the short to medium term. Such treatments are generally well received by patients and their carers and can have a significant impact on the burden of the disorder. The necessary skills are not always available, so that access to these types of treatment way well be quite limited, especially in locations where clinical psychologists are few in numbers. Training of mental health staff, especially psychiatric nurses, in the skills to disseminate these interventions has not necessarily been as easy or as successful as was once hoped for [48]. Planners of mental health services need to prioritize the training of those with psychological knowledge and treatment skills so that psychosocial interventions become more available and accessible to those suffering from schizophrenia and their carers.

Acknowledgments. The family intervention study [11], cognitive-behavioral therapy study [29,30], and dual diagnosis study [45] were funded by the Department of Health; the Manchester cognitive-behavioral therapy study [31] was funded by the Wellcome Trust; and the SoCRATES study was funded by the Medical Research Council.

References

1. NHS Centre for Reviews and Dissemination (1999) Drug treatment for schizophrenia. Effective Health Care 5:1–12
2. Brown GW, Birley JLT, Wing JK (1972) The influence of family life on the course of schizophrenic disorders: a replication. Br J Psychiatry 121:241–258
3. Vaughn CE, Leff JP (1976) The influence of family factors and social factors on the course of psychiatric illness: a comparison of schizophrenic and depressed neurotic patients. Br J Psychiatry 129:125–137
4. Leff JP, Vaughn CE (1985) Expressed emotion in families. Guilford, New York
5. Kavanagh D (1992) Recent developments in expressed emotion and schizophrenia. Br J Psychiatry 160:601–620
6. Butzlaff RL, Hooley JM (1998) Expressed emotion and psychiatric relapse: a meta analysis. Arch Gen Psychiatry 55:547–552
7. Mari JJ, Streiner DL (1994) An overview of family intervention and relapse on schizophrenia: meta analysis of research findings. Psychol Med 24:565–578
8. Penn DL, Mueser KT (1996) Research update on the psychosocial treatment of schizophrenia. Am J Psychiatry 153:607–617
9. Tarrier N (1996) A psychological approach to the management of schizophrenia. In: Moscarelli M, Sartorius N (eds) The economics of schizophrenia. Wiley, Chichester
10. Barrowclough C, Tarrier N (1992, reprinted 1997) Families of schizophrenic patients: a cognitive-behavioural intervention. Chapman & Hall, London
11. Tarrier N, Barrowclough C, Vaughn C, et al (1988) The community management of schizophrenia: a controlled trial of a behavioural intervention with families. Br J Psychiatry 153:532–542
12. Tarrier N, Barrowclough C, Vaughn C, et al (1989) The community management of schizophrenia: a controlled trial of a behavioural intervention with families: two year follow-up. Br J Psychiatry 154:625–628
13. Tarrier N, Barrowclough C, Porceddu K, et al (1994) The Salford Family Intervention project for schizophrenic relapse prevention: five and eight year accumulating relapses. Br J Psychiatry 165:829–832
14. Tarrier N (1987) An investigation of residual psychotic symptoms in discharged schizophrenic patients. Br J Clin Psychol 26:141–143
15. Falloon IRH, Talbot RE (1981) Persistent auditory hallucinations: coping mechanisms and implications for management. Psychol Med 11:329–339
16. Breier A, Strauss JS (1983) Self-control in psychotic disorders. Arch Gen Psychiatry 40:1141–1145
17. Cohen CI, Beck BS (1985) Personal coping styles of schizophrenic outpatients. Hosp Commun Psychiatry 36:407–410

18. Carr V (1988) Patient's techniques for coping with schizophrenia: an exploratory study. Br J Med Psychol 61:339–352
19. Romme M, Escher A (1989) Hearing voices. Schizophr Bull 15:209–216
20. Kinney CF (1999) Coping with schizophrenia: the significance of appraisal. Unpublished PhD thesis, Faculty of Medicine, University of Manchester
21. Zeidner M, Endler NS (1996) Handbook of coping: theory, research and applications. Wiley, Chichester
22. Bandura A (1977) Self-efficacy: towards a unifying theory of behavior change. Psychol Rev 84:191–215
23. Nuechterlein KH (1987) Vulnerability models: state of the art. In: Hafner H, Gattaz W, Jangerick W (eds) Searches for the cause of schizophrenia. Springer-Verlag, Berlin
24. Kanfer FH, Saslow G (1965) Behavioral analysis: an alternative to diagnostic classification. Arch Gen Psychiatry 12:529–538
25. Haddock G, Tarrier N (1998) Assessment and formulation in the cognitive behavioural treatment of psychosis. In: Tarrier N, Wells A, Haddock G (eds) Treating complex cases: the cognitive behavioural therapy approach. Wiley, Chichester
26. Lowe CF, Higson PJ (1981) Self-instructional training and cognitive behaviour modification: a behavioural analysis. In: Davey G (ed) Applications of conditioning theory. Methuen, London, pp 162–188
27. Karoly P, Kanfer FH (1982) Self-management and behaviour change: from theory to practice. Pergamon, New York
28. Haddock G, Tarrier N, Spaulding W, et al (1998) Individual cognitive-behaviour therapy in the treatment of schizophrenia: a review. Clin Psychol Rev 18:821–838
29. Tarrier N, Beckett R, Harwood S, et al (1993) A controlled trial of two cognitive behavioural methods of treating drug-resistant residual psychotic symptoms in schizophrenic patients: 1. Outcome. Br J Psychiatry 162:524–532
30. Tarrier N, Sharpe L, Beckett R, et al (1993) A controlled trial of two cognitive behavioural methods of treating drug-resistant residual psychotic symptoms in schizophrenic patients: II. Treatment specific changes in coping and problem solving. Soc Psychiatry Psychiatr Epidemiol 28:5–10
31. Tarrier N, Yusupoff L, Kinney C, et al (1998) A randomized controlled trial of intensive cognitive behaviour therapy for chronic schizophrenia. BMJ 317:303–307
32. Sackett D, Richardson WS, Rosenberg W, et al (1997) Evidence-based medicine. Churchill-Livingstone, Edinburgh
33. Tarrier N, Kinney C, McCarthy E, et al (2001) The cognitive-behavioural treatment of persistent symptoms in chronic schizophrenia: are some types of psychotic symptoms more responsive to cognitive-behaviour therapy? Behav Cogn Psychother 29:45–55
34. Tarrier N, Yusupoff L, McCarthy E, et al (1998) Some reasons why patients suffering from chronic schizophrenia fail to continue in psychological treatment. Behav Cogn Psychother 26:177–181
35. Tarrier N, Wittkowski A, Kinney C, et al (1999) The durability of the effects of cognitive behaviour therapy in the treatment of chronic schizophrenia: twelve months follow-up. Br J Psychiatry 174:500–504
36. Tarrier N, Kinney C, McCarthy E, et al (2000) Two year follow-up of cognitive behaviour therapy and supportive counseling in the treatment of persistent symptoms in chronic schizophrenia. J Consul Clin Psychol 68:917–922
37. Kuipers E, Garety P, Fowler D, et al (1997) The London-East Anglia randomized controlled trial of cognitive-behaviour therapy for psychosis. Br J Psychiatry 171:319–325
38. Kuipers E, Fowler D, Garety P, et al (1998) London-East Anglia randomized controlled trial of cognitive-behavioural therapy for psychosis. III: Follow-up and economic evaluation. Br J Psychiatry 173:61–69
39. Sensky T, Turkington D, Kingdon D, et al (2000) Cognitive-behavioural treatment for persistent symptoms in schizophrenia. Arch Gen Psychiatry 57:165–173

40. Drury V, Birchwood M, Cochrane R, et al (1996) Cognitive therapy and recovery from acute psychosis: I. Impact on psychotic symptoms. Br J Psychiatry 169:593–601
41. Drury V, Birchwood M, Cochrane R, et al (1996) Cognitive therapy and recovery from acute psychosis: I. Impact on recovery time. Br J Psychiatry 169:602–607
42. Haddock G, Tarrier N, Morrison AP, et al (1999) A pilot study evaluating the effectiveness of individual inpatient cognitive-behavioural therapy in early psychosis. Soc Psychiatry Psychiatr Epidemiol 34:254–258
43. Lewis SW, Tarrier N, Haddock G, et al (2000) A randomized controlled trial of cognitive-behavioural therapy in acute early schizophrenia: the SoCRATES trial. Submitted for publication
44. Smith J, Hucker S (1994) Schizophrenia and substance abuse. Br J Psychiatry 165:13–21
45. Barrowclough C, Haddock G, Tarrier N, et al (2001) Randomised controlled trial of motivational interviewing and cognitive behavioural intervention for schizophrenic patients with associated drug and alcohol misuse. Am J Psychiatr (in press)
46. Miller WR, Rollnick S (1991) Motivational interviewing; preparing people to change addictive behaviour. Guilford Press, New York
47. Rollnick S, Miller WR (1995) What is motivational interviewing? Behav Cogn Psychother 23:325–334
48. Tarrier N, Barrowclough C, Haddock G, et al (1999) The dissemination of innovative cognitive-behavioural psychosocial treatments for schizophrenia. Journal of Mental Health 8:569–582

Subject Index